Myelodysplastic Syndromes

Guest Editor

BENJAMIN L. EBERT, MD, PhD

HEMATOLOGY/ONCOLOGY CLINICS OF NORTH AMERICA

www.hemonc.theclinics.com

Consulting Editors

GEORGE P. CANELLOS, MD
NANCY BERLINER, MD

April 2010 • Volume 24 • Number 2

SAUNDERS an imprint of ELSEVIER, Inc.

W.B. SAUNDERS COMPANY
A Division of Elsevier Inc.

1600 John F. Kennedy Blvd. • Suite 1800 • Philadelphia, PA 19103-2899

http://www.theclinics.com

HEMATOLOGY/ONCOLOGY CLINICS OF NORTH AMERICA Volume 24, Number 2
April 2010 ISSN 0889-8588, ISBN 13: 978-1-4377-2203-1

Editor: Kerry Holland

Hematology/Oncology Clinics (ISSN 0889-8588) is published bimonthly by Elsevier Inc., 360 Park Avenue South, New York, NY 10010-1710. Months of issue are February, April, June, August, October, and December. Business and Editorial Offices: 1600 John F. Kennedy Blvd., Ste. 1800, Philadelphia, PA 19103–2899. Customer Service Office: 3251 Riverport Lane, Maryland Heights, MO 63043. Periodicals postage paid at New York, NY and at additional mailing offices. Subscription prices are $306.00 per year (domestic individuals), $483.00 per year (domestic institutions), $152.00 per year (domestic students/residents), $347.00 per year (Canadian individuals), $591.00 per year (Canadian institutions) $413.00 per year (international individuals), $591.00 per year (international institutions), and $206.00 per year (international and Canadian students/residents). International air speed delivery is included in all *Clinics* subscription prices. All prices are subject to change without notice. **POSTMASTER:** Send address changes to *Hematology/Oncology Clinics of North America*, Elsevier Health Sciences Division, Subscription Customer Service, 3251 Riverport Lane, Maryland Heights, MO 63043. Customer Service (orders, claims, online, change of address): Elsevier Health Sciences Division, Subscription Customer Service, 3251 Riverport Lane, Maryland Heights, MO 63043. Tel: 1-800-654-2452 (U.S. and Canada); 314-447-8871 (outside U.S. and Canada). Fax: 314-447-8029. E-mail: journalscustomerservice-usa@elsevier.com (for print support); journalsonlinesupport-usa@elsevier.com (for online support).

Reprints. For copies of 100 or more, of articles in this publication, please contact the Commercial Reprints Department, Elsevier Inc., 360 Park Avenue South, New York, New York 10010-1710; Tel.: 212-633-3813, Fax: 212-462-1935, E-mail: reprints@elsevier.com.

Hematology/Oncology Clinics of North America is covered in *MEDLINE/PubMed (Index Medicus), EMBASE/ Excerpta Medica, and BIOSIS.*

Printed and bound by CPI Group (UK) Ltd, Croydon, CR0 4YY

Transferred to Digital Print 2011

Contributors

CONSULTING EDITORS

GEORGE P. CANELLOS, MD
William Rosenberg Professor of Medicine, Department of Medical Oncology,
Dana-Farber Cancer Institute, Boston, Massachusetts

NANCY BERLINER, MD
Chief, Division of Hematology, Brigham and Women's Hospital; Professor of Medicine,
Harvard Medical School, Boston, Massachusetts

GUEST EDITOR

BENJAMIN L. EBERT, MD, PhD
Assistant Professor, Department of Medicine, Brigham and Women's
Hospital; Dana-Farber Cancer Institute, Department of Medical Oncology, Harvard
Medical School, Boston; and Harvard Stem Cell Institute, Cambridge, Massachusetts

AUTHORS

PETER D. APLAN, MD
Senior Investigator, Genetics Branch, Center for Cancer Research, National Cancer
Institute, National Institutes of Health, Bethesda, Maryland

A.J. BARRETT, MD
Section Chief, Bone Marrow Transplantation, Hematology Branch, Division of Intramural
Research, National Heart, Lung and Blood Institute, Bethesda, Maryland

MATTHIAS BARTENSTEIN, MD
Post Doctoral Research Fellow, Clinical Research Division, Fred Hutchinson Cancer
Research Center, Seattle, Washington

SARAH H. BEACHY, PhD
Postdoctoral Fellow, Genetics Branch, Center for Cancer Research, National Cancer
Institute, National Institutes of Health, Bethesda, Maryland

RAFAEL BEJAR, MD, PhD
Department of Medicine, Brigham and Women's Hospital; Dana-Farber Cancer Institute,
Department of Medical Oncology, Harvard Medical School, Boston, Massachusetts

JOHN M. BENNETT, MD
James P. Wilmot Cancer Center, Strong Memorial Hospital, Rochester, New York

MARIO CAZZOLA, MD
Professor of Hematology, Department of Hematology Oncology, Medical School,
University of Pavia, Pavia, Italy

COREY CUTLER, MD, MPH, FRCP(C)
Assistant Professor of Medicine, Harvard Medical School, Dana-Farber Cancer Institute, Boston, Massachusetts

H. JOACHIM DEEG, MD
Member, Clinical Research Division, Fred Hutchinson Cancer Research Center; Professor, Department of Medicine, University of Washington School of Medicine, Seattle, Washington

BENJAMIN L. EBERT, MD, PhD
Assistant Professor, Department of Medicine, Brigham and Women's Hospital; Dana-Farber Cancer Institute, Department of Medical Oncology, Harvard Medical School, Boston; and Harvard Stem Cell Institute, Cambridge, Massachusetts

JEAN-PIERRE ISSA, MD
Department of Leukemia and Center for Cancer Epigenetics, The University of Texas M. D. Anderson Cancer Center, Houston, Texas

ALY KARSAN, MD
Genome Sciences Centre; Terry Fox Laboratory, BC Cancer Research Centre; Department of Pathology and Laboratory Medicine, University of British Columbia; Department of Pathology and Laboratory Medicine, BC Cancer Agency, Vancouver, British Columbia, Canada

RAMI S. KOMROKJI, MD
Clinical Director, Department of Malignant Hematology, H. Lee Moffitt Cancer Center and Research Institute; Assistant Professor of Oncologic Sciences, University of South Florida, Tampa, Florida

ALAN F. LIST, MD
Executive Vice President, Physician-in-Chief, H. Lee Moffitt Cancer Center and Research Institute; Professor of Oncologic Sciences, University of South Florida, Tampa, Florida

LUCA MALCOVATI, MD
Professor of Hematology, Department of Hematology Oncology, Medical School, University of Pavia, Pavia, Italy

MIKKAEL A. SEKERES, MD, MS
Department of Hematologic Oncology and Blood Disorders; Associate Professor of Medicine; Director, Leukemia Program, Cleveland Clinic Taussig Cancer Institute, Cleveland, Ohio

ELAINE M. SLOAND, MD
Senior Clinical Investigator, Hematology Branch, Division of Intramural Research, National Heart, Lung and Blood Institute, Bethesda, Maryland

DANIEL T. STARCZYNOWSKI, PhD
Genome Sciences Centre; Terry Fox Laboratory, BC Cancer Research Centre; Department of Pathology and Laboratory Medicine, University of British Columbia, Vancouver, British Columbia, Canada

DAVID P. STEENSMA, MD, FACP
Associate Professor of Medicine, Harvard Medical School; Department of Hematologic Malignancies, Dana-Farber Cancer Institute, Boston, Massachusetts

RICHARD M. STONE, MD
Professor of Medicine, Harvard Medical School; Department of Hematologic Malignancies, Dana-Farber Cancer Institute, Boston, Massachusetts

LING ZHANG, MD
H. Lee Moffitt Cancer Center and Research Institute, Tampa, Florida

Contributors

DAVID P. STEENSMA, MD, FACP
Associate Professor of Medicine, Harvard Medical School, Department of Hematologic Malignancies, Dana-Farber Cancer Institute, Boston, Massachusetts

RICHARD M. STONE, MD
Professor of Medicine, Harvard Medical School, Department of Hematologic Malignancies, Dana-Farber Cancer Institute, Boston, Massachusetts

LING ZHANG, MD
H. Lee Moffitt Cancer and Research Institute, Tampa, Florida

Contents

The incidence of the myelodysplastic syndromes (MDS) in the United States is reported as 3.4 per 100,000 people, translating to over 10,000 new diagnoses annually. This figure is considered to be an underestimate as our data capture techniques improve, and probably translates to a prevalence of approximately 60,000 people or more living with the disease. Patients are in their seventh or eighth decades at diagnosis, typically present with cytopenias, and have substantive transfusion requirements. The most common risk factors for developing MDS include advanced age, male gender, previous exposure to chemotherapy or radiation therapy, smoking, or, in rare cases, exposure to industrial chemicals.

Myelodysplastic syndrome (MDS) disorders are clonal diseases that often carry stereotypic chromosomal abnormalities. A smaller proportion of cases harbor point mutations that activate oncogenes or inactivate tumor suppressor genes. New technologies have accelerated the pace of discovery and are responsible for the identification of novel genetic mutations associated with MDS and other myeloid neoplasms. These discoveries have identified novel mechanisms in the pathogenesis of MDS. This article touches on the better known genetic abnormalities in MDS and explains in greater detail those that have been discovered more recently. Understanding how mutations lead to MDS and how they might cooperate with each other has become more complicated as the number of MDS-associated genetic abnormalities has grown. In some cases, these mutations have prognostic significance that could improve upon the various prognostic scoring systems in common clinical use.

Epigenetic mechanisms, such as DNA methylation and histone modifications, drive stable, clonally propagated changes in gene expression and can therefore serve as molecular mediators of pathway dysfunction in neoplasia. Myelodysplastic syndrome (MDS) is characterized by frequent epigenetic abnormalities, including the hypermethylation of genes that control proliferation, adhesion, and other characteristic features of this leukemia. Aberrant DNA hypermethylation is associated with a poor prognosis in MDS that can be accounted for by more rapid progression to acute myeloid leukemia. In turn, treatment with drugs that modify epigenetic pathways (DNA methylation and histone deacetylation inhibitors) induces durable remissions and prolongs life in MDS, offering some hope and direction in the future management of this deadly disease.

Laboratory evidence and clinical evidence suggest that some patients with myelodysplastic syndrome (MDS) have immunologically mediated disease. This article describes the laboratory evidence supporting a role for the immune system in the marrow failure of MDS and clinical trials using IST in these patients.

Myelodysplastic syndromes (MDS) are heterogeneous clonal hematologic malignancies characterized by cytopenias caused by ineffective hematopoiesis and propensity to progress to acute myeloid leukemia. Innate immunity provides immediate protection against pathogens by coordinating activation of signaling pathways in immune cells. Given the prominent role of the innate immune pathway in regulating hematopoiesis, it is not surprising that aberrant signaling of this pathway is associated with hematologic malignancies. Increased activation of the innate immune pathway may contribute to dysregulated hematopoiesis, dysplasia, and clonal expansion in myelodysplastic syndromes.

Three general approaches have been used to model myelodysplastic syndrome (MDS) in mice, including treatment with mutagens or carcinogens, xenotransplantation of human MDS cells, and genetic engineering of mouse hematopoietic cells. This article discusses the phenotypes observed in available mouse models for MDS with a concentration on a model that leads to aberrant expression of conserved homeobox genes that are important regulators of normal hematopoiesis. Using these models of MDS should allow a more complete understanding of the disease process and provide a platform for preclinical testing of therapeutic approaches.

Lenalidomide was approved by the US Food and Drug Administration (FDA) for treatment of transfusion-dependent lower-risk myelodysplastic syndrome patients with deletion (del) (5q) alone or with additional karyotype abnormalities. The approval was based on high rates of prolonged transfusion independence and complete cytogenetic response in this subset. In lower-risk non-del(5q) patients, meaningful erythroid responses also were reported with a low frequency of cytogenetic improvement, although inferior to that observed in the del(5q) patients. There is now a better understanding of the mechanism of the karyotype-dependent drug action, explaining the disparate response rates and frequency of myelosuppression. In del(5q) patients, lenalidomide suppresses the clone by inhibiting the nuclear sequestration of the haplodeficient cell cycle regulatory protein cdc25c, thereby promoting selective G2 arrest and apoptosis. In non-del(5q) patients, lenalidomide enhances erythropoietin receptor signaling. Future directions include use of biologic and molecular markers as predictive tools to select patients and use of combination strategies to overcome resistance to lenalidomide in del(5q) patients or enhance erythropoeisis in non-del 5 patients.

Practical Recommendations for Hypomethylating Agent Therapy of Patients With Myelodysplastic Syndromes

David P. Steensma and Richard M. Stone

Clinicians commonly administer one or the other of the two hypomethylating agents currently approved in the United States—azacitidine or decitabine—to patients with aggressive forms of myelodysplastic syndromes (MDS). However, there continues to be uncertainty about the optimal choice of agent, the best initial dose and treatment schedule, the role of hypomethylating agents in patients with more indolent disease, the most appropriate management of treatment-associated adverse events, and the most desirable approach to maintain responses. The evidence base supporting clinical decisions around these questions varies widely in depth and quality. This article discusses practical considerations for clinicians who use hypomethylating agents to treat patients with MDS.

Hematopoietic Stem Cell Transplantation for MDS

Matthias Bartenstein and H. Joachim Deeg

Hematopoietic stem cell transplantation (HSCT) offers potentially curative therapy for patients with myelodysplastic syndromes (MDS). However, as the majority of patients with MDS are in the seventh or eighth decade of life, conventional transplant regimens have been used only infrequently, and only with the development of reduced-intensity conditioning has transplantation been applied more broadly to older patients. Dependent upon disease status at the time of transplantation, 30% to 70% of patients can be expected to be cured of their disease and survive long term. However, posttransplant relapse and graft-versus-host disease (GVHD) remain problems and further investigations are needed.

Novel Therapies for Myelodysplastic Syndromes

David P. Steensma

Preliminary therapeutic successes have prompted a new wave of clinical trials enrolling patients with myelodysplastic syndromes (MDS), using compounds with a broad range of potential mechanisms of action. This article discusses several of the agents currently in development for MDS, reviewing clinical trial data related to five classes of novel therapeutics: clofarabine, a halogenated purine nucleoside analog; ezatiostat (TLK199), a glutathione analog that indirectly activates c-Jun kinase;

tipifarnib, a farnesyltransferase inhibitor; laromustine (cloretazine), an alkylating agent with a metabolite that inhibits one mechanism of DNA damage
repair; and eight drugs that inhibit histone deacetylase. Although MDS are
still difficult clinical problems, and most patients with MDS still succumb to
disease-related complications within 3 to 5 years of diagnosis, ongoing
development of novel agents promises that there will be new treatment
options for patients within the next 5 to 10 years.

Myelodysplastic syndromes (MDS) are spectrum of bone marrow failure
disorders that share a common pathologic feature: cytologic dysplasia.
The classification of MDS reflects the understanding of the disease. It is
hoped that in the future classification and risk stratification will be based
on underlying pathobiology of different disease subsets and molecular signatures where the pathologic classification represents their phenotype.
This article reviews MDS classification and risk stratification highlighting
differences between the various systems.

The clinical heterogeneity of myelodysplastic syndromes (MDS) is best illustrated by the observation that these disorders range from indolent conditions with a near-normal life expectancy to forms approaching acute
myeloid leukemia (AML). A risk-adapted treatment strategy is mandatory
for conditions showing a highly variable clinical course, and definition of
the individual risk has been based so far on the use of prognostic
scoring systems. The authors have developed a prognostic model that accounts for the World Health Organization (WHO) categories, cytogenetics,
transfusion dependency, and bone marrow fibrosis. This WHO classification-based Prognostic Scoring System (WPSS) is able to classify patients
into five risk groups showing different survivals and probabilities of leukemic evolution. WPSS predicts survival and leukemia progression at any
time during follow-up, and may therefore be used for implementing risk-
adapted treatment strategies.

Allogeneic hematopoietic stem cell transplantation remains the only
known curative procedure for the myelodysplastic syndromes (MDS). Because the median age at diagnosis for MDS is in the late seventh decade of
life, despite the curative potential, transplantation is not undertaken routinely, and careful consideration must be made regarding the appropriateness of the transplant recipient. This article focuses on appropriate patient
selection for transplantation for MDS.

THE CLINICS ARE NOW AVAILABLE ONLINE!

Access your subscription at:
www.theclinics.com

Preface
The Biology and Treatment
of Myelodysplastic Syndrome

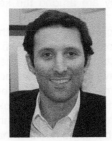

Benjamin L. Ebert, MD, PhD
Guest Editor

Myelodysplastic syndrome (MDS) has been a challenging disease to study because of the heterogeneity of clinical phenotype, a dearth of cell culture or animal models, relatively poor insight into the molecular pathology compared with other neoplastic disorders, and limited effective therapeutic options. Recently, however, major strides have been made in the treatment and understanding of this disease. The US Food and Drug Administration (FDA) has approved 3 new drugs for the treatment of MDS, new disease genes have been discovered, major insights have been made into the biology of the disorder, and animal models of MDS have been developed. The articles in this issue of *Hematology/Oncology Clinics of North America* review the progress in this rapidly developing field and highlight open questions that remain to be addressed.

MDS is a common disease that is likely dramatically underdiagnosed. The incidence of MDS has been tracked by the US Surveillance, Epidemiology and End Results (SEER) program since 2001.[1] The 2004 SEER data indicate that approximately 15,000 new cases of MDS are diagnosed per year in the United States. The number of patients who present with unexplained anemia, leukopenia, or thrombocytopenia is much higher, indicating that many MDS patients go undiagnosed.[2]

Diagnosing MDS is now of greater importance, with evidence that azacytidine changes the natural history of the disease. Azacytidine and decitabine, both of which decrease DNA methylation, and lenalidomide, an analog of thalidomide, are now approved by the FDA because of their efficacy in the treatment of MDS.[3–6] In a randomized phase III clinical trial of higher-risk MDS patients, azacytidine significantly prolonged survival compared with conventional care.[3] Lenalidomide has particular activity in low-risk patients with del(5q), leading to transfusion independence and cytogenetic remissions. A host of additional therapeutic agents are now under investigation, including histone deacetylase inhibitors, the farnesyltransferase inhibitor tipifarnib, the purine nucleoside clofarabine, the novel alkylating agent laromustine (cloretazine), and the glutathione S-transferase analog ezatiostat (TLK199).

Hematol Oncol Clin N Am 24 (2010) xiii–xvi
doi:10.1016/j.hoc.2010.02.014   hemonc.theclinics.com
0889-8588/10/$ – see front matter © 2010 Elsevier Inc. All rights reserved.

Bone marrow transplantation remains the sole therapeutic approach with the proven potential to cure MDS, but the procedure has high morbidity and mortality in the population of patients who develop MDS.[7] The development of reduced-intensity conditioning regimens makes bone marrow transplantation a possibility for older patients, but disease relapse and graft-versus-host disease remain major causes of posttransplant morbidity and mortality.[8,9] Patient selection, timing of transplant, incorporation of hypomethylating agents, and immunotherapy are among the key parameters that are currently under intensive investigation.

The identification of molecular abnormalities in MDS holds the potential for the development of a genetic taxonomy of MDS, improved prognostic scoring systems, and the identification of novel therapeutic targets. The characterization of balanced translocations and activating mutations in tyrosine kinases have led to tremendous insights into the biology and treatment of acute myeloid leukemia and myeloproliferative neoplasms, but neither of these molecular lesions are common in MDS. Approximately 50% of patients have cytogenetic abnormalities that are evident by standard karyotyping, and a higher percentage have smaller copy number abnormalities that can be detected by more sensitive approaches, such as single nucleotide polymorphism microarrays.[10] Most of the cytogenetic lesions involve the gain or loss of large amounts of chromosomal material. Functional approaches are now leading to the identification of critical genes within heterozygous deletions, particularly on chromosome 5q.[11,12]

Somatically acquired point mutations also play a major role in the pathophysiology of MDS. Mutations occur in several well-established oncogenes and tumor suppressor genes, including NRAS, JAK2, and TP53.[13–15] Germline mutations in RUNX1 cause familial thrombocytopenia with predisposition to acute myeloid leukemia and are also acquired somatically in MDS.[16–18] Recently, mutations have been identified in TET2, c-CBL, and ASXL1.[19–21] Some of these mutations appear to have prognostic significance, although they are not part of the current classification or prognostic scoring schemes.

Epigenetic modifications, including aberrant DNA methylation, have emerged as an important aspect of MDS biology. Methylation of cytosine residues within CpG islands in promoters results in silencing of gene expression. Whole genome analysis of DNA methylation in MDS has revealed recurrent methylation of several key genes, including CDKN2A, CDKN2B, CDH1, and DAPK1.[22] In addition, a subset of MDS patients has a hypermethylator phenotype, with extensive DNA methylation throughout the genome. Therapeutic efficacy of azacytidine and decitabine, which decrease DNA methylation, further highlights the importance of epigenetic abnormalities in MDS.

The immune system has emerged as a central player in the biology and treatment of MDS. Components of the immune system, including cytotoxic T cells and elevated levels of tumor necrosis factor α, cause ineffective hematopoiesis in some cases of MDS, and immunosuppressive therapy benefits a subset of patients. In addition, it has recently been reported that haploinsufficiency for 2 micro-RNAs on chromosome 5q, miR-145 and miR-146a, suppresses the innate immune system.

This issue of Hematology/Oncology Clinics of North America reviews the state of the field and key open questions in each of the areas of study described earlier. Dr Sekeres discusses the epidemiology of MDS. Somatic genetic abnormalities in MDS are reviewed by Drs Bejar and Ebert, and epigenetic abnormalities are discussed by Dr Issa. Drs Sloand and Barrett review the role of the immune system and immunosuppressive therapy in MDS, and Drs Starczynowski and Karsan review the role of the innate immune system in the 5q- syndrome. Murine models with an MDS phenotype are surveyed by Drs Beachy and Aplan. Therapeutic approaches to MDS are reviewed in 3 individual articles: lenalidomide is reviewed by Drs Komrokji and List, clinical use of hypomethylating agents is reviewed by Drs Steensma and Stone, and bone marrow transplantation for MDS is reviewed by Drs Bartenstein and Joachim Deeg. In addition, novel therapeutic agents that are currently being examined in clinical trials are reviewed by Dr Steensma. The stratification of MDS patients is also discussed in 3 separate articles: classification schemes for MDS are discussed by Drs Komrokji, Zhang, and Bennett; prognostic scoring strategies are reviewed by Drs Cazzola and Malcovati; and selection of patients for bone marrow transplantation is reviewed by Dr Cutler. Scientific and therapeutic progress of MDS has historically lagged behind the study of other hematologic malignancies, such as acute leukemia and myeloproliferative neoplasms. The articles in this issue of *Hematology/Oncology Clinics of North America* illustrate the rapid progress in MDS research, from molecular pathophysiology to improved therapies. Insights into the biology of MDS, the development of model systems to study MDS, and the application of new technologies with unprecedented power to interrogate the cancer genome promise to increase the rate of discovery, transforming our understanding of MDS and leading to improvements in the treatment this disease.

Benjamin L. Ebert, MD, PhD
Brigham and Women's Hospital
Harvard Medical School
1 Blackfan Circle, Karp 5.210
Boston, MA 02445, USA

E-mail address:
bebert@partners.org

REFERENCES

1. Ma X, Does M, Raza A, et al. Myelodysplastic syndromes: incidence and survival in the United States. Cancer 2007;109:1536–42.
2. Guralnik J, Eisenstaedt R, Ferrucci L, et al. Prevalence of anemia in persons 65 years and older in the United States: evidence for a high rate of unexplained anemia. Blood 2004;104:2263–8.
3. Fenaux P, Mufti GJ, Hellstrom-Lindberg E, et al. Efficacy of azacitidine compared with that of conventional care regimens in the treatment of higher-risk myelodysplastic syndromes: a randomised, open-label, phase III study. Lancet Oncol 2009;10:223–32.
4. Kantarjian H, Issa JP, Rosenfeld CS, et al. Decitabine improves patient outcomes in myelodysplastic syndromes: results of a phase III randomized study. Cancer 2006;106:1794–803.
5. List A, Dewald G, Bennett J, et al. Lenalidomide in the myelodysplastic syndrome with chromosome 5q deletion. N Engl J Med 2006;355:1456–65.
6. Silverman LR, Demakos EP, Peterson BL, et al. Randomized controlled trial of azacitidine in patients with the myelodysplastic syndrome: a study of the cancer and leukemia group B. J Clin Oncol 2002;20:2429–40.
7. Nachtkamp K, Kundgen A, Strupp C, et al. Impact on survival of different treatments for myelodysplastic syndromes (MDS). Leuk Res 2009;33:1024–8.
8. Alyea EP, Kim HT, Ho V, et al. Impact of conditioning regimen intensity on outcome of allogeneic hematopoietic cell transplantation for advanced acute myelogenous leukemia and myelodysplastic syndrome. Biol Blood Marrow Transplant 2006;12:1047–55.

9. Martino R, Iacobelli S, Brand R, et al. Retrospective comparison of reduced-intensity conditioning and conventional high-dose conditioning for allogeneic hematopoietic stem cell transplantation using HLA-identical sibling donors in myelodysplastic syndromes. Blood 2006;108:836–46.

10. Haase D, Germing U, Schanz J, et al. New insights into the prognostic impact of the karyotype in MDS and correlation with subtypes: evidence from a core dataset of 2124 patients. Blood 2007;110:4385–95.

11. Ebert BL, Pretz J, Bosco J, et al. Identification of RPS14 as a 5q- syndrome gene by RNA interference screen. Nature 2008;451:335–9.

12. Ebert BL. Deletion 5q in myelodysplastic syndrome: a paradigm for the study of hemizygous deletions in cancer. Leukemia 2009;23:1252–6.

13. Lyons J, Janssen JW, Bartram C, et al. Mutation of Ki-ras and N-ras oncogenes in myelodysplastic syndromes. Blood 1988;71:1707–12.

14. Christiansen DH, Andersen MK, Pedersen-Bjergaard J. Mutations with loss of heterozygosity of p53 are common in therapy-related myelodysplasia and acute myeloid leukemia after exposure to alkylating agents and significantly associated with deletion or loss of 5q, a complex karyotype, and a poor prognosis. J Clin Oncol 2001;19:1405–13.

15. Hellstrom-Lindberg E, Cazzola M. The role of JAK2 mutations in RARS and other MDS. Hematology Am Soc Hematol Educ Program 2008;52–9.

16. Song WJ, Sullivan MG, Legare RD, et al. Haploinsufficiency of CBFA2 causes familial thrombocytopenia with propensity to develop acute myelogenous leukaemia. Nat Genet 1999;23:166–75.

17. Harada H, Harada Y, Tanaka H, et al. Implications of somatic mutations in the AML1 gene in radiation-associated and therapy-related myelodysplastic syndrome/acute myeloid leukemia. Blood 2003;101:673–80.

18. Christiansen DH, Andersen MK, Pedersen-Bjergaard J. Mutations of AML1 are common in therapy-related myelodysplasia following therapy with alkylating agents and are significantly associated with deletion or loss of chromosome arm 7q and with subsequent leukemic transformation. Blood 2004;104:1474–81.

19. Sanada M, Suzuki T, Shih LY, et al. Gain-of-function of mutated C-CBL tumour suppressor in myeloid neoplasms. Nature 2009;460:904–8.

20. Delhommeau F, Dupont S, Della Valle V, et al. Mutation in TET2 in myeloid cancers. N Engl J Med 2009;360:2289–301.

21. Gelsi-Boyer V, Trouplin V, Adelaide J, et al. Mutations of polycomb-associated gene ASXL1 in myelodysplastic syndromes and chronic myelomonocytic leukaemia. Br J Haematol 2009;145:788–800.

22. Boultwood J, Wainscoat JS. Gene silencing by DNA methylation in haematological malignancies. Br J Haematol 2007;138:3–11.

The Epidemiology of Myelodysplastic Syndromes

Mikkael A. Sekeres, MD, MS[a,b,*]

KEYWORDS

• Myelodysplastic syndromes • Epidemiology • Risk factors
• Incidence • Characteristics

Patients with a blood picture compatible with the myelodysplastic syndromes (MDS) were first described at the beginning of the 20th Century, whereas the first MDS case series was published approximately 35 years ago.[1,2] This timing places the recognition of MDS and development of effective therapies a full 50 to100 years behind what has occurred for other hematologic malignancies. Similarly, the depth of understanding of MDS epidemiology lags behind that of other cancers.

Within the past decade three drugs, azacitidine, lenalidomide, and decitabine,[3–5] have been approved by the US Food and Drug Administration (FDA) specifically for MDS. Other active therapies used off-label for treating MDS include hematopoietic growth factors used to treat cytopenias associated with MDS (particularly erythropoiesis stimulating agents [ESAs])[6,7]; cytotoxic drugs, such as cytarabine and clofarabine; and those with immune modulating mechanisms of action, such as thalidomide and antithymocyte globulin. The availability of such therapies, along with their acknowledged differential activity in various MDS subtypes, has in part spurred the maturation rate of epidemiologic knowledge to quantify the societal impact of MDS and ascertain numbers of patients responsive to specific therapies and to identify risk factors for developing MDS.

This article reviews the most recent published incidence rates and characteristics of patients with MDS, and known risk factors for developing this collection of diseases.

MYELODYSPLASTIC SYNDROMES: INCIDENCE AND PREVALENCE

In 2001 in the United States, the Surveillance, Epidemiology, and End Results (SEER) program of the National Cancer Institute and the Centers for Disease Control and

[a] Department of Hematologic Oncology and Blood Disorders, Cleveland Clinic Taussig Cancer Institute, Desk R35, 9500 Euclid Avenue, Cleveland, OH 44195, USA
[b] Leukemia Program, Cleveland Clinic Taussig Cancer Institute, Desk R35, 9500 Euclid Avenue, Cleveland, OH, 44195 USA
* Department of Hematologic Oncology and Blood Disorders, Cleveland Clinic Taussig Cancer Institute, Desk R35, 9500 Euclid Avenue, Cleveland, OH 44195.
E-mail address: sekerem@ccf.org

Hematol Oncol Clin N Am 24 (2010) 287–294
doi:10.1016/j.hoc.2010.02.011
0889-8588/10/$ – see front matter © 2010 Elsevier Inc. All rights reserved.

hemonc.theclinics.com

Prevention started to track incidence rates of MDS, alongside other cancers. Based on these SEER data, collected from 2001 to 2003, the age-adjusted incidence rate of MDS in the United States was estimated to be 3.4 per 100,000 people, which translates to approximately 10,000 new cases per year.[8] Over this 3-year period, the incidence rate increased from approximately 3.3 per 100,000 people in 2001 to 3.4 in 2002 and then to 3.6 in 2003, not from an epidemic of MDS over this time period but because cancer registries were still fine tuning their identification and classification of the disease.[9] In 2004, the incidence rate was estimated at 3.8 per 100,000 people, cresting the rate of acute myeloid leukemia (AML) and potentially making MDS the most common type of leukemia, with new yearly diagnoses estimated to be close to 15,000 citizens in the United States. Rates were lowest for people younger than 40 years, at 0.14 per 100,000, and highest with increasing age, at 36 per 100,000 for patients 80 years and older. As these data derive from cancer registries, they do not include detailed patient information other than age at diagnosis, gender, race, French-American-British (FAB) classification at diagnosis, and survival. The incidence rate in the United States is similar to that reported in England/Wales and Sweden (3.6 per 100,000), Germany (4.1 per 100,000), and France (3.2 per 100,000), but higher than is seen in Japan (1.0 per 100,000).[10–13]

Defining prevalence rates (numbers of people living with MDS, as opposed to new diagnoses) has been elusive. Preliminary data from Germany reveals a prevalence rate of 20.7 per 100,000 people.[14] If we assume that incidence, and thus prevalence rates, between the United States and Germany are similar, this would translate to approximately 60,000 people living with MDS in the United States. However, even this is thought to be a gross underestimate because of failure to diagnose the disease.

In a study by Guralnik and colleagues in 2004, the prevalence of anemia in the United States was estimated from 2000 blood samples collected from people 65 years of age or older as part of the third National Health and Nutrition Examination Survey.[15] The overall prevalence was 10.6%, divided approximately equally into three categories: people with nutrient-deficiency anemia (ie, anemia associated with vitamin or iron deficiency); people with anemia of chronic inflammation with or without renal insufficiency; and unexplained anemia. Within this last category, 17% of people had macrocytic anemia, leucopenia, or thrombocytopenia (ie, peripheral blood findings typical of MDS). This percentage would in turn translate to a prevalence of 170,000 people. Complicating the matter further, these data were derived from an era before the approval of MDS therapies by the FDA. As at least one of these therapies (azacitidine) has prospectively demonstrated a survival advantage in higher-risk patients with MDS,[16] prevalence rates can be expected to increase because of case finding. Thus, although a prevalence rate of 170,000 people with MDS can be assumed to be an overestimate, a rate of 60,000 people is almost assuredly underestimating the impact of the disease.

MYELODYSPLASTIC SYNDROMES CHARACTERISTICS

What is the clinical picture of MDS in the United States? This question can be answered from data derived from SEER and the North American Association of Cancer Registries (NAACR),[9] and from a recent study characterizing patients with MDS that was based on over 4500 surveys completed by 101 physicians.[17]

The SEER/NAACR study is based on data from 24,798 subjects over the years 2001 to 2003 and encompassing approximately 82% of the population in the United States. In addition to age-dependent incidence rates discussed earlier, men have higher age-adjusted rates per 100,000 people than women (4.4 vs 2.5), as do whites compared with blacks (3.3 vs 2.4), though one study that uses Veterans Administration data belies this latter difference.[18] The 3-year relative survival rates for all participants is 45%.

In the survey study of 4514 subjects, 670 were newly diagnosed, of whom 38% were women, whereas the remainder were established patients. The median age at diagnosis was 71 years and among established patients was 72 to 75 years. Secondary MDS was seen in approximately 10% of all subjects, most following chemotherapy (76%).

Among recently diagnosed subjects with MDS, the majority had some degree of pancytopenia: the median hemoglobin value was 9.1 g/dL (interquartile range 8–10 g/dL); the median platelet count was 100,000/mm^3 (interquartile range 56,000–150,500/mm^3); and the median absolute neutrophil count was 1780/mm^3 (interquartile range 1070–2800/mm^3). A minority of subjects had circulating blasts: a mean of 16% had 1% to 5% blasts, whereas a mean of 10% had more than 5% blasts.

Lower-risk MDS (FAB categories of refractory anemia [RA] and RA with ring sideroblasts [RARS]; World Health Organization [WHO] categories of RA, RARS, refractory cytopenia with multilineage dysplasia, refractory cytopenia with multilineage dysplasia and ring sideroblasts, MDS with deletion of chromosome 5q [del (5q)], and MDS unclassified; and International/Prognostic Scoring System (IPSS) scores of low and intermediate-1) was more common in established than in recently diagnosed cases, comprising 60% to 69% of established versus 50% of recently diagnosed subjects with MDS using FAB criteria; 56% to 66% versus 51%, respectively, using WHO criteria; and 75% to 79% versus 64%, respectively, using IPSS criteria.

Among lower-risk, newly diagnosed subjects with MDS, 22% were dependent on red blood cell transfusions, whereas 57% had ever received a red blood cell transfusion. Only 5.5% were dependent on platelet transfusions, whereas 37% had ever received a platelet transfusion. Corresponding percentages were much higher in higher-risk subjects. Among those newly diagnosed, 68% were dependent on red blood cell transfusions, whereas 88% had ever received a transfusion; and 33% were dependent on platelet transfusions, whereas 58% had ever received such a transfusion. Regardless of timing of diagnosis, or severity of MDS, ESAs were used by more than 50% of this MDS population. The only potentially curative therapy for MDS, bone marrow transplantation, had been performed or was even being considered in less than 5% of all subjects, even in the era of reduced intensity transplantation.

RISK FACTORS FOR DEVELOPING MYELODYSPLASTIC SYNDROMES

As discussed in the first section of this article, the single greatest risk factor for developing MDS is advancing age, with yearly incidence rates increasing tenfold for octogenarians compared with the rest of the population.

The majority of secondary MDS cases arise following chemotherapy for other cancers, particularly alkylating agents or topoisomerase inhibitors, and following radiation therapy.[10,17] The typical latency period for secondary MDS after exposure to alkylating agents or radiation therapy is 5 to 10 years, and the risk appears to be dose dependent.[19,20] These specific types of secondary MDS are characterized by unbalanced translocations involving chromosome 5 or chromosome 7, or complex cytogenetics.[21] MDS following exposure to topoisomerase inhibitors is much less common, with a latency period of approximately 2 years.[22] It is more often characterized by a balanced translocation often involving 11q23 (the mixed lineage leukemia gene); long-term prognosis is poor for either type of secondary MDS.[23,24]

For example, two recent studies have explored the rates of secondary myeloid malignancies (MDS and AML) among patients with non-Hodgkin lymphoma who have undergone autologous bone marrow transplantation.[25,26] In both series, subjects were heavily pretreated with alkylating agents and topoisomerase inhibitors, and received Cytoxan/total body irradiation or busulfan/Cytoxan preparative regimens for their transplantation. Rates of secondary MDS/AML approached 7% at 10 years, or 20% at 20 years of follow-up. MDS has also been reported at definable, lower rates following alkylating, topoisomerase-inhibitor, or radiation therapy for breast and other solid tumor cancers, and following exposure to purine analogs for lymphoid malignancies.[20,27–38] Specific polymorphisms in the methylene tetrahydrofolate reductase gene (involved in DNA synthesis) may predict for a higher risk for secondary MDS/AML after treatment with cyclophosphamide, particularly in patients with breast cancer.[39]

Other therapies examined for a subsequent risk for developing MDS include radio-immunotherapy (eg, with I^{131}-tositumomab), which does not appear to have an association.[40] The use of granulocyte colony-stimulating factor (G-CSF) in children may increase the incidence of secondary MDS and AML,[41–43] which has also been reported as a possible complication following breast cancer therapy.[33] MDS may also evolve from an antecedent hematologic disorder, particularly polycythemia vera after treatment with P^{32} or busulfan.[44]

Though several other risk factors have been proposed for de novo MDS development, few have been confirmed by epidemiologic studies. One of the more common established risk factors, in addition to age and male gender, is environmental and occupational exposure to organic solvents, such as benzene and its derivatives. The association of benzene exposure to MDS development may be greater in those with specific nicotinamide adenine dinucleotide phosphate (NADPH): quinine oxidoreductase (NQO1) polymorphisms.[45] Case-control studies confirm an increasing risk for MDS in association with family history of hematopoietic cancer and exposure to agricultural chemicals (insecticides, pesticides, herbicides, or fertilizer); solvents; and radiation exposure.[46,47] One such study in the United States found the odds ratios for an MDS association and environmental factors to be 4.55 for agricultural chemical exposure, 2.05 for solvent exposure, and 3.22 for smokers who were also exposed to agricultural chemicals or solvents.[47] Other studies have linked the development of MDS to exposure to genotoxic industrial agents, including radiation, halogenated organics, metals, and petroleum products, in addition to pesticides and solvents.[48,49]

A recent meta-analysis examined the association between smoking or alcohol intake and the development of MDS.[50] Across 10 studies, composed of 2105 cases and 3363 controls, the odds ratio for MDS developing in smokers was 1.45 (95% CI 1.21, 1.74), indicating a 45% increase in risk. The association between alcohol intake and MDS was examined in five studies, composed of 745 cases and 1642 controls. The overall association was 1.31 (95% CI 0.79–2.18), indicating a possible increase in risk of 31%, though confidence intervals crossed parity.

MDS is not considered a familial or congenital disorder. This being said, rare cases of familial MDS and AML have been reported, mostly in association with loss of 5q and or 7q,[51–53] or with familial platelet disorders[54] in which there appears to be differential expression of genes involved in signal transduction.[55] MDS has also been associated with a family history of hematologic cancers, with an odds ratio of 1.92.[47] A rare G-CSF receptor polymorphism may also predispose to high-risk MDS, also through altered signal transduction.[56]

SUMMARY

The epidemiology of MDS is the next frontier in understanding the population impact of the disease, including numbers and types of patients affected and the societal impact of their transfusion and therapeutic needs. As our knowledge regarding risk factors for developing the disease and pathobiologic correlates grow, so too will our ability to design individual-specific, rather than disease-specific therapies, and hopefully reverse the growth of MDS with the aging population in the United States.

REFERENCES

1. Nageli O: d Spez. Pathol u.Therop. 2nd edition. Vienna; 1913, vol. 8.
2. Saarni MI, Linman JW. Preleukemia. The hematologic syndrome preceding acute leukemia. Am J Med 1973;55:38.
3. Kantarjian H, Issa JP, Rosenfeld CS, et al. Decitabine improves patient outcomes in myelodysplastic syndromes: results of a phase III randomized study. Cancer 2006;106:1794.
4. List A, Dewald G, Bennett J, et al. Lenalidomide in the myelodysplastic syndrome with chromosome 5q deletion. N Engl J Med 2006;355:1456.
5. Silverman LR, Demakos EP, Peterson BL, et al. Randomized controlled trial of azacitidine in patients with the myelodysplastic syndrome: a study of the cancer and leukemia group B. J Clin Oncol 2002;20:2429.
6. Kantarjian H, Fenaux P, Sekeres MA, et al. Phase 1/2 Study of AMG 531 in thrombocytopenic patients (pts) with low-risk Myelodysplastic Syndrome (MDS): update including extended treatment. Blood ASH Annual Meeting Abstracts 2007;110:250.
7. Kantarjian H, Giles F, Greenberg P, et al. Effect of romiplostim in patients (pts) with Low or Intermediate Risk Myelodysplastic Syndrome (MDS) Receiving Azacytidine. Blood ASH Annual Meeting Abstracts 2008;112:224.
8. Ma X, Does M, Raza A, et al. Myelodysplastic syndromes: incidence and survival in the United States. Cancer 2007;109:1536.
9. Rollison DE, Howlader N, Smith MT, et al. Epidemiology of myelodysplastic syndromes and chronic myeloproliferative disorders in the United States, 2001–2004, using data from the NAACCR and SEER programs. Blood 2008;112:45.
10. Aul C, Gattermann N, Schneider W. Age-related incidence and other epidemiological aspects of myelodysplastic syndromes. Br J Haematol 1992;82:358.
11. Maynadie M, Verret C, Moskovtchenko P, et al. Epidemiological characteristics of myelodysplastic syndrome in a well-defined French population. Br J Cancer 1996;74:288.
12. McNally RJ, Rowland D, Roman E, et al. Age and sex distributions of hematological malignancies in the U.K. Hematol Oncol 1997;15:173.
13. Radlund A, Thiede T, Hansen S, et al. Incidence of myelodysplastic syndromes in a Swedish population. Eur J Haematol 1995;54:153.
14. Schoonen W, Strupp C, Aul C, et al. Incidence and prevalence of myelodysplastic syndromes (MDS) in Duesseldorf 1996–2005. Leuk Res 2009;33:S62.
15. Guralnik JM, Eisenstaedt RS, Ferrucci L, et al. Prevalence of anemia in persons 65 years and older in the United States: evidence for a high rate of unexplained anemia. Blood 2004;104:2263.
16. Fenaux P, Mufti GJ, Hellstrom-Lindberg E, et al. Efficacy of azacitidine compared with that of conventional care regimens in the treatment of higher-risk myelodysplastic syndromes: a randomised, open-label, phase III study. Lancet Oncol 2009;10:223.
17. Sekeres MA, Schoonen WM, Kantarjian H, et al. Characteristics of US patients with myelodysplastic syndromes: results of six cross-sectional physician surveys. J Natl Cancer Inst 2008;100:1542.

18. Komrokji RS, Matacia-Murphy GM, Ali NH, et al. Outcome of patients with myelodysplastic syndromes in the Veterans Administration population. Leuk Res 2009; 13:13.

19. Pedersen-Bjergaard J, Specht L, Larsen SO, et al. Risk of therapy-related leukaemia and preleukaemia after Hodgkin's disease. Relation to age, cumulative dose of alkylating agents, and time from chemotherapy. Lancet 1987;2: 83.

20. Smith RE, Bryant J, DeCillis A, et al. Acute myeloid leukemia and myelodysplastic syndrome after doxorubicin-cyclophosphamide adjuvant therapy for operable breast cancer: the National Surgical Adjuvant Breast and Bowel Project Experience. J Clin Oncol 2003;21:1195.

21. Pedersen-Bjergaard J, Rowley JD. The balanced and the unbalanced chromosome aberrations of acute myeloid leukemia may develop in different ways and may contribute differently to malignant transformation. Blood 1994;83:2780.

22. Rowley JD, Olney HJ. International workshop on the relationship of prior therapy to balanced chromosome aberrations in therapy-related myelodysplastic syndromes and acute leukemia: overview report. Genes Chromosomes Cancer 2002;33:331.

23. Pedersen-Bjergaard J. Therapy-related myelodysplasia and acute leukemia. Leuk Lymphoma 1995;15(Suppl 1):11.

24. Pedersen-Bjergaard J, Pedersen M, Roulston D, et al. Different genetic pathways in leukemogenesis for patients presenting with therapy-related myelodysplasia and therapy-related acute myeloid leukemia. Blood 1995;86:3542.

25. Friedberg JW, Neuberg D, Stone RM, et al. Outcome in patients with myelodysplastic syndrome after autologous bone marrow transplantation for non-Hodgkin's lymphoma. J Clin Oncol 1999;17:3128.

26. Kalaycio M, Rybicki L, Pohlman B, et al. Risk factors before autologous stem-cell transplantation for lymphoma predict for secondary myelodysplasia and acute myelogenous leukemia. J Clin Oncol 2006;24:3604.

27. Barnard DR, Lange B, Alonzo TA, et al. Acute myeloid leukemia and myelodysplastic syndrome in children treated for cancer: comparison with primary presentation. Blood 2002;100:427.

28. Bhatia S, Krailo MD, Chen Z, et al. Therapy-related myelodysplasia and acute myeloid leukemia after Ewing sarcoma and primitive neuroectodermal tumor of bone: A report from the Children's Oncology Group. Blood 2007;109:46.

29. Blayney DW, Longo DL, Young RC, et al. Decreasing risk of leukemia with prolonged follow-up after chemotherapy and radiotherapy for Hodgkin's disease. N Engl J Med 1987;316:710.

30. Franklin J, Pluetschow A, Paus M, et al. Second malignancy risk associated with treatment of Hodgkin's lymphoma: meta-analysis of the randomised trials. Ann Oncol 2006;17:1749.

31. Franklin JG, Paus MD, Pluetschow A, et al. Chemotherapy, radiotherapy and combined modality for Hodgkin's disease, with emphasis on second cancer risk. Cochrane Database Syst Rev 2005;(4):CD003187.

32. Josting A, Wiedenmann S, Franklin J, et al. Secondary myeloid leukemia and myelodysplastic syndromes in patients treated for Hodgkin's disease: a report from the German Hodgkin's Lymphoma Study Group. J Clin Oncol 2003;21: 3440.

33. Le Deley MC, Suzan F, Cutuli B, et al. Anthracyclines, mitoxantrone, radiotherapy, and granulocyte colony-stimulating factor: risk factors for leukemia and myelodysplastic syndrome after breast cancer. J Clin Oncol 2007;25:292.

34. Leleu X, Soumerai J, Roccaro A, et al. Increased incidence of transformation and myelodysplasia/acute leukemia in patients with Waldenstrom macroglobulinemia treated with nucleoside analogs. J Clin Oncol 2009;27:250.
35. McLaughlin P, Estey E, Glassman A, et al. Myelodysplasia and acute myeloid leukemia following therapy for indolent lymphoma with fludarabine, mitoxantrone, and dexamethasone (FND) plus rituximab and interferon alpha. Blood 2005;105: 4573.
36. Pedersen-Bjergaard J. Insights into leukemogenesis from therapy-related leukemia. N Engl J Med 2005;352:1591.
37. Smith SM, Le Beau MM, Huo D, et al. Clinical-cytogenetic associations in 306 patients with therapy-related myelodysplasia and myeloid leukemia: the University of Chicago series. Blood 2003;102:43.
38. Wheeler C, Khurshid A, Ibrahim J, et al. Incidence of post transplant myelodysplasia/acute leukemia in non-Hodgkin's lymphoma patients compared with Hodgkin's disease patients undergoing autologous transplantation following cyclophosphamide, carmustine, and etoposide (CBV). Leuk Lymphoma 2001; 40:499.
39. Guillem VM, Collado M, Terol MJ, et al. Role of MTHFR (677, 1298) haplotype in the risk of developing secondary leukemia after treatment of breast cancer and hematological malignancies. Leukemia 2007;21:1413.
40. Bennett JM, Kaminski MS, Leonard JP, et al. Assessment of treatment-related myelodysplastic syndromes and acute myeloid leukemia in patients with non-Hodgkin lymphoma treated with tositumomab and iodine I131 tositumomab. Blood 2005;105:4576.
41. Freedman MH, Alter BP. Risk of myelodysplastic syndrome and acute myeloid leukemia in congenital neutropenias. Semin Hematol 2002;39:128.
42. Relling MV, Boyett JM, Blanco JG, et al. Granulocyte colony-stimulating factor and the risk of secondary myeloid malignancy after etoposide treatment. Blood 2003;101:3862.
43. Rosenberg PS, Alter BP, Bolyard AA, et al. The incidence of leukemia and mortality from sepsis in patients with severe congenital neutropenia receiving long-term G-CSF therapy. Blood 2006;107:4628.
44. Finazzi G, Caruso V, Marchioli R, et al. Acute leukemia in polycythemia vera: an analysis of 1638 patients enrolled in a prospective observational study. Blood 2005;105:2664.
45. Larson RA, Wang Y, Banerjee M, et al. Prevalence of the inactivating 609C–T polymorphism in the NAD(P)H:quinone oxidoreductase (NQO1) gene in patients with primary and therapy-related myeloid leukemia. Blood 1999;94:803.
46. Nisse C, Haguenoer JM, Grandbastien B, et al. Occupational and environmental risk factors of the myelodysplastic syndromes in the North of France. Br J Haematol 2001;112:927.
47. Strom SS, Gu Y, Gruschkus SK, et al. Risk factors of myelodysplastic syndromes: a case-control study. Leukemia 1912;19:2005.
48. Goldberg H, Lusk E, Moore J, et al. Survey of exposure to genotoxic agents in primary myelodysplastic syndrome: correlation with chromosome patterns and data on patients without hematological disease. Cancer Res 1990;50: 6876.
49. West RR, Stafford DA, Farrow A, et al. Occupational and environmental exposures and myelodysplasia: a case-control study. Leuk Res 1995;19:127.
50. Du Y, Fryzek J, Sekeres MA, et al. Smoking and alcohol intake as risk factors for myelodysplastic syndromes (MDS). Leuk Res 2009;9:9.

51. Gao Q, Horwitz M, Roulston D, et al. Susceptibility gene for familial acute myeloid leukemia associated with loss of 5q and/or 7q is not localized on the commonly deleted portion of 5q. Genes Chromosomes Cancer 2000;28:164.
52. Grimwade DJ, Stephenson J, De Silva C, et al. Familial MDS with 5q- abnormality. Br J Haematol 1993;84:536.
53. Smith ML, Cavenagh JD, Lister TA, et al. Mutation of CEBPA in familial acute myeloid leukemia. N Engl J Med 2004;351:2403.
54. Buijs A, Poddighe P, van Wijk R, et al. A novel CBFA2 single-nucleotide mutation in familial platelet disorder with propensity to develop myeloid malignancies. Blood 2001;98:2856.
55. Pradhan A, Mijovic A, Mills K, et al. Differentially expressed genes in adult familial myelodysplastic syndromes. Leukemia 2004;18:449.
56. Wolfler A, Erkeland SJ, Bodner C, et al. A functional single-nucleotide polymorphism of the G-CSF receptor gene predisposes individuals to high-risk myelodysplastic syndrome. Blood 2005;105:3731.

The Genetic Basis of Myelodysplastic Syndromes

Rafael Bejar, MD, PhD[a,c], Benjamin L. Ebert, MD, PhD[b,c,d],*

KEYWORDS

- Myelodysplastic syndromes • Genetic mutations
- Myeloid neoplasms • Karyotypic abnormalities

Myelodysplastic syndromes (MDS) represent a broad group of hematologic disorders characterized by ineffective hematopoiesis, cytopenias, and in many cases, progression to acute myeloid leukemia (AML). Recurrent somatic genomic abnormalities include gains or losses of chromosomal segments, balanced translocations, point mutations, and epigenetic modifications. These lesions alter the differentiation, self-renewal, or proliferation of an MDS stem cell and its progeny. A complete description of the molecular lesions in MDS will enable more accurate prognostic predictions, a molecular taxonomy of MDS, and the identification of novel therapeutic targets in MDS.

Approximately 50% of patients with MDS have diseased cells with an abnormal karyotype.[1] The most common of these cytogenetic alterations are loss of the long arm of chromosome 5 (-5q), loss of chromosome 7 or 7q (-7/7q-), deletion of chromosome arm 20q (20q-), and gain of chromosome 8 (+8) (**Fig. 1**). The International Prognostic Scoring System (IPSS) for MDS incorporates the most common karyotypic abnormalities into its risk score, attributing the worst risk to patients that carry three or more chromosomal irregularities. Less is known about how these large regions contribute to disease pathogenesis at a molecular level, but some insights have been made recently.

The analysis of mononuclear cell karyotypes is currently the only genetic test in routine clinical use for MDS diagnosis. However, many cases harbor submicroscopic deletions or amplifications, acquired uniparental disomy, and point mutations that can

[a] Department of Medicine, Brigham and Women's Hospital, Harvard Medical School, 75 Francis Street, Boston, MA 02115, USA
[b] Department of Medicine, Brigham and Women's Hospital, Harvard Medical School, Karp Research Building, CHRB 05.211, 1 Blackfan Circle, Boston, MA 02115, USA
[c] Dana-Farber Cancer Institute, Department of Medical Oncology, Harvard Medical School, 44 Binney Street, Boston, MA 02115, USA
[d] Harvard Stem Cell Institute, 42 Church Street, Cambridge, MA 02138, USA
* Corresponding author. Department of Medicine, Brigham and Women's Hospital, Harvard Medical School, Karp Research Building, CHRB 05.211, 1 Blackfan Circle, Boston, MA 02115.
E-mail address: Benjamin_Ebert@dfci.harvard.edu

Hematol Oncol Clin N Am 24 (2010) 295–315
doi:10.1016/j.hoc.2010.02.001
0889-8588/10/$ – see front matter © 2010 Elsevier Inc. All rights reserved.

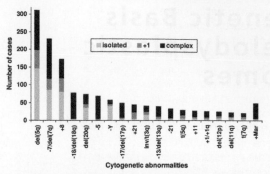

Fig. 1. Relative frequencies of the most common cytogenetic anomalies in MDS subdivided into isolated, with one additional anomaly, and complex anomalies (three or more abnormalities). Of the 2072 subjects evaluated in this study, 988 (48%) had a normal metaphase karyotype. (*Reproduced from* Haase D, Germing U, Schanz J, et al. New insights into the prognostic impact of the karyotype in MDS and correlation with subtypes: evidence from a core dataset of 2124 patients. Blood 2007;110:4385–95. © The American Society of Hematology; with permission.)

have prognostic significance. The IPSS, although slightly outdated, is the most commonly used prognostic index clinically.[2] The IPSS includes a subset of common chromosomal abnormalities, but does not take into account these more cryptic mutations. For example, point mutations causing the activation of *RAS* genes or the inactivation of *RUNX1* or *P53* are well described in MDS cases with normal and abnormal cytogenetics. As the list of genes found to be recurrently mutated in MDS has grown, the biologic and clinical consequences of these mutations has not been fully elucidated. Thus, they are not yet considered in clinical practice. Similarly, the role of epigenetic modifications in the pathogenesis of MDS has been highlighted by the clinical efficacy of hypomethylating agents.[3] However, molecular predictors of response are not yet established. With the genomic analysis of larger patient cohorts, stronger clinical correlations may be possible and more detailed molecular analysis of patients with MDS may become clinical useful.

With an increasingly extensive catalog of genetic lesions that MDS cells can harbor, a framework is emerging that helps explain how mutations cooperate to create the clonally expanded, dysplastic hematopoiesis characteristic of MDS. Genetic lesions contribute, to varying extents, to a survival advantage for abnormal hematopoietic stem cells over their normal counterparts or the acquisition of stem cell like self-renewal in a committed myeloid progenitor, dysplastic development of one or more cell lines, increased apoptosis of differentiating cells, or changes in genomic instability. Ultimately, mutations lead to the increase in proliferation and more complete block in differentiation associated with progression to acute myeloid leukemia.

This article focuses on our understanding of the genetic basis of MDS to date, with more attention given to recent discoveries in this field and the novel technologies that have made them possible.

CHROMOSOMAL AMPLIFICATIONS AND DELETIONS

The large chromosomal deletions found in patients with MDS contain many protein coding genes and several less well-characterized noncoding genes. The large range of potential targets has made it difficult to identify the mechanisms by which gene loss leads to MDS. However, the search for MDS-associated genes has been helped by comparing chromosomal deletions across many patients. Mapping of the proximal and distal breakpoints from different patients has been used to create and narrow the boundaries of commonly deleted regions (CDRs). The long arm of chromosome 5 is the most common chromosomal deletion in MDS and has been found to contain two distinct CDRs. The more distal of these lies in 5q33.1 and was defined by analyzing deletions in patients with the clinical phenotype described by the 5q- syndrome - refractory anemia, thrombocythemia, and low risk of progression to AML. This CDR contains 40 protein coding genes, three known micro RNAs, and at least two lincRNA genes.

Because only one allele is deleted in 5q- MDS, initial efforts focused on the identification of genes that are inactivated on the intact allele, consistent with homozygous inactivation of a tumor suppressor. No mutations or microdeletions on the intact allele have been identified.[4] An alternative hypothesis is that loss of a single allele, leading to a quantitative decline of its gene product, could contribute to the development of MDS.

By targeting each of the 40 known genes in the 5q- syndrome CDR with short-hairpin RNAs (shRNAs), we identified the ribosomal protein S14 (*RPS14*) gene as a causal gene for the 5q- syndrome, capable of reproducing in vitro the profound block in erythroid differentiation seen in patients with this MDS variant. The introduction of an exogenous *RPS14* gene rescued the block in erythroid differentiation in cultured CD34[+] cells from 5q- syndrome MDS patients.[5] Of note, congenital mutations in one allele of other ribosomal proteins have been identified in Diamond Blackfan Anemia, a rare disorder with a strikingly similar erythroid phenotype as the 5q- syndrome.[6] The mechanism of erythroid failure appears to involve activation of the p53 pathway.[7–9]

Most patients with 5q deletions do not have the clinical features of the 5q- syndrome and carry more proximal breakpoints that result in the loss of both 5q CDRs. The proximal common deleted region contains many genes, including *CTNNA1,* which is epigenetically silenced in some cases of 5q-, *EGR1*, and *HSPA9*.[10,11] Heterozygous inactivation of EGR1 increases hematopoietic stem cell self-renewal, and may therefore contribute to clonal advantage of cells with deletion of this region.[12] The full phenotype of 5q- MDS is likely caused by the integrated effects of haploinsufficiency for multiple genes as reviewed recently.[4,13]

Several genes that lie outside of the 5q- CDRs have also been implicated in myeloid malignancies and are often lost in patients who have MDS with large 5q deletions. These genes include *NPM1* and the tumor suppressor *APC*. *NPM1* mutations are the most commonly identified mutations in patients with cytogenetically normal AML. Inactivation of one allele of *NPM1* in a murine model results in an MDS-like phenotype.[14,15]

Patients with low risk MDS and 5q- have a striking response to lenalidomide, a derivative of thalidomide, with 67% achieving transfusion independence and 45% achieving a cytogenetic response in a Phase II clinical trial.[16] Two phosphatases, *CDC25C* and *PP2A*, are located on 5q and have been implicated in the response to lenalidomide.[17] *CDC25C* is located within the proximal 5q CDR and is directly inhibited by lenalidomide in vitro. Knockdown of these phosphatases sensitizes cells to lenalidomide-mediated apoptosis. Similarly, the *SPARC* gene is located in the distal common deleted region, and treatment with lenalidomide increases *SPARC* gene expression.[18]

Genes from other commonly deleted regions have not been as clearly implicated in the pathogenesis of MDS. Multiple CDRs on chromosome 7q have been described that include several candidate genes, but most patients with 7q deletions have lost two or more of these regions.[19,20] Unlike the favorable prognosis associated with an isolated 5q deletion, the presence of any chromosome 7 abnormality, including uniparental disomy, has been shown to be a marker of poor outcomes in MDS.[21] Which gene or genes are responsible for this negative prognosis have yet to be well characterized.

Isolated deletion of the long arm of chromosome 20 (20q-) is the third most common recurrent chromosomal loss in MDS after deletion of 5q and 7q. This abnormality is also found in AML and represents the most frequent chromosomal deletion in myeloproliferative neoplasms (MPN). The common deleted region of 20q has been mapped to a segment between 20q11 and 20q13.[22,23] This smallest CDR contains 19 genes, none of which have been found to be mutated or otherwise directly implicated in myeloid diseases to date. Isolated loss of 20q is incorporated into the IPSS risk score and is considered a positive prognostic marker. However, there is evidence that late emergence of 20q- during disease progression is an indicator of genomic instability and may be associated with poor outcome.[24]

Trisomy 8 (+8) is the only common chromosomal amplification recurrently associated with MDS. It can be found in other hematologic malignancies and in some solid tumors. Gene expression analyses of leukemic cells have shown increased transcription of genes from chromosome 8 from patients with trisomy 8 AML. Comparison of this expression pattern to that of normal CD34$^+$ cells revealed upregulation of antiapoptotic genes.[25] Similar studies with CD34$^+$ cells from patients with MDS demonstrated increased expression of pro- and antiapoptotic genes. When tested in culture, trisomy 8 CD34$^+$ cells were resistant to irradiation and were able to form hematopoietic colonies despite expression of apoptotic proteins normally associated with rapid senescence and cell death.[26] The clinical correlate of this cellular phenotype is decreased survival seen in patients with +8 MDS (22 months mean survival compared with 53 months for normal karyotype MDS) and a lower response to chemotherapy in patients with +8 AML.

A subset of patients with MDS and trisomy 8 as their sole cytogenetic abnormality are notable for their clinical response to immune suppression. These patients tend to be younger, have refractory anemia of short duration, and are more likely to carry HLA DR15.[27] Studies have shown expansion of Vβ-restricted CD8$^+$ positive T-cells in patients with +8 MDS and a return to more normal polyclonal Vβ expression after successful treatment with immunosuppressants.[28] Patients who respond to immunosuppression can achieve transfusion independence and even normalization of their red blood cell count. However, successful treatment does not abolish the +8 clone, which can actually expand in the bone marrow of responders after immunosuppression. These findings suggest that the +8 clone is resistant to killing by cytotoxic T-cells and likely has a growth advantage compared with normal hematopoietic precursors that are enhanced in the setting of autoimmunity. This immune mechanism may play a role in cases of MDS without +8, as the response to immunotherapy is not exclusive to this group.

Isolated loss of chromosome Y (-Y) in hematologic cells is an age-related phenomenon and most often is not associated with a myeloid disorder. In patients with MDS, loss of Y in the majority of cells can be a useful marker of disease burden, but likely has no bearing on the mechanism of disease.[29,30] Like patients with a normal karyotype, those with -Y are considered to have prognostically favorable cytogenetics in the IPSS.

BALANCED TRANSLOCATIONS

Analysis of gene partners in balanced translocations can be very informative, since it identifies genes likely to be involved in the pathogenesis of the underlying disease.

This has been a particularly fruitful approach in chronic and acute myeloid leukemias. However, unlike AML, recurrent chromosomal translocations in MDS are rare.[31] Recurrent translocations do occur involving the MDS1-EVI1 locus on chromosome 3q and between partners on chromosomes 6p and 9q.[32-34] Other genes that are involved in rarer translocations include RUNX1, TEL, MEL1, NUP98, and IER3.[35-39] Many translocations in MDS occur in the setting of a more widely disturbed cytogenetic profile, making it unclear if these represent disease modifying changes or incidental rearrangements in a highly unstable genome.

The MDS1-EVI1 gene locus is unusual in that it encodes two related proteins with partially opposing functions. Alternative splicing of transcripts results in either expression of the full length MDS1-EVI1 gene product or just the Evi1 protein alone.[40] Evi1 can repress the function of Gata1 and thus alter normal hematopoietic differentiation. It can also down-regulate activity of the Mds1-Evi1 fusion protein.[41] The MDS1-EVI1 locus is one of the most common translocation partners in myeloid malignancies and has been identified as a common site for retroviral insertional oncogenesis.[32,42,43] Presence of a 3q translocation is typically associated with a poor prognosis. In patients with MDS or AML without a 3q translocation, overexpression of EVI1 often occurs and also confers a poor prognosis.[44,45] Finally, EVI1 overexpression in a mouse bone marrow transplant model generates an MDS like phenotype.[46] Although translocations involving this locus on 3q are typically associated with AML, they are frequent enough in MDS that they can be used as evidence to support a diagnosis of MDS in patients with equivocal evidence of dysplasia.[33]

Translocations between chromosomes 6p and 9q are also considered presumptive evidence of MDS in patients with unexplained anemia and little evidence of marrow dysplasia.[33] In AML, where this translocation is more common, it is a marker of poor prognosis. The genes involved in this translocation are DEK (on 6p21) and NUP214 on 9q34. DEK encodes a DNA binding protein and can inhibit histone acyltransferase activity and modulate transcript splicing. NUP214 encodes a member of the nuclear pore complex. The DEK/NUP214 fusion protein up-regulates protein synthesis in myeloid cells, but how it might contribute to leukemogenesis or dysplasia is not yet clear.

A novel MDS-related gene was recently discovered because of its involvement in a slightly different 6p to 9q translocation. In this case, the IER3 gene from 6p21 was fused to a transcript-poor region of 9q34, resulting is loss of expression of the IER3 gene product. IER3 is an immediate early response gene involved in proapoptotic signaling. Evidence for IER3 rearrangements was found in several other patients and expression of IER3 was dysregulated in more than half of patients who have MDS without 6p abnormalities.[37]

UNIPARENTAL DISOMY AND COPY NUMBER VARIATION

Several recently developed technologies are capable of genome-wide assessment of DNA copy number, identifying amplifications and deletions in an unbiased manner that are not apparent by standard cytogenetic analysis. These techniques include high-density comparative genome hybridization (aCGH), single nucleotide polymorphism (SNP) microarrays and copy number variation (CNV) genotyping, and next-generation DNA resequencing technologies. Genome-wide sequencing using next-generation technologies has not yet been applied to MDS, although aCGH and SNP array studies have been performed extensively. These studies have already highlighted novel MDS disease alleles and loci.

SNP microarrays were initially designed to genotype single nucleotide polymorphisms, but they can also detect changes in DNA copy number, including small chromosomal deletions or amplifications, that are unrecognized by traditional karyotyping. A commonly used version of these chips, the Affymetrix 6.0 array, has probes dedicated solely to the determination of copy number at nearly one million loci on the human genome.[47,48] Areas of acquired copy number neutral, uniparental disomy (aUPD) are also detectable with these instruments and can point to disease-related abnormalities that would otherwise go unnoticed. Several groups have used SNP-arrays to examine DNA from MDS bone marrow samples. One of their common findings is that more than half of the patients who have MDS with normal cytogenetics by metaphase karyotyping harbor cryptic copy number changes or aUPD.[49–51] Some of these changes are microdeletions or aUPD at the loci of known MDS karyotypic abnormalities, such as on the long arm of chromosome 7. More importantly, these findings appear to have prognostic importance in MDS and AML.[21,52] In addition, SNP array studies have highlighted genes that were subsequently found to be mutated in a substantial portion of cases, including the *TET2* gene and *CBL* described below.

POINT MUTATIONS IN MYELODYSPLASTIC SYNDROME GENES
TET2 Mutations

The *TET1* gene was identified as a rare translocation partner with the mixed-lineage leukemia gene (MLL) in a fraction of patients with AML.[53] Neither this gene, nor the other two genes it shares homology with, *TET2* and *TET3*, had previously been associated with malignancy. In the last year, *TET2* was reported to be mutated at high frequency in several myeloid malignancies, including MDS. Using SNP-arrays, analysis of DNA samples from patients with MDS, MDS/MPN, and AML revealed recurrent acquired uniparental disomy and small deletions in chromosomal segment 4q24.[54,55] The only open reading frame in the smallest commonly altered region was the *TET2* gene and mutations of highly conserved codons in *TET2* were identified in these patients. *TET2* mutations were not limited to a single class of myeloid disorders. Many patients with MPN (∼10%) had *TET2* mutations (often associated with loss of heterozygosity of 4q24) as did a large fraction of unselected patients with MDS (∼20%), chronic myelomonocytic leukemia (CMML) (∼30%), and secondary AML (∼25%), including those without obvious alterations of the 4q24 locus. Subsequent studies have confirmed that *TET2* mutations are not exclusive of several genetic abnormalities and are found alongside *PML-RAR, FLT3-ITD, JAK2 V617F, MPL W515L/K, KIT D816V, NRAS*, and *NPM1* mutations and in myeloid malignancies with no known mutations.[56–59] Point mutations of *TET1* or *TET3* were not found in a large set of MPN samples and have not been reported in other myeloid malignancies to date.[56]

No other recurring gene mutation has been identified in such a broad spectrum of myeloid neoplasms at such high frequency, which prompts the speculation that impairment of *TET2* function promotes a common element in the pathogenesis of all of these diseases, namely the establishment or maintenance of clonal hematopoiesis.[60–62] Mutations of this gene could not be the sole cause of the dysplasia seen in patients with MDS because patients with polycythemia vera (PV) carrying *TET2* mutations have normal (albeit amplified) erythroid differentiation. Nor does *TET2* seem to promote transformation to acute leukemia in isolation. In a study of 96 subjects with MDS, *TET2* mutations were no more likely to be found in those with high risk disease nor were any new mutations seen during disease progression.[63] In another study, *TET2* mutations were found more frequently in low and intermediate-1 risk groups.[64]

Instead, it appears that impairment of *TET2* function may provide a survival advantage to early hematopoietic progenitors without profound effects on differentiation or proliferation. Single colony assays of CD34$^+$ cells from the bone marrow of patients with *JAK2 V617F* and *TET2* mutations support this view.[54] A subset of more primitive CD34$^+$CD38$^-$ cells from these patients often carried *TET2* mutations without associated *JAK2* mutations. The proportion of *TET2*-only mutant cells was greater in this CD34$^+$CD38$^-$ group than in more mature CD34$^+$CD38$^+$ cells. In the five subjects studied, no cells carrying the *JAK2 V617F* mutation were found to have wild-type *TET2*. CD34+ stem cells from two subjects with *TET2* mutated/*JAK2 V617F* positive neoplasms could repopulate the bone marrow of sub-lethally irradiated NOD-SCID mice, whereas cells from three subjects with the *JAK2* mutation and wild-type *TET2* could not. Fifteen weeks after engraftment, single colony assays of surviving cells revealed that the population of *TET2* mutated, *JAK2* wild-type cells had grown at the expense of those cells carrying mutations in both genes. This finding suggests that the *TET2* mutation might have preceded the *JAK2 V617F* mutation in these subjects and that it resides in a more primitive hematopoietic stem cell.

Evidence for mutations in TET2 as an early event in myeloid disorders is not universal, however. Saint-Martin and colleagues[58] studied four family cohorts with a strong inherited predisposition for MPNs and AML. These subjects did not carry germline *JAK2* mutations, but often acquired them when they presented with myeloid malignancies. Many of the affected members of these cohorts developed *TET2* mutations, but several others did not, and no two related subjects acquired the same *TET2* mutation. In one subject with *JAK2 V617F/TET2*-mutant PV for which several bone marrow samples were available, it was noted that the subject had mostly *JAK2 V617F*-positive clones that were *TET2* negative at an early stage of the disease. The remaining clones were either completely wild-type or contained the *JAK2 V617F* mutation and a single *TET2* mutation. When the subject progressed to acute leukemia, almost all bone marrow mononuclear cells contained biallelic *TET2* mutations in addition to *JAK2 V617F*. These findings demonstrate that *TET2* mutations can be either primary or secondary events and are consistent with impaired *TET2* function creating a selective growth advantage for disease stem cells.

Less is known about the role of *TET2* mutations in MDS. In a study of 96 subjects with MDS, Kosmider and colleagues[63] found mutation of *TET2* to be a positive prognostic factor independent of IPSS risk group. There was no difference in clinical markers at the time of presentation in the mutated compared with the non-mutated group. In contrast, other groups have found that patients with AML or CMML that carry *TET2* mutations have decreased overall survival.[56,65] It is not clear why *TET2* mutations appear to be protective in MDS, but are unfavorable in more proliferative myeloid diseases. It is possible that patients who have MDS with TET2 mutations as the basis of their disease lack other, less favorable genetic lesions, and hence have better outcomes. But for the subset of patients with more aggressive diseases, the lack of *TET2* function could enhance the effect of the additional mutations they have acquired or impart a relative resistance to treatment. Studies with a much larger number of subjects are needed to better understand the prognostic implications of *TET2* mutations.

The mechanism through which *TET2* mutations promote diverse myeloid malignancies is not well understood. However, a recent study on the function of its homolog *TET1* suggests that *TET2* may affect epigenetic modulation of gene expression.[66] *TET1* encodes a 2-oxoglutarate and Fe(II)-dependent enzyme that catalyzes the conversion of 5-methylcytosine (5-mC) to 5-hydroxymethylcytosine (5-hmC). This modified base was found to comprise roughly 5% of all CpG islands in mouse embryonic stem cells. The authors speculate that 5-hmC could be a chemical intermediate in the demethylation of cytosine residues, either by spontaneous or enzyme-mediated conversion. Alternatively, DNA methyltransferases may not recognize 5-hmC, and therefore, may not methylate cytosines on newly synthesized DNA strands complementary to regions with these epigenetic marks. The result would be a net loss of cytosine methylation mediated by *TET* proteins. MDS and AML are disorders whose pathogenesis involves hypermethylation of several tumor suppressor genes, and are diseases for which inhibitors of DNA methyltransferases have shown efficacy. It is intriguing to have identified a frequently mutated gene whose likely mechanism of action could explain the basis for these observations. Of particular interest will be the analysis of whether *TET2*-mutation status predicts response to therapy with the hypomethylating agents 5-azacytidine and decitabine.

ASXL1 Mutations

The *ASXL1* gene is another example of a gene that has recently been found to carry mutations in a variety of myeloid disorders including MDS. This gene encodes a chromatin-binding protein that functions as a ligand-dependent coactivator of the retinoic acid receptor. It regulates the response to retinoic acid in a cell-type specific manner and is thought to mediate its effects through a direct interaction with the histone acyltransferase *NCOA1* (also known as *SRC-1*) or the histone demethylase *LSD1*.[67,68] *ASXL1* is located in 20q11, but is proximal to the 20q common deleted region in patients with MDS.

ASXL1 was identified as a myeloid disease gene from aCGH experiments analyzing germline and CD34[+]-cell DNA from a small set of patients with MDS/AML. One individual had a small, atypical deletion on chromosome 20 that encompassed the *ASXL1* locus. Subsequent sequencing identified mutations of this gene in 16% of subjects with MDS/AML and in 43% with CMML.[69] Most of these samples were studied to see if they carried mutations in several other MDS associated genes, including *HRAS*, *KRAS*, *NRAS*, *RUNX1*, *NFIA*, *CTNNB1*, and *TET2*. In this small sample set, mutations in *RUNX1* and *TET2* were identified in subjects with MDS and these did not coexist with *ASXL1* mutations. In CMML cases, *RUNX1* and *TET2* mutations were not exclusive of *ASXL1* mutations. In contrast, *ASXL1* mutations were found in several MPN samples, but none of these were from subjects with PV and none carried the *JAK2 V617F* mutation.[70] This finding suggests that loss of *ASXL1* activity might replace the pathogenicity of the constitutively activated *JAK2* oncogene in a subset of *JAK2* wild-type myeloproliferative diseases. As was the case with CMML samples, *TET2* mutations were not exclusive of *ASXL1* mutations in these MPNs. Mutations in *ASXL1* were also identified in 20% of a group of subjects with AML, most of which had normal cytogenetics. Although nearly half of these subjects had *NPM1* mutations, *ASXL1* and *NPM1* mutations were epistatic.[71] In this study, the investigators suggest that this mutual exclusivity could mean that *ASXL1* and *NPM1* contribute to the same pathogenic pathway. The alternative interpretation is that these genes represent completely independent mechanisms of transformation because many of the *ASXL1* mutated AML cases arose from chronic myeloid diseases, whereas most *NPM1*-mutated cases did not.

Exactly how *ASXL1* contributes to the development of MDS and other myeloid disorders is not clear. *ASXL1* deficient mice do not have a dramatic myeloerythroid phenotype or gross changes in their stem cell compartment.[72] The higher incidence of *ASXL1* mutations in CMML and AML compared with MDS and its mutual exclusivity with *JAK2* in MPNs prompts the speculation that *ASXL1* mutations may drive cell proliferation with few effects on morphology or differentiation. Finally, the clinical implications of *ASXL1* mutations in patients with MDS are not yet known.

CBL Mutations

The *CBL* gene encodes an E3 ubiquitin ligase and contains a tyrosine kinase binding domain. It negatively regulates tyrosine kinase activity by promoting ubiquitination of these proteins, leading to their degradation.[73–75] Using the same approach that led to the discovery of *TET2* mutations, mutations of the *CBL* gene were found in a large fraction of patients with myeloid disorders who were noted to have acquired uniparental disomy of 11q.[76] Most of these patients had CMML or atypical chronic myelocytic leukemia (aCML), but *CBL* mutations were found in a few patients with refractory anemia with excess blasts. In several *CBL* mutants without 11q UPD, a second inactivating mutation in *CBL* was identified. Although some mutations appear to cause loss of function, other evidence indicates that *CBL* may function as an oncogene. Mutations in *CBL* occur almost exclusively in a short segment of the protein coding region and maintain the reading frame of the gene. The mutated protein product has impaired ubiquitin ligase activity and can impair the function of wild-type *CBL* in a dominant negative fashion.[77] Expression of mutant *CBL* in 3T3 cells enhances their ability to form colonies in agar and tumors in nude mice. In this sense, *CBL* appears to be an oncogene and not a tumor suppressor. The answer is that it may be a little of each. Mice deficient for *cbl* have an expanded hematopoietic progenitor pool and some degree of hypersensitivity to cytokine signaling, but do not develop MDS or MPN. When a mutant *CBL* gene is inserted into hematopoietic cells from these mice, they show dramatic hypersensitivity to cytokine stimulation and proliferate much more. It appears that *CBL* mutants gain the ability to promote tyrosine kinase signaling that is separate from their loss of ubiquitin ligase activity, possibly through dominant negative inhibition of its homolog *CBLB*.[77]

CBL mutations have previously been identified in rare cases of de novo AML, and are most frequently associated with core-binding factor leukemias.[78–80] Most *CBL* mutant samples from patients with AML are negative for mutations in *FLT3, KIT, NPM1, CEBPA,* and *RAS* genes, implying that loss of *CBL* function can substitute for the growth advantage conveyed by these oncogenic mutations more commonly associated with AML. *CBL* mutations are also found at high frequency (17%) in cases of juvenile myelomonocytic leukemia (JMML).[81] These mutations are exclusive of *RAS* and *PTPN11* mutations, which are associated with 25% to 35% of JMML cases.

Although *CBL* mutations have been found in patients with MDS, it is primarily associated with the monocytic myeloproliferative disorders JMML, CMML, and aCML. Its mechanism of action and lack of association with other pro-proliferative oncogene mutations suggest that mutation of *CBL* has an effect comparable to that caused by constitutive activation of tyrosine kinases. It remains to be seen whether *CBL* mutations play a role In lower risk MDS or whether loss of this protein function confers a worse prognosis in this disease.

Receptor Tyrosine Kinase and RAS Pathway Mutations

Activating mutations in the *RAS* family of oncogenes were among the first frequently recurring point mutations identified in patients with MDS.[82,83] They are present in roughly 15% of MDS cases and are associated with an increased risk for progression to AML.[84,85] Various missense mutations in codon 12 of *NRAS* are the most common *RAS* mutations in MDS, with mutations at other sites or in *KRAS* occurring at lower frequency.[86] Like *CBL* mutations, oncogenic *RAS* mutations are more common in patients with CMML (~50%) and JMML (~30%).[81]

RAS proteins are mediators of signal pathways downstream of receptor tyrosine kinases, such as those that mediate cytokine sensitivity in hematopoietic cells. These include receptors for thrombopoietin, erythropoietin, stem cell factor, Flt-3 ligand, platelet-derived growth factors, several interleukins, insulin and insulin-like growth factors, and the colony stimulating factors. Some of these receptors have been found to have activating mutations in advanced cases of MDS or CMML, including *FLT3*, *CSF1R* (aka *c-FMS*), and *KIT*, although these are more commonly associated with AML.[87] Other *RTK-RAS* pathway genes mutated in myeloid disorders include *BRAF* and *PTPN11*, both of which are rare in MDS.[88,89]

TP53 Mutations

Mutations of the critical cell-cycle checkpoint gene *TP53* are among the most common genetic abnormalities in malignancies. In MDS, *TP53* mutations occur in 10% to 15% of patients, but this frequency can be higher in those with prior exposure to alkylating agents or radiation.[90–93] Inactivating mutations of *TP53* are associated with advanced disease, complex karyotype, and resistance to treatment; all of which portend a poor prognosis.[94] The presence of *TP53* mutations may even be an independent risk factor after accounting for IPSS risk score.[95,96] As the sensitivity of molecular diagnostics improve, it will be feasible to determine if patients carry *TP53* mutations in diseased subclones at low frequency. This treatment resistant *TP53*-mutant population may drive progression of disease and expand after therapy even in patients who otherwise appear to have a good prognostic profile.[97]

RUNX1 Mutations

RUNX1 is a member of the core-binding factor family of proteins and an important regulator of normal hematopoiesis.[98] Like *TET2*, *RUNX1* abnormalities are found in many myeloid disorders. In MDS, mutations are present in 7% to 15% of cases of de novo disease, but appear to be more frequent in therapy-related MDS.[92,99–102] Patients who have MDS with *RUNX1* mutations are more likely to have advanced disease and carry a poor prognosis.[99,102,103]

The *RUNX1* protein contains two primary domains important for its function: a proximal Runt DNA binding domain and a distal activation domain. Mutations are found throughout the length of the gene in patients with de novo MDS, but tend to cluster in the DNA binding domain in patients with AML and therapy-related MDS.[103] Heterozygous Runt domain mutations can act as dominant negatives, severely limiting *RUNX1* activity, and may be partially responsible for the poorer outcome of patients with therapy-related disease.[104,105]

Manipulation of *RUNX1* in mice has helped explain how acquired *RUNX1* mutations could lead to MDS and AML. Complete *RUNX1* knockout results in embryonic lethality without evidence of definitive hematopoiesis. However, selective *RUNX1* excision in adult animals does not block hematopoiesis. Instead, these mice show lymphoid defects, expansion of the myeloid progenitor pool, inefficient platelet production, and extramedullary hematopoiesis, but not progression to AML.[98] In contrast, mice transplanted with bone marrow cells overexpressing *RUNX1* with a Runt domain mutation developed increasing bone marrow blast counts, splenomegaly, and often died of an AML-like disease.[106] Mice transplanted with cells expressing *RUNX1* with a more distal frameshift mutation instead developed a more MDS-like phenotype with marked erythroid dysplasia and pancytopenia with a lower rate of progression to AML.

Further evidence of the role of *RUNX1* in myelodysplasia and progression to AML comes from the rare autosomal dominant disease known as the familial platelet disorder with propensity to acute leukemia (FPD). Affected persons with FPD often have an MDS-like disease characterized by low number of platelets that may function abnormally. About 35% of patients with FPD will develop AML, often by acquiring a second *RUNX1* mutation in their remaining wild-type allele.[107,108]

In the mouse models and human cases of congenital *RUNX1* mutations, progression of disease occurs only after a long latency and likely requires cooperating mutations. In patients with MDS and patients with AML arising from MDS, *RUNX1* mutations have been associated with activating mutations in the receptor tyrosine kinase-RAS pathway and the presence of chromosome 7 deletions, [93,102,109] which suggests that these abnormalities are complementary, each driving a distinct step in the pathogenesis of more advanced disease.

JAK2 Mutations

Activating mutations of *JAK2* are the defining genetic lesion of PV and are found in roughly half of patients with essential thrombocythemia (ET) or primary myelofibrosis.[110] In MDS, the mutation rate is much lower with the *JAK2 V617F* mutation reported in approximately 5% of unselected patients with MDS.[111] This frequency is higher in a subset of patients. More than half of patients with refractory anemia with ringed sideroblasts and thrombocytosis (RARS-T) carry the *JAK2 V617F* mutation and a smaller number contain activating mutations of *MPL*.[112,113] These patients typically have low risk disease and rarely progress to acute leukemia. This mutation frequency is comparable to that seen in essential thrombocytosis, prompting the speculation that some cases of RARS-T could be considered to be the frustrated expression of a myeloproliferative disorder and not always a subcategory of MDS.[114] The alternative view is that the acquisition of a *JAK2 V617F* mutation in the setting of RARS leads to thrombocytosis, but patients retain the risk of progression associated with RARS.[115]

There remains a population of *JAK2 V617F* positive patients who have MDS without ringed sideroblasts.[116] Whether these patients have an MDS/MPN overlap syndrome or simply MDS is less clear. Analysis of a 5q- MDS cohort demonstrated the *JAK2* mutation in 6% of these patients.[117] Those positive for *JAK2 V617F* had higher peripheral white blood cell counts, a trend toward a higher platelet count, but no excess blasts in their bone marrow. One patient sample was subject to clonal analysis, identifying the 5q- abnormality in 91% of metaphases. However, single colony assays revealed the *JAK2 V617F* mutation in closer to 50% of cells, which suggests that the *JAK2* mutation developed in a subclone that had already acquired the 5q- deletion. In this genetic background, constitutive *JAK2* activity may provide a clonal advantage without being able to drive the proliferation of terminally differentiated cells seen in PV and ET. It also suggests that targeting *JAK2* activity in patients who have MDS with *JAK2 V617F* mutations might do little to ameliorate the risk of subsequent disease progression.

EPIGENETICS

Patterns of gene expression are commonly altered in MDS and can occur as a consequence of genetic mutations and from epigenetic chromatin modifications that do not alter the underlying DNA sequence. There is considerable evidence that epigenetic changes play a role in the pathogenesis of myeloid disorders and are targets for therapeutic intervention. Furthermore, many of the genes that are frequently mutated or deleted in MDS, including *TET2*, *ASXL1*, and *RUNX1*, have direct roles in chromatic remodeling.

The most common epigenetic mark associated with myeloid malignancies is DNA methylation of cytosine residues. Typically, cytosine methylation in CpG islands of promoter regions negatively regulates the expression of nearby genes. Examples of genes that are silenced by DNA methylation in myeloid disorders include *CDH1*,

CDKN2A (p14, p16), CDKN2B (p15), CTNNA1, MEG3, and SNRPN.[10,118-121]Genes that are commonly silenced by DNA methylation in MDS and AML have rarely been found to be inactivated by mutation in these disorders.[122,123] However, increased promoter DNA methylation is associated with MDS progression to AML.[124]

A more detailed exploration into the role of DNA methylation and other epigenetic modifications in MDS can be found in the accompanying article by Jean Pierre Issa.

INTEGRATION OF GENETIC ABNORMALITIES

Technical advances in the ability to query the genome have created a growing list of genetic alterations associated with MDS and other myeloid disorders. Each of these abnormalities is likely implicated in one or more of the steps necessary to convert a normal early hematopoietic cell into a greatly expanded diseased clone. However, there has been less progress in our ability to integrate the large number of potential MDS-related genetic abnormalities into well-characterized pathologic mechanisms. This is, in part, made more difficult by the heterogeneity of diseases encompassed within MDS. In-depth analyses of a large numbers of subjects, with well-characterized clinical phenotypes, are needed to have the power to make correlations between genetic abnormalities. Studies of smaller numbers of subjects have uncovered sets of mutations and deletions that either occur more frequently with each other or seem to be mutually exclusive. This information has been used to create a framework for understanding mechanisms responsible for the development of MDS.

One view considers the preleukemic nature of MDS and ascribes to disease cells a subset of the genetic abnormalities needed for transformation. Progression of disease is assumed to come from the acquisition of additional mutations that then lead to AML. In its simplest form, two major classes of mutations are required for leukemogenesis: Class I mutations that drive proliferation and Class II mutations that impair differentiation.[125] Activating mutations of NRAS or JAK2 are considered Class I mutations, whereas mutations of transcription factors like RUNX1 are considered class II mutations. Large chromosomal deletions are also considered Class II mutations. In this model, preleukemic cases of MDS should only harbor Class II mutations. The acquisition of Class I mutations would be presumed to quickly lead to leukemia. However, most cases of MDS are low risk and do not have a high risk for progression to leukemia. This may be because they would take a long time to acquire additional mutations or because some gene mutations associated with MDS might exert a weaker phenotype compared with the more severe mutations seen in AML.

A more detailed approach considers several independent pathways that could lead to MDS and progression to AML, using therapy-related MDS/AML cases to support the model.[93,102] This still leaves many cases of MDS without detectable genetic abnormalities to explain their pathogenesis. Most identified mutations are associated with more advanced disease and confer a poor prognosis (Table 1). Yet most patients with MDS have low risk disease, and hence, are more likely to have few or no pathogenic mutations. These patients may have disease caused by stromal deficiencies or epigenetic changes, but more likely, they carry genetic mutations that have yet to be identified. Analyses of these apparently genetically normal cases have yielded several of the recent discoveries in the field.

For example, the discoveries of ASXL1 and TET2 mutations have not only expanded the repertoire of genetic alterations that can occur in MDS but they have revealed some of the mechanisms that may generate the epigenetic dysregulation that is associated with MDS and AML. These DNA modifying enzymes represent a separate class of proteins implicated in the pathogenesis of myeloid disorders, joining the ranks of

Table 1
Reported frequency of MDS-related gene mutations in various myeloid disorders and association with prognosis relative to disease category

Mutated Genes	Myeloid Disorder				
	MDS	CMML	JMML	MPN	AML
TET2	+++	+++	−	++	+++
RUNX1	++	+++	?	+	++
NRAS/KRAS	++	+++	+++	R	++
ASXL1	++	+++	?	++	++
TP53	++	−	?		++
CBL	+	+++	++	+	+
JAK2	+	+	?	+++	+
PTPN11	R	R	+++	?	+
CEBPA	R	++	?	?	+
NPM1	R	+	?		+++
FLT3	R		R		++

Keys: ?, not reported; −, not detected; R, <5% rare; +, 5%–10%; ++, 10%–20%; +++, >20%; ▨, associated with poor prognosis; ▢, associated with better prognosis.

transcription factors, tyrosine kinase pathway members, cell-cycle inhibitors, and anti-apoptotic proteins. There are likely more members of this class waiting to be discovered.

Whole genome sequencing has emerged as a powerful tool in the search for novel disease-related genetic mutations. The sequencing of an AML genome led to the identification of several gene candidates, including the recurrently mutated gene *IDH1*.[126] This study also shed light on the genetic context in which these mutations arise. Extrapolating from the number of potential mutations that were validated, it is estimated that the leukemic cells carried about 750 somatic mutations, the vast majority of which were in noncoding, nonconserved areas of the genome and unlikely to be pathogenic. In fact, the ratio of normal to mutant alleles suggests that almost all of these mutations were present in every diseased cell, which implies that they may have been acquired before clonal expansion and not necessarily picked up along the way because of disease-related genomic instability or defects in DNA repair. Normal hematopoietic stem cells from older adults likely harbor hundreds of similarly inconsequential mutations, all of which could be detected as potential candidates in a whole-genome analysis were one of these cells to transform into a malignant clone. Identifying the disease-related abnormalities requires assigning a likely impact to each mutation and looking for its presence in other patients. Eventually, sequencing of multiple disease genomes will create a less biased filtering system by characterizing which sites or genes are mutated more often than chance.

The promise of these types of techniques extends beyond their unbiased nature. Comprehensive strategies, such as whole genomic sequencing of diseased cells, epigenetic profiling, and expression analysis, will allow us to understand how several disease-causing mutations interact when applied to a larger number of samples. The ability to make correlations between multiple genetic changes is particularly important in MDS, where no single, extremely high frequency or disease-defining mutation exists. Studying samples of patients who have MDS with these broad genomic tools at different points in time will enable us to identify the collection of genetic alterations associated with disease progression. We may find that certain mutations are detected primarily at the time of diagnosis, suggesting that these represent disease initiating events, whereas other mutations might be uniquely found at the time of transformation. Alternatively, it may be that a particular set of genetic lesions are required for disease progression and the order in which they are acquired does not matter. By identifying those mutations that are mutually exclusive, we will learn more about the molecular mechanisms and pathways that give rise to these disorders.

Finally, it will be necessary to integrate the clinical implications of the mutations identified in patients with MDS. As the cost of testing falls and the necessary analytical tools mature, comprehensive genetic analyses could be employed at the individual level, genotyping the pathogenome of each patient with MDS to better define their prognosis and help select their optimal therapy.

REFERENCES

1. Haase D, Germing U, Schanz J, et al. New insights into the prognostic impact of the karyotype in MDS and correlation with subtypes: evidence from a core dataset of 2124 patients. Blood 2007;110(13):4385–95.
2. Greenberg P, Cox C, LeBeau MM, et al. International scoring system for evaluating prognosis in myelodysplastic syndromes. Blood 1997;89(6):2079–88.
3. Garcia-Manero G. Demethylating agents in myeloid malignancies. Curr Opin Oncol 2008;20(6):705–10.
4. Graubert TA, Payton MA, Shao J, et al. Integrated genomic analysis implicates haploinsufficiency of multiple chromosome 5q31.2 genes in de novo myelodysplastic syndromes pathogenesis. PLoS One 2009;4(2):e4583.
5. Ebert BL, Pretz J, Bosco J, et al. Identification of RPS14 as the 5q- syndrome gene by RNA interference screen. Nature 2008;451(7176):335–9.
6. Draptchinskaia N, Gustavsson P, Andersson B, et al. The gene encoding ribosomal protein S19 is mutated in Diamond-Blackfan anaemia. Nat Genet 1999; 21(2):169–75.
7. McGowan KA, Li JZ, Park CY, et al. Ribosomal mutations cause p53-mediated dark skin and pleiotropic effects. Nat Genet 2008;40(8):963–70.
8. Fumagalli S, Di Cara A, Neb-Gulati A, et al. Absence of nucleolar disruption after impairment of 40S ribosome biogenesis reveals an rpL11-translation-dependent mechanism of p53 induction. Nat Cell Biol 2009;11(4):501–8.
9. Barlow JL, Drynan LF, Hewett DR, et al. A p53-dependent mechanism underlies macrocytic anemia in a mouse model of human 5q- syndrome. Nat Med 2010; 16:59–66.
10. Liu TX, Becker MW, Jelinek J, et al. Chromosome 5q deletion and epigenetic suppression of the gene encoding alpha-catenin (CTNNA1) in myeloid cell transformation. Nat Med 2007;13(1):78–83.
11. Xie H, Hu Z, Chyna B, et al. Human mortalin (HSPA9): a candidate for the myeloid leukemia tumor suppressor gene on 5q31. Leukemia 2000;14(12): 2128–34.
12. Joslin JM, Fernald AA, Tennant TR, et al. Haploinsufficiency of EGR1, a candidate gene in the del(5q), leads to the development of myeloid disorders. Blood 2007;110(2):719–26.
13. Ebert BL. Deletion 5q in myelodysplastic syndrome: a paradigm for the study of hemizygous deletions in cancer. Leukemia 2009;23(7):1252–6.
14. Grisendi S, Bernardi R, Rossi M, et al. Role of nucleophosmin in embryonic development and tumorigenesis. Nature 2005;437(7055):147–53.

15. Sportoletti P, Grisendi S, Majid SM, et al. Npm1 is a haploinsufficient suppressor of myeloid and lymphoid malignancies in the mouse. Blood 2008;111(7): 3859–62.

16. List A, Dewald G, Bennett J, et al. Lenalidomide in the myelodysplastic syndrome with chromosome 5q deletion. N Engl J Med 2006;355(14):1456–65.

17. Wei S, Chen X, Rocha K, et al. A critical role for phosphatase haplodeficiency in the selective suppression of deletion 5q MDS by lenalidomide. Proc Natl Acad Sci U S A 2009;106(31):12974–9.

18. Pellagatti A, Jadersten M, Forsblom AM, et al. Lenalidomide inhibits the malignant clone and up-regulates the SPARC gene mapping to the commonly deleted region in 5q- syndrome patients. Proc Natl Acad Sci U S A 2007; 104(27):11406–11.

19. Beau MM, Espinosa R, Davis EM, et al. Cytogenetic and molecular delineation of a region of chromosome 7 commonly deleted in malignant myeloid diseases. Blood 1996;88(6):1930–5.

20. Liang H, Fairman J, Claxton DF, et al. Molecular anatomy of chromosome 7q deletions in myeloid neoplasms: evidence for multiple critical loci. Proc Natl Acad Sci U S A 1998;95(7):3781–5.

21. Gondek LP, Tiu R, O'Keefe CL, et al. Chromosomal lesions and uniparental disomy detected by SNP arrays in MDS, MDS/MPD and MDS-derived AML. Blood 2008;111(3):1534–42.

22. Roulston D, Espinosa R, Stoffel M, et al. Molecular genetics of myeloid leukemia: identification of the commonly deleted segment of chromosome 20. Blood 1993; 82(11):3424–9.

23. Wang PW, Eisenbart JD, Espinosa R, et al. Refinement of the smallest commonly deleted segment of chromosome 20 in malignant myeloid diseases and development of a PAC-based physical and transcription map. Genomics 2000;67(1): 28–39.

24. Liu Y-C, Ito Y, Hsiao H-H, et al. Risk factor analysis in myelodysplastic syndrome patients with del(20q): prognosis revisited. Cancer Genet Cytogenet 2006; 171(1):9–16.

25. Virtaneva K, Wright FA, Tanner SM, et al. Expression profiling reveals fundamental biological differences in acute myeloid leukemia with isolated trisomy 8 and normal cytogenetics. Proc Natl Acad Sci U S A 2001;98(3):1124–9.

26. Sloand EM, Pfannes L, Chen G, et al. CD34 cells from patients with trisomy 8 myelodysplastic syndrome (MDS) express early apoptotic markers but avoid programmed cell death by up-regulation of antiapoptotic proteins. Blood 2007;109(6):2399–405.

27. Barrett AJ, Sloand E. Autoimmune mechanisms in the pathophysiology of myelodysplastic syndromes and their clinical relevance. Haematologica 2009;94(4): 449–51.

28. Sloand EM, Mainwaring L, Fuhrer M, et al. Preferential suppression of trisomy 8 compared with normal hematopoietic cell growth by autologous lymphocytes in patients with trisomy 8 myelodysplastic syndrome. Blood 2005;106(3):841–51.

29. Wiktor A, Rybicki BA, Piao ZS, et al. Clinical significance of Y chromosome loss in hematologic disease. Genes Chromosomes Cancer 2000;27(1):11–6.

30. Wong AK, Fang B, Zhang L, et al. Loss of the Y chromosome: an age-related or clonal phenomenon in acute myelogenous leukemia/myelodysplastic syndrome? Arch Pathol Lab Med 2008;132(8):1329–32.

31. Look AT. Molecular pathogenesis of MDS. Hematology Am Soc Hematol Educ Program 2005;2005:156–60.

32. Poppe B, Dastugue N, Vandesompele J, et al. EVI1 is consistently expressed as principal transcript in common and rare recurrent 3q26 rearrangements. Genes Chromosomes Cancer 2006;45(4):349–56.

33. Vardiman JW, Thiele J, Arber DA, et al. The 2008 revision of the World Health Organization (WHO) classification of myeloid neoplasms and acute leukemia: rationale and important changes. Blood 2009;114(5):937–51.

34. Shapira MY, Hirshberg B, Amir G, et al. 6;9 translocation in myelodysplastic syndrome. Cancer Genet Cytogenet 1999;112(1):57–9.

35. Nucifora G, Begy CR, Kobayashi H, et al. Consistent intergenic splicing and production of multiple transcripts between AML1 at 21q22 and unrelated genes at 3q26 in (3;21)(q26;q22) translocations. Proc Natl Acad Sci U S A 1994;91(9): 4004–8.

36. Raza-Egilmez SZ, Jani-Sait SN, Grossi M, et al. NUP98-HOXD13 gene fusion in therapy-related acute myelogenous leukemia. Cancer Res 1998;58(19): 4269–73.

37. Steensma DP, Neiger JD, Porcher JC, et al. Rearrangements and amplification of IER3 (IEX-1) represent a novel and recurrent molecular abnormality in myelo-dysplastic syndromes. Cancer Res 2009;69(19):7518–23.

38. Lahortiga I, Agirre X, Belloni E, et al. Molecular characterization of a t(1;3)(p36;q21) in a patient with MDS. MEL1 is widely expressed in normal tissues, including bone marrow, and it is not overexpressed in the t(1;3) cells. Oncogene 2004;23(1):311–6.

39. Xinh PT, Tri NK, Nagao H, et al. Breakpoints at 1p36.3 in three MDS/AML(M4) patients with t(1;3)(p36;q21) occur in the first intron and in the 5′ region of MEL1. Genes Chromosomes Cancer 2003;36(3):313–6.

40. Bordereaux D, Fichelson S, Tambourin P, et al. Alternative splicing of the Evi-1 zinc finger gene generates mRNAs which differ by the number of zinc finger motifs. Oncogene 1990;5(6):925–7.

41. Soderholm J, Kobayashi H, Mathieu C, et al. The leukemia-associated gene MDS1/EVI1 is a new type of GATA-binding transactivator. Leukemia 1997; 11(3):352–8.

42. Morishita K, Parker DS, Mucenski ML, et al. Retroviral activation of a novel gene encoding a zinc finger protein in IL-3-dependent myeloid leukemia cell lines. Cell 1988;54(6):831–40.

43. Du Y, Jenkins NA, Copeland NG. Insertional mutagenesis identifies genes that promote the immortalization of primary bone marrow progenitor cells. Blood 2005;106(12):3932–9.

44. Russell M, List A, Greenberg P, et al. Expression of EVI1 in myelodysplastic syndromes and other hematologic malignancies without 3q26 translocations. Blood 1994;84(4):1243–8.

45. Barjesteh van Waalwijk van Doorn-Khosrovani S, Erpelinck C, van Putten WLJ, et al. High EVI1 expression predicts poor survival in acute myeloid leukemia: a study of 319 de novo AML patients. Blood 2003;101(3):837–45.

46. Buonamici S, Li D, Chi Y, et al. EVI1 induces myelodysplastic syndrome in mice. J Clin Invest 2004;114(5):713–9.

47. Maresso K, Broeckel U, Rao DC, et al. Genotyping platforms for mass-throughput genotyping with snps, including human genome-wide scans, in advances in genetics. Adv Genet 2008;60:107–39.

48. Nishida N, Koike A, Tajima A, et al. Evaluating the performance of Affymetrix SNP Array 6.0 platform with 400 Japanese individuals. BMC Genomics 2008; 9:431.

49. Gondek LP, Dunbar AJ, Szpurka H, et al. SNP array karyotyping allows for the detection of uniparental disomy and cryptic chromosomal abnormalities in MDS/MPD-U and MPD. PLoS One 2007;2(11):e1225.

50. Heinrichs S, Kulkarni RV, Bueso-Ramos CE, et al. Accurate detection of uniparental disomy and microdeletions by SNP array analysis in myelodysplastic syndromes with normal cytogenetics. Leukemia 2009;23(9):1605–13.

51. Mohamedali A, Gaken J, Twine NA, et al. Prevalence and prognostic significance of allelic imbalance by single-nucleotide polymorphism analysis in low-risk myelodysplastic syndromes. Blood 2007;110(9):3365–73.

52. Tiu RV, Gondek LP, O'Keefe CL, et al. New lesions detected by single nucleotide polymorphism array-based chromosomal analysis have important clinical impact in acute myeloid leukemia. J Clin Oncol 2009;27(31):5219–26.

53. Lorsbach RB, Moore J, Mathew S, et al. TET1, a member of a novel protein family, is fused to MLL in acute myeloid leukemia containing the t(10;11)(q22;q23). Leukemia 2003;17(3):637–41.

54. Delhommeau F, Dupont S, Valle VD, et al. Mutation in TET2 in myeloid cancers. N Engl J Med 2009;360(22):2289–301.

55. Jankowska AM, Szpurka H, Tiu RV, et al. Loss of heterozygosity 4q24 and TET2 mutations associated with myelodysplastic/myeloproliferative neoplasms. Blood 2009;113(25):6403–10.

56. Abdel-Wahab O, Mullally A, Hedvat C, et al. Genetic characterization of TET1, TET2, and TET3 alterations in myeloid malignancies. Blood 2009;114(1):144–7.

57. Mohamedali AM, Smith AE, Gaken J, et al. Novel TET2 mutations associated with UPD4q24 in myelodysplastic syndrome. J Clin Oncol 2009;27(24):4002–6.

58. Saint-Martin C, Leroy G, Delhommeau F, et al. Analysis of the Ten-Eleven Translocation 2 (TET2) gene in familial myeloproliferative neoplasms. Blood 2009; 114(8):1628–32.

59. Tefferi A, Levine RL, Lim KH, et al. Frequent TET2 mutations in systemic mastocytosis: clinical, KITD816V and FIP1L1-PDGFRA correlates. Leukemia 2009; 23(5):900–4.

60. Tefferi A, Lim KH, Abdel-Wahab O, et al. Detection of mutant TET2 in myeloid malignancies other than myeloproliferative neoplasms: CMML, MDS, MDS/MPN and AML. Leukemia 2009;23(7):1343–5.

61. Mullighan CG. TET2 mutations in myelodysplasia and myeloid malignancies. Nat Genet 2009;41(7):766–7.

62. Levine RL, Carroll M. A common genetic mechanism in malignant bone marrow diseases. N Engl J Med 2009;360(22):2355–7.

63. Kosmider O, Gelsi-Boyer V, Cheok M, et al. TET2 mutation is an independent favorable prognostic factor in myelodysplastic syndromes (MDSs). Blood 2009;114(15):3285–91.

64. Langemeijer SM, Kuiper RP, Berends M, et al. Acquired mutations in TET2 are common in myelodysplastic syndromes. Nat Genet 2009;41(7):838–42.

65. Kosmider O, Gelsi-Boyer V, Ciudad M, et al. TET2 gene mutation is a frequent and adverse event in chronic myelomonocytic leukemia. Haematologica 2009; 94(12):1676–81.

66. Tahiliani M, Koh KP, Shen Y, et al. Conversion of 5-methylcytosine to 5-hydroxymethylcytosine in mammalian DNA by MLL partner TET1. Science 2009; 324(5929):930–5.

67. Cho Y-S, Kim E-J, Park U-H, et al. Additional Sex Comb-like 1 (ASXL1), in cooperation with SRC-1, acts as a ligand-dependent coactivator for retinoic acid receptor. J Biol Chem 2006;281(26):17588–98.

68. Lee S-W, Cho Y-S, Na J-M, et al. Additional sex comb-like 1 represses RAR-mediated transcription through associating with heterochromatin protein 1 and lysine-specific demethylase 1. J Biol Chem 2010;285(1):18–29.

69. Gelsi-Boyer V, Trouplin V, Adelaide J, et al. Mutations of polycomb-associated gene ASXL1 in myelodysplastic syndromes and chronic myelomonocytic leukaemia. Br J Haematol 2009;145(6):788–800.

70. Carbuccia N, Murati A, Trouplin V, et al. Mutations of ASXL1 gene in myeloproliferative neoplasms. Leukemia 2009;23(11):2183–6.

71. Carbuccia N, Trouplin V, Gelsi-Boyer V, et al. Mutual exclusion of ASXL1 and NPM1 mutations in a series of acute myeloid leukemias. Leukemia 2010;24(2):469–73.

72. Fisher CL, Pineault N, Brookes C, et al. Loss-of-function additional sex combs-like1 mutations disrupt hematopoiesis but do not cause severe myelodysplasia or leukemia. Blood 2010;115(1):38–46.

73. Sargin B, Choudhary C, Crosetto N, et al. Flt3-dependent transformation by inactivating c-Cbl mutations in AML. Blood 2007;110(3):1004–12.

74. Saur SJ, Sangkhae V, Geddis AE, et al. Ubiquitination and degradation of the thrombopoietin receptor c-Mpl. Blood 2010;115(6):1254–63.

75. Thien CB, Langdon WY. Cbl: many adaptations to regulate protein tyrosine kinases. Nat Rev Mol Cell Biol 2001;2(4):294–307.

76. Dunbar AJ, Gondek LP, O'Keefe CL, et al. 250K single nucleotide polymorphism array karyotyping identifies acquired uniparental disomy and homozygous mutations, including novel missense substitutions of c-Cbl, in myeloid malignancies. Cancer Res 2008;68(24):10349–57.

77. Sanada M, Suzuki T, Shih L-Y, et al. Gain-of-function of mutated C-CBL tumour suppressor in myeloid neoplasms. Nature 2009;460(7257):904–8.

78. Caligiuri MA, Briesewitz R, Yu J, et al. Novel c-CBL and CBL-b ubiquitin ligase mutations in human acute myeloid leukemia. Blood 2007;110(3):1022–4.

79. Abbas S, Rotmans G, Lowenberg B, et al. Exon 8 splice site mutations in the gene encoding the E3-ligase CBL are associated with core binding factor acute myeloid leukemias. Haematologica 2008;93(10):1595–7.

80. Reindl C, Quentmeier H, Petropoulos K, et al. CBL exon 8/9 mutants activate the FLT3 pathway and cluster in core binding factor/11q deletion acute myeloid leukemia/myelodysplastic syndrome subtypes. Clin Cancer Res 2009;15(7):2238–47.

81. Loh ML, Sakai DS, Flotho C, et al. Mutations in CBL occur frequently in juvenile myelomonocytic leukemia. Blood 2009;114(9):1859–63.

82. Hirai H, Kobayashi Y, Mano H, et al. A point mutation at codon 13 of the N-ras oncogene in myelodysplastic syndrome. Nature 1987;327(6121):430–2.

83. Lyons J, Janssen JW, Bartram C, et al. Mutation of Ki-ras and N-ras oncogenes in myelodysplastic syndromes. Blood 1988;71(6):1707–12.

84. Paquette RL, Landaw EM, Pierre RV, et al. N-ras mutations are associated with poor prognosis and increased risk of leukemia in myelodysplastic syndrome. Blood 1993;82(2):590–9.

85. Constantinidou M, Chalevelakis M, Economopoulos T, et al. Codon 12 ras mutations in patients with myelodysplastic syndrome: incidence and prognostic value. Ann Hematol 1997;74(1):11–4.

86. Nakagawa T, Saitoh S, Imoto S, et al. Multiple point mutation of N- ras and K- ras oncogenes in myelodysplastic syndrome and acute myelogenous leukemia. Oncology 1992;49(2):114–22.

87. Shih LY, Huang CF, Wang PN, et al. Acquisition of FLT3 or N-ras mutations is frequently associated with progression of myelodysplastic syndrome to acute myeloid leukemia. Leukemia 2004;18(3):466–75.

88. Loh ML, Martinelli S, Cordeddu V, et al. Acquired PTPN11 mutations occur rarely in adult patients with myelodysplastic syndromes and chronic myelomonocytic leukemia. Leuk Res 2005;29(4):459–62.

89. Christiansen DH, Andersen MK, Desta F, et al. Mutations of genes in the receptor tyrosine kinase (RTK)/RAS-BRAF signal transduction pathway in therapy-related myelodysplasia and acute myeloid leukemia. Leukemia 2005; 19(12):2232–40.

90. Christiansen DH, Andersen MK, Pedersen-Bjergaard J. Mutations with loss of heterozygosity of p53 are common in therapy-related myelodysplasia and acute myeloid leukemia after exposure to alkylating agents and significantly associated with deletion or loss of 5q, a complex karyotype, and a poor prognosis. J Clin Oncol 2001;19(5):1405–13.

91. Wattel E, Preudhomme C, Hecquet B, et al. p53 mutations are associated with resistance to chemotherapy and short survival in hematologic malignancies. Blood 1994;84(9):3148–57.

92. Harada H, Harada Y, Tanaka H, et al. Implications of somatic mutations in the AML1 gene in radiation-associated and therapy-related myelodysplastic syndrome/acute myeloid leukemia. Blood 2003;101(2):673–80.

93. Pedersen-Bjergaard J, Christiansen DH, Desta F, et al. Alternative genetic pathways and cooperating genetic abnormalities in the pathogenesis of therapy-related myelodysplasia and acute myeloid leukemia. Leukemia 2006;20(11): 1943–9.

94. Kaneko H, Misawa S, Horiike S, et al. TP53 mutations emerge at early phase of myelodysplastic syndrome and are associated with complex chromosomal abnormalities. Blood 1995;85(8):2189–93.

95. Horiike S, Kita-Sasai Y, Nakao M, et al. Configuration of the TP53 gene as an independent prognostic parameter of myelodysplastic syndrome. Leuk Lymphoma 2003;44(6):915–22.

96. Kita-Sasai Y, Horiike S, Misawa S, et al. International prognostic scoring system and TP53 mutations are independent prognostic indicators for patients with myelodysplastic syndrome. Br J Haematol 2001;115(2):309–12.

97. Jadersten M, Saft L, Pellagatti A, et al. Clonal heterogeneity in the 5q- syndrome: p53 expressing progenitors prevail during lenalidomide treatment and expand at disease progression. Haematologica 2009;94(12):1762–6.

98. Growney JD, Shigematsu H, Li Z, et al. Loss of Runx1 perturbs adult hematopoiesis and is associated with a myeloproliferative phenotype. Blood 2005;106(2): 494–504.

99. Steensma DP, Gibbons RJ, Mesa RA, et al. Somatic point mutations in RUNX1/ CBFA2/AML1 are common in high-risk myelodysplastic syndrome, but not in myelofibrosis with myeloid metaplasia. Eur J Haematol 2005;74(1):47–53.

100. Chen CY, Lin LI, Tang JL, et al. RUNX1 gene mutation in primary myelodysplastic syndrome—the mutation can be detected early at diagnosis or acquired during disease progression and is associated with poor outcome. Br J Haematol 2007;139(3):405–14.

101. Christiansen DH, Andersen MK, Pedersen-Bjergaard J. Mutations of AML1 are common in therapy-related myelodysplasia following therapy with alkylating agents and are significantly associated with deletion or loss of chromosome arm 7q and with subsequent leukemic transformation. Blood 2004;104(5):1474–81.

102. Pedersen-Bjergaard J, Andersen MK, Andersen MT, et al. Genetics of therapy-related myelodysplasia and acute myeloid leukemia. Leukemia 2008;22(2): 240–8.

103. Harada H, Harada Y, Niimi H, et al. High incidence of somatic mutations in the AML1/RUNX1 gene in myelodysplastic syndrome and low blast percentage myeloid leukemia with myelodysplasia. Blood 2004;103(6):2316–24.

104. Harada Y, Harada H. Molecular pathways mediating MDS/AML with focus on AML1/RUNX1 point mutations. J Cell Physiol 2009;220(1):16–20.

105. Matheny CJ, Speck ME, Cushing PR, et al. Disease mutations in RUNX1 and RUNX2 create nonfunctional, dominant-negative, or hypomorphic alleles. EMBO J 2007;26(4):1163–75.

106. Watanabe-Okochi N, Kitaura J, Ono R, et al. AML1 mutations induced MDS and MDS/AML in a mouse BMT model. Blood 2008;111(8):4297–308.

107. Preudhomme C, Renneville A, Bourdon V, et al. High frequency of RUNX1 biallelic alteration in acute myeloid leukemia secondary to familial platelet disorder. Blood 2009;113(22):5583–7.

108. Owen CJ, Toze CL, Koochin A, et al. Five new pedigrees with inherited RUNX1 mutations causing familial platelet disorder with propensity to myeloid malignancy. Blood 2008;112(12):4639–45.

109. Niimi H, Harada H, Harada Y, et al. Hyperactivation of the RAS signaling pathway in myelodysplastic syndrome with AML1/RUNX1 point mutations. Leukemia 2006;20(4):635–44.

110. Levine RL, Gilliland DG. Myeloproliferative disorders. Blood 2008;112(6):2190–8.

111. Steensma DP, Dewald GW, Lasho TL, et al. The JAK2 V617F activating tyrosine kinase mutation is an infrequent event in both "atypical" myeloproliferative disorders and myelodysplastic syndromes. Blood 2005;106(4):1207–9.

112. Malcovati L, Della Porta MG, Pietra D, et al. Molecular and clinical features of refractory anemia with ringed sideroblasts associated with marked thrombocytosis. Blood 2009;114(17):3538–45.

113. Boissinot M, Garand R, Hamidou M, et al. The JAK2-V617F mutation and essential thrombocythemia features in a subset of patients with refractory anemia with ring sideroblasts (RARS). Blood 2006;108(5):1781–2.

114. Wardrop D, Steensma DP. Is refractory anaemia with ring sideroblasts and thrombocytosis (RARS-T) a necessary or useful diagnostic category? Br J Haematol 2009;144(6):809–17.

115. Hellstrom-Lindberg E, Cazzola M. The role of JAK2 mutations in RARS and other MDS. Hematology 2008;2008(1):52–9.

116. Steensma DP, Tefferi A. JAK2 V617F and ringed sideroblasts: not necessarily RARS-T. Blood 2008;111(3):1748.

117. Ingram W, Lea NC, Cervera J, et al. The JAK2 V617F mutation identifies a subgroup of MDS patients with isolated deletion 5q and a proliferative bone marrow. Leukemia 2006;20(7):1319–21.

118. Boultwood J, Wainscoat JS. Gene silencing by DNA methylation in haematological malignancies. Br J Haematol 2007;138(1):3–11.

119. Mahmud M, Stebbing J. Epigenetic modifications in AML and MDS. Leuk Res 2010;34(2):139–40.

120. Ye Y, McDevitt MA, Guo M, et al. Progressive chromatin repression and promoter methylation of CTNNA1 associated with advanced myeloid malignancies. Cancer Res 2009;69(21):8482–90.

121. Benetatos L, Hatzimichael E, Dasoula A, et al. CpG methylation analysis of the MEG3 and SNRPN imprinted genes in acute myeloid leukemia and myelodysplastic syndromes. Leuk Res 2010;34(2):148–53.

122. Daskalakis M, Nguyen TT, Nguyen C, et al. Demethylation of a hypermethylated P15/INK4B gene in patients with myelodysplastic syndrome by 5-aza-2'-deoxycytidine (decitabine) treatment. Blood 2002;100(8):2957–64.
123. Nakamaki T, Bartram C, Seriu T, et al. Molecular analysis of the cyclin-dependent kinase inhibitor genes, p15, p16, p18 and p19 in the myelodysplastic syndromes. Leuk Res 1997;21(3):235–40.
124. Jiang Y, Dunbar A, Gondek LP, et al. Aberrant DNA methylation is a dominant mechanism in MDS progression to AML. Blood 2009;113(6):1315–25.
125. Kelly LM, Gilliland DG. Genetics of myeloid leukemias. Annu Rev Genomics Hum Genet 2002;3:179–98.
126. Mardis ER, Ding L, Dooling DJ, et al. Recurring mutations found by sequencing an acute myeloid leukemia genome. N Engl J Med 2009;361(11):1058–66.

Epigenetic Changes in the Myelodysplastic Syndrome

Jean-Pierre Issa, MD[a,b,]*

KEYWORDS

- Myelodysplastic syndrome • Acute myelogenous leukemia
- Epigenetic changes • DNA methyltransferase

The myelodysplastic syndromes (MDSs) are a group of diverse and heterogeneous syndromes characterized by clonal proliferation, bone marrow failure, and an increased risk of development of acute myelogenous leukemia (AML).[1] The natural course of the disease ranges from slow progression to rapid evolution into AML. There are several classification systems for MDS, such as the International Prognostic Scoring System,[2] the World Health Organization classification,[3] and more recent clinical schemes,[4] but none captures the full heterogeneity of the disease. Heterogeneity and progression are likely related to molecular changes that drive the disease phenotype and biology, but these remain incompletely understood. Insights into the pathogenesis of cancer has come from studying genetic changes in neoplastic cells.[5,6] In MDS, several cytogenetic abnormalities have been identified that characterize subgroups of patients, such as deletions of chromosome 5 or 7 in patients with poor prognosis, isolated deletion of 5q, or trisomy 8. Mutations of several genes also characterize subsets of cases, including RAS, TET2, RUNX1, and other genes. Despite these advances, the molecular causes of MDS and its peculiar clinical features remain poorly understood. Epigenetic changes have been recognized in the past decade as major drivers of the malignant phenotype.[7] Epigenetics refers to the study of clonally inherited changes in gene expression without accompanying genetic changes. There are 3 general molecular mechanisms carrying epigenetic information—DNA methylation, histone modifications, and RNA interference.[8,9] In cancer, there is particular recent interest in the involvement

Relevant work in the author's laboratory is supported by National Institutes of Health grants CA100632, CA098006, and CA121104. The author is an American Cancer Society Clinical Research professor supported by a generous gift from the F. M. Kirby Foundation.

[a] Department of Leukemia, The University of Texas M. D. Anderson Cancer Center, Unit 428, 1515 Holcombe, Unit 428, Houston, TX 77030, USA

[b] Center for Cancer Epigenetics, The University of Texas M. D. Anderson Cancer Center, Unit 428, 1515 Holcombe, Houston, TX 77030, USA

* Department of Leukemia, The University of Texas M. D. Anderson Cancer Center, Unit 428, 1515 Holcombe, Houston, TX 77030.

E-mail address: jpissa@mdanderson.org

Hematol Oncol Clin N Am 24 (2010) 317–330

doi:10.1016/j.hoc.2010.02.007

0889-8588/10/$ – see front matter © 2010 Elsevier Inc. All rights reserved.

of aberrant DNA methylation and histone modifications in gene silencing that then mediate altered physiology.[10,11] They may be particularly relevant to MDS pathogenesis given that the disease responds well to drugs that affect DNA methylation,[12] a major epigenetic modulator. In this article, recent progress in MDS epigenetics and epigenetic-based therapies is reviewed.

DNA METHYLATION IN EPIGENETIC REGULATION

DNA methylation is a covalent modification of cytosines resulting in the formation of 5-methylcytosine (5mC), a base that changes the interactions between protein and DNA. In adult mammalian cells, DNA methylation normally affects cytosine when it is part of the cytosine-phospho-guanine (CpG) dinucleotide. CpG methylation can occur anywhere in the genome but is particularly relevant when it involves CpG rich regions called CpG islands. In turn, these can be present in about half of human gene promoters. CpG island methylation is associated with absent transcription from the involved promoter, and this silencing is stably transmitted through mitosis, thus ensuring clonal inheritance.[13] This association between CpG island methylation and absent transcription is most striking when considering the 2 physiologic conditions where this process was described, X-chromosome inactivation[14] and imprinting.[15] In both cases, 1 of the 2 copies of the involved genes is transcriptionally silent in association with promoter methylation, despite continued normal expression of the unmethylated allele. Evidence for a direct role of methylation in maintaining the silenced state is from studies where methylation was relieved via pharmacologic[16] or genetic[17] reduction in DNA methyltransferase (DNMT) activity. In most such studies, biallelic expression could be restored, in association with decreased methylation of the affected promoters.

The mechanism whereby CpG island methylation suppresses gene transcription recently was partially elucidated (**Fig. 1**), at least in vitro.[18] Methylated CpG islands

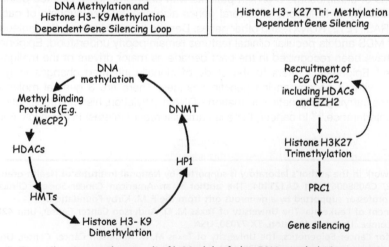

Fig. 1. Two silencing pathways. (*Left*) Model of the DNA methylation associated gene-silencing loop. The cascade of events may start with DNA methylation triggering histone modifications or with H3K9 methylation triggering silencing, which then promotes DNA methylation. (*Right*) PcG-based silencing. Targeting PRC2 to a given promoter results in histone deacetylation and H3K27 trimethylation, which triggers PRC1 binding, a closed chromatin structure and gene silencing. In turn, H3K27 trimethylation may also recruit PRC2 binding to sustain silencing through mitosis.

form excellent binding sites for methylated DNA-binding proteins (often with transcriptional repression properties), such as MeCp2. MeCp2 binding is followed by the recruitment of a protein complex that includes histone deacetylases (HDACs) and eventually leads to a closed chromatin configuration. This closed chromatin configuration results in exclusion of transcription factors, thus ensuring allele-specific inactivation. Methylation-related epigenetic silencing also is associated with histone H3 lysine 9 (H3K9) methylation.[9] Evidence suggests that H3K9 methylation is a critical modification that is associated with closed chromatin at DNA methylation sites, and it was proposed that a cascade of events follows DNA methylation (MeCP2 binding, H3K9 deacetylation, and H3K9 methylation) and ensures transcriptional suppression (see **Fig. 1**).[19,20,21] Separately, DNMT1 can directly suppress transcription (without DNA methylation) through interactions with HDACs.[22,23] H3K9 methylation itself seems to set up a silencing loop by attracting more DNA methylation[24] and may sometimes precede hypermethylation.[25]

DNA METHYLATION CHANGES IN CANCER

There are complex changes in DNA methylation in cancer. For the most part, these changes involve simultaneous global demethylation, increased expression of DNMTs, and de novo methylation at previously unmethylated CpG islands. Demethylation was first discovered by studying overall 5mC content in tumors and seems to involve primarily satellite DNA, repetitive sequences, and CpG sites located in introns.[26,27] The cause of this demethylation remains unclear, although it could be related to alterations in proliferation or cell-cycle control.[28] The functional consequences of hypomethylation are not entirely clear, but there is mounting evidence that gene-specific hypomethylation can cause increased expression of various genes that could contribute to the neoplastic phenotype.[29] An increased mutation rate was demonstrated in cells in which severe hypomethylation (>75%) was achieved by homozygous deletion of DNMT1,[30] but it is not clear whether or not this degree of hypomethylation is ever achieved in neoplasms.[31]

Increased enzymatic DNMT activity is a property of nearly all transformed cells.[32] Increased mRNA levels for DNMT1, DNMT3a, and DNMT3b also are described in some neoplasms, including leukemias,[33,34,35] and these 3 DNMT genes probably account for the observed increase in activity. The causes and functional significance of these increases remain unclear. DNMTs seem to be cell-cycle regulated,[36] and it is argued that DNMT levels reflect the physiologic state of increased proliferation in neoplasia.[37] Alternatively, DNMT1 is reported to increase after oncogene activation,[38,39] and it is possible that its levels in neoplasia reflect the various molecular defects seen in tumors. The functional significance of increased DNMT activity is also poorly defined. In several systems, increased DNMT activity has been found to be transforming,[38,40] but it is not clear whether or not this is due to increased CpG island methylation and tumor-suppressor gene silencing or to direct effects on the cell cycle. The facts that in primary tumors and cell lines no correlation was found between DNMT activity and gene silencing[41,42] and that DNMT-related transformation is reversible when the oncogenic stimulus is removed[38] support the latter possibility. Nevertheless, simultaneous inhibition of several DNMTs does inhibit cancer cell growth,[43] making them potential therapeutic targets.

In parallel to global hypomethylation and increased DNMT activity, there also are distinct and frequent localized increases in methylation, often involving CpG islands.[10,11] Because CpG island methylation is associated with repressed transcription that is stably inherited through mitosis, this de novo methylation in transformed cells is proposed as an alternate mechanism for inactivating tumor-suppressor genes.[7] Several genes are shown to be transcriptionally silent in neoplasia in association with CpG island methylation, including in leukemias. The most convincing evidence for CpG island methylation as a true alternative to mutations in neoplasia is from studies of *RB1*,[44] *p16*,[45] *VHL*,[46] and *MLH1*.[47] For each of these genes, the tumor-spectrum of methylation events is virtually the same as that for mutations, and there are described cases where 1 allele of the gene is inactivated by methylation whereas the other is mutated, suggesting an equivalent growth advantage for each event in neoplasia. For example, in colorectal cancer, the HCT116 cell line carries 1 mutated unmethylated *p16* allele whereas the second allele is unmutated but densely hypermethylated and transcriptionally silent.[45] Moreover, the *MLH1* mismatch repair gene is unmutated but densely methylated in the mismatch repair deficient cell line RKO, and nearly normal levels of mismatch repair can be restored by inhibiting DNMT activity.[48]

HISTONE MODIFICATIONS AND THE HISTONE CODE

Histones are small proteins that form a core around which DNA is wrapped, forming nucleosomes. Nucleosomes are the basic in vivo structural unit of DNA and consist of 8 histone molecules (2 each of histones H2A, H2B, H3, and H4) around which a loop of DNA is wrapped.[49] Although H2A and H2B are thought to play primarily a structural role, it has become apparent that histones H3 and H4 are key integrators of a variety of signals that regulate gene transcription.[9,50,51] In particular, these 2 histone proteins have histone tails, or strings of amino acids, that protrude outside the basic nucleosomal structure and make contact with DNA. Specific post-translational modifications of the amino acids in these histone tails (eg, methylation, acetylation, phosphorylation, ubiquitination, and sumoylation) interact with other proteins to create nucleosomes that are relaxed and promote transcription or nucleosomes that are closed, exclude transcription factors, and result in gene silencing. These histone modifications occur dynamically and are mediated by specific histone-modifying proteins. Targeting of these histone modifiers to specific gene promoters in turn is achieved by transcriptional activator/coactivator complexes in response to physiologic stimuli. Thus, histone modifications form a code that integrates gene activation/inactivation/silencing signals, such that the transcriptional activity of a given promoter can be predicted by looking at the specific histone modifications.[9]

Currently, the best understood histone modifications are acetylation and methylation of specific residues, although it is clear that other modifications also play a role in the process.[9] Acetylation of specific residues on histones H3 and H4 is typically associated with active gene transcription.[52] Methylation of specific residues can be associated with activation of transcription (H3 lysine 4 [H3K4]) or silencing (H3K9 and H3K27).[50] The different modifications also significantly interact. Thus, H3K4 methylation promotes H3K9 acetylation. Moreover, H3K9 can be acetylated or methylated (but not both), and the switch from acetylation to methylation at this residue seems to be a key element of silencing across many organisms. H3K9 promotes silencing by recruiting HP1 and a silencing complex that changes chromatin structure locally and results in exclusion of transcription factors. An added complexity to the process was demonstrated when residues were shown to have several possible methylation states.[53,54,55] For H3K9, mono- and dimethylation are associated with euchromatin silencing, and trimethylation is associated with pericentromeric heterochromatin silencing. The H3K9 methylation/silencing switch seems conserved across evolution and is active in mammalian cells.[50] H3K27 methylation seems distinct from H3K9 methylation; H3K27 trimethylation is reported to occur early in X-chromosome inactivation[56] and leads to silencing by recruitment of polycomb group (PCG) proteins.[57] In contrast, H3K9 trimethylation is primarily a mark of heterochromatin and leads to silencing by recruitment of HP1 proteins.[50] Thus, these 2 processes, which are mediated by different enzymes, are potentially functionally distinct. There is considerable interest in the involvement of the histone code in stemness and differentiation. A bivalent chromatin domain is described in embryonic stem cells,[58] whereby some unexpressed genes have coexistence of activating (H3K4Me) and silencing marks (H3K27Me). On differentiation, this bivalency resolves into the activated or the suppressed state.

Although histone modifications are stable, histones are eventually degraded, and the nucleosome structure is substantially altered during DNA synthesis.[59] Moreover, histone acetylation and methylation can be directly reversed by many HDACs and histone demethylases. Thus, for histone modifications to retain epigenetic memory, some form of targeting has to be operative. DNA methylation is one such form of targeting as is persistent expression of transcription factors. It also is argued that the histone modifications themselves could be a form of epigenetic memory in the absence of DNA methylation or other proteins to direct the process.[60]

HISTONE MODIFICATIONS AND CANCER

Histone modifications are implicated in the neoplastic process in a variety of ways. Indirectly, several genes that are altered in cancer affect gene expression via recruitment of histone-modifying enzymes and resulting changes in gene expression. For example, the PML-RARalpha gene translocation in acute promyelocytic leukemia recruits HDACs to inhibit the expression of target genes, thus contributing to malignant transformation.[61] More directly, several histone-modifying enzymes are molecularly altered in cancer. For example, the histone acetyltransferase CBP is mutated in some acute leukemias[62]; the MLL gene, an H3K4 methylase, is rearranged in a significant portion of acute leukemias[63]; the RIZ1 gene, a putative histone methylase, is silenced in some cancers[64]; and EZH2, an H3K27 trimethylase, is overexpressed in various malignancies,[65] which also exhibit de novo H3K27triM mediated silencing.[66] Another mechanism modifying the histone code in cancer is aberrant promoter methylation.[67] Such DNA methylation may lead to silencing via recruitment of histone-modifying enzymes that ultimately alter the histone code in favor of gene silencing.

EPIGENETIC CHANGES IN MDS

Most studies of epigenetics in MDS thus far have focused on DNA methylation. Several genes are transcriptionally silenced in association with promoter DNA methylation in this disease (**Table 1**). These include genes involved in cell-cycle regulation (CDKN2A), apoptosis (DAPK1 and RIL), adhesion and motility (CDH1 and CDH13) and other pathways. Some of these genes clearly have minimal functional impact on the disease, because they are not expressed in normal hematopoietic cells. MDS cases often show hypermethylation of several genes simultaneously.[80] Thus, hypermethylation can be viewed in a similar way as mismatch repair deficiency and microsatellite instability in cancer: many loci are affected simultaneously, a few of which likely have functional consequences.

In MDS, CDKN2B (P15) is the most extensively studied gene. CDKN2B was reported methylated in 30% to 80% of the cases, with the variability likely due to different methods of measurement as well as inclusion of different types of MDS. Thus, CDKN2B methylation is reported as frequent in therapy-related MDS and in

Table 1
Aberrant promoter CpG island hypermethylation in MDS

Gene	Methylation Frequency (%)	Function	Note
Calcitonin[68]	50	Differentiation	
CDKN2B[69]	23–80	Cyclin-dependent kinase inhibitor; cell cycle/proliferation	Tumor-suppressor; methylation correlates with poor prognosis and progression to AML[70]
DAPK[71]	50	Proapoptotic serine/threonine kinase	
RASSF1[72]	9	Negative regulator of RAS signaling	Tumor-suppressor
FHIT[73]	50	Purine metabolism	Putative tumor-suppressor; methylation correlates with poor prognosis and progression to AML[74]
HIC1[75]	32	Transcriptional repressor	Tumor-suppressor
CDH1[75]	15–27	Adhesion and motility	Methylation correlates with poor prognosis and progression to AML[76]
CTNNA1[77]	10	Alpha catenin	
ERα[75]	7–19	Estrogen receptor	Methylation as part of a panel of genes (also including CDH1 and CDKN2A) correlates with poor prognosis and progression to AML[78]
RIL[79]	36–70	Proapoptotic, tumor suppressor	
CDH13[78]	21	Adhesion and motility	
NOR1[78]	15	Oxidored-nitro domain-containing protein	
NPM2[78]	20	Nucleophosmin/nucleoplasmin 2, involved in development	
OLIG2[78]	41	Basic helix-loop-helix transcription factor	
PGRA[78]	45	Progesterone receptor	
PGRB[78]	45	Progesterone receptor	

chronic myelomonocytic leukemia , refractory anemia with excess blasts in transformation, or AML arising from MDS.[69,70,81,82,83] CDKN2B methylation in MDS also is associated with older age, deletions of 5q and 7q, and a poor prognosis.[69,70,81,82,83] When present, CDKN2B methylation in MDS affects several lineages from clonogenic cells to circulating mononuclear cells.[84] In a mouse model, loss of CDKN2B was associated with enhanced myeloid progenitor and reduced erythroid progenitor formation,[85] suggesting that its inactivation plays a functional role in MDS.

In a recent study focusing on quantitative analysis of the methylation status of 10 separate genes, a hypermethylator phenotype was identified that marks a subset of cases with MDS.[80] This phenomenon, first described in colon cancer,[42] results in the simultaneous inactivation of several genes by an unknown mechanism. In MDS, this form of intense hypermethylation is associated with rapid progression to AML and a shortened survival in multivariate analyses.[80] This explains in part why the methylation of so many genes is reported as prognostic in MDS (see **Table 1**): in all likelihood, all these studies of individual genes are pointing to a common subset of cases affected by the hypermethylator phenotype.

Whole genome scans for DNA methylation are beginning to reveal the complexity of the disease at an epigenetic level.[86,87] Hundreds of genes are frequently hypermethylated in MDS, with evidence for enrichment of WNT pathway genes.[86] As indicated by studies of individual genes, hypermethylation across the genome is associated with poor prognostic features and transformation to AML. There was a distinct methylation pattern in MDS and related AMLs compared with de novo AML, pointing to distinct pathogenic mechanisms.[86] Thus, a consensus has emerged that DNA methylation is abnormal early on in MDS and that progression of the disease is associated with accumulation of additional epigenetic events.

In contrast to DNA methylation, detailed studies of histone modifications in MDS remain to be described. A few cases of AML have chromosomal translocations involving MLL1, a known epigenetic modifier. Recently, mutations in the polycomb-related gene ASXL1 were described in about 10% of cases,[88] and mutations in the TET2 gene were found in about 25% of cases. TET2 is related to TET1, a gene that converts 5mC to 5-hydroxymethylcytosine, and thus may be involved in regulation of DNA methylation. It is not known whether or not MDS cases with abnormalities in MLL1, ASXL1, or TET2 have characteristic epigenetic patterns.

EPIGENETIC THERAPY

Treatment of cancer by targeting epigenetic pathways is referred to as epigenetic therapy.[89] The principle of this approach is to reverse pathologic gene expression changes in malignant cells, which is presumed to elicit a therapeutic effect that culminates in tumor responses. The specific therapeutic effect induced by these agents is a matter of debate, and there are data favoring many differing pathways affected by this therapy, including differentiation, senescence, apoptosis, immune recognition, and other pathways.[12] In addition, many epigenetic drugs show dose-dependent cytotoxicity,[90,91] which could also be a factor in responses. The therapeutic index of this approach lies, in principle, in the fact that cancer cells are more dependent on continued silencing of tumor-suppressor genes and like molecules than normal cells. There are concerns that epigenetic therapy could have dramatic effects on normal cells through reactivating, for example, imprinted genes, and may even lead to cancer formation. In vivo, however, these fears have not been substantiated in studies so far, with no evidence of unusual side effects, new chromosomal defects, or secondary malignancies.[31] It is likely that the doses of drugs that elicit such effects are not achievable in vivo.

Targeting epigenetics at the present time essentially equates to targeting silencing pathways in cancer and their potential interactions. A central pathway (see **Fig. 1**) involves DNA methylation, methyl-binding proteins, histone deacetylation, histone (H3K9) methylation, and eventual binding of a silencing protein complex that, itself, may trigger more methylation.[92] This silencing loop is stable, as evidenced by imprinted genes and the inactive X chromosome, which remain turned off for decades in adult cells. There is also a distinct silencing mechanism in development and cancer that involves the PCG complexes PRC1 and PRC2, resulting in H3K27me3 modification. These complexes also involve HDACs. Each step in these silencing cascades is a potential target for therapeutic intervention. Combining inhibition of several epigenetic targets will likely be synergistic, as demonstrated for DNA methylation and HDAC inhibition.[93] There are 2 epigenetic targets for which drugs are available in clinical trials—DNA methylation and histone deacetylation.

5-Azacytidine (azacitidine) and 5-aza-2'-deoxycytidine (decitabine) (DAC) are 2 hypomethylating cytosine analogs with activity in leukemia.[94,95] Both drugs were synthesized in the 1960s as cytosine analogs and were shown in the early 1980s to be potent DNA methylation inhibitors and in vitro differentiation inducers.[96] DNA methylation inhibition is related to the shared modified structure of the cytosine ring with a C to N substitution at the 5 position, resulting in trapping and eventual degradation of DNA methyltransferases. Azacitidine incorporates into RNA and, after intracellular conversion to DAC, incorporates into DNA and inhibits DNA methylation. Unlike azacitidine, DAC does not incorporate into RNA and is directly incorporated into DNA, resulting in 10-fold higher demethylating activity at equimolar concentrations in vitro.[96] Both drugs have activity in MDS demonstrated in randomized studies,[94,97,98] and both are approved by the United States Food and Drug Administration. A feature of azacitidine and DAC studies in MDS is delayed clearance of blasts, delayed myelosuppression, slow responses (median number of cycles to best response was >3), and eventual cytogenetic responses. A similar phenomenon is reported in patients with chronic myelogenous leukemia treated with DAC.[99] These clinical studies have suggested that the mechanism of action of these drugs is not cytotoxicity, although the exact mechanism of achieving complete remissions is not known.

There are a variety of HDAC inhibitors (HDIs) in clinical trials currently.[100] These include drugs discovered through activity in the National Cancer Institute's NCI-60 cell line panel (romidepsin), drugs discovered through in vitro differentiation screens (vorinostat), or drugs discovered to be HDIs serendipitously (valproic acid[101]). For all these drugs, in vitro inhibition of HDAC activity was demonstrated as well as gene reactivation and induction of apoptosis. Again, the mechanism of downstream action of these drugs is unclear, with recent data pointing toward DNA damage and effects on reactive oxygen species[102] (in addition to gene expression activation). Clinically, several of these drugs are in phase I/II studies, with activity demonstrated for romidepsin and vorinostat in lymphomas,[103] and both drugs are approved for the treatment of cutaneous T-cell lymphoma. Less data are available in MDS and AML, though anecdotal responses are reported.[104,105]

Drugs targeting other epigenetic pathways are currently in development or preclinical studies. There is particular interest in drugs that can inhibit the activity of various histone methyltransferases,[106,107] because these could work independently of (and complement) DNA methylation and HDIs. It is likely that several drugs targeting epigenetic pathways will enter clinical trials in MDS in the next few years.

SUMMARY

Epigenetic pathways mediate cancer-specific gene expression abnormalities in several genes involved in determining the neoplastic phenotype. MDS is characterized by several epigenetic abnormalities that can help determine prognosis and risk of progression to AML. Drugs that target epigenetic pathways have changed the natural history of MDS and offer some hope that the disease could be treated successfully in the next decade.

REFERENCES

1. Steensma DP, Tefferi A. The myelodysplastic syndrome(s): a perspective and review highlighting current controversies. Leuk Res 2003;27(2):95–120.
2. Greenberg P, Cox C, LeBeau MM, et al. International scoring system for evaluating prognosis in myelodysplastic syndromes. Blood 1997;89(6):2079–88.
3. Bennett JM, Kouides PA, Forman SJ. The myelodysplastic syndromes: morphology, risk assessment, and clinical management (2002). Int J Hematol 2002;76(Suppl):2228–38.

4. Kantarjian H, O'Brien S, Ravandi F, et al. Proposal for a new risk model in myelodysplastic syndrome that accounts for events not considered in the original International Prognostic Scoring System. Cancer 2008;113(6): 1351–61.
5. Hirai H. Molecular mechanisms of myelodysplastic syndrome. Jpn J Clin Oncol 2003;33(4):153–60.
6. Pederson-Bjergaard J, Christiansen DH, Andersen MK, et al. Causality of mye-lodysplasia and acute myeloid leukemia and their genetic abnormalities. Leukemia 2002;16(11):2177–84.
7. Jones PA, Baylin SB. The epigenomics of cancer. Cell 2007;128(4):683–92.
8. Cedar H. DNA methylation and gene activity. Cell 1988;53(1):3–4.
9. Jenuwein T, Allis CD. Translating the histone code. Science 2001;293(5532): 1074–80.
10. Baylin SB, Herman JG, Graff JR, et al. Alterations in DNA methylation—a funda-mental aspect of neoplasia. Adv Cancer Res 1998;72:141–96.
11. Jones PA, Laird PW. Cancer epigenetics comes of age. Nat Genet 1999;21: 163–7.
12. Issa JP, Kantarjian HM. Targeting DNA methylation. Clin Cancer Res 2009; 15(12):3938–46.
13. Bird A. DNA methylation patterns and epigenetic memory. Genes Dev 2002; 16(1):6–21.
14. Heard E, Clerc P, Avner P. X-chromosome inactivation in mammals. Annu Rev Genet 1997;31:571–610.
15. Barlow DP. Gametic imprinting in mammals. Science 1995;270(5242):1610–3.
16. Jones PA. Altering gene expression with 5-azacytidine. Cell 1985;40(3):485–6.
17. Li E, Beard C, Jaenisch R. Role for DNA methylation in genomic imprinting. Nature 1993;366(6453):362–5.
18. Jones PL, Wolffe AP. Relationships between chromatin organization and DNA meth-ylation in determining gene expression. Semin Cancer Biol 1999;9(5):339–47.
19. Fahrner JA, Eguchi S, Herman JG, et al. Dependence of histone modifications and gene expression on DNA hypermethylation in cancer. Cancer Res 2002; 62(24):7213–8.
20. Kondo Y, Shen L, Issa JP. Critical role of histone methylation in tumor suppressor gene silencing in colorectal cancer. Mol Cell Biol 2003;23(1):206–15.
21. Nguyen CT, Weisenberger DJ, Velicescu M, et al. Histone H3-lysine 9 methyla-tion is associated with aberrant gene silencing in cancer cells and is rapidly reversed by 5-aza-2'-deoxycytidine. Cancer Res 2002;62(22):6456–61.
22. Fuks F, Burgers WA, Brehm A, et al. DNA methyltransferase dnmt1 associates with histone deacetylase activity. Nat Genet 2000;24(1):88–91 [In Process Citation].
23. Rountree MR, Bachman KE, Baylin SB. DNMT1 binds HDAC2 and a new co-repressor, DMAP1, to form a complex at replication foci. Nat Genet 2000; 25(3):269–77.
24. Tamaru H, Selker EU. A histone H3 methyltransferase controls DNA methylation in Neurospora crassa. Nature 2001;414(6861):277–83.
25. Bachman KE, Park BH, Rhee I, et al. Histone modifications and silencing prior to DNA methylation of a tumor suppressor gene. Cancer Cell 2003;3(1):89–95.
26. Feinberg AP, Vogelstein B. Hypomethylation distinguishes genes of some human cancers from their normal counterparts. Nature 1983;301(5895):89–92.
27. Ji W, Hernandez R, Zhang XY, et al. DNA demethylation and pericentromeric re-arrangements of chromosome 1. Mutat Res 1997;379(1):33–41.

28. Goodman JI, Counts JL. Hypomethylation of dna: a possible nongenotoxic mechanism underlying the role of cell proliferation in carcinogenesis. Environ Health Perspect 1993;101(Suppl 5):169–72.
29. Ehrlich M. DNA methylation in cancer: too much, but also too little. Oncogene 2002;21(35):5400–13.
30. Chen RZ, Pettersson U, Beard C, et al. DNA hypomethylation leads to elevated mutation rates. Nature 1998;395(6697):89–93.
31. Yang AS, Estecio MR, Garcia-Manero G, et al. Comment on "Chromosomal instability and tumors promoted by DNA hypomethylation" and "Induction of tumors in nice by genomic hypomethylation". Science 2003;302(5648):1153.
32. Kautiainen TL, Jones PA. DNA methyltransferase levels in tumorigenic and non-tumorigenic cells in culture. J Biol Chem 1986;261(4):1594–8.
33. Eads CA, Danenberg KD, Kawakami K, et al. CpG island hypermethylation in human colorectal tumors is not associated with DNA methyltransferase overexpression. Cancer Res 1999;59(10):2302–6.
34. Issa JP, Vertino PM, Wu J, et al. Increased cytosine DNA-methyltransferase activity during colon cancer progression. J Natl Cancer Inst 1993;85(15):1235–40.
35. Robertson KD, Uzvolgyi E, Liang G, et al. The human DNA methyltransferases (DNMTs) 1, 3a and 3b: coordinate mRNA expression in normal tissues and overexpression in tumors. Nucleic Acids Res 1999;27(11):2291–8.
36. Szyf M, Kaplan F, Mann V, et al. Cell cycle-dependent regulation of eukaryotic DNA methylase level. J Biol Chem 1985;260(15):8653–6.
37. Lee PJ, Washer LL, Law DJ, et al. Limited up-regulation of DNA methyltransferase in human colon cancer reflecting increased cell proliferation. Proc Natl Acad Sci U S A 1996;93(19):10366–70.
38. Bakin AV, Curran T. Role of DNA 5-methylcytosine transferase in cell transformation by fos. Science 1999;283(5400):387–90.
39. Rouleau J, MacLeod AR, Szyf M. Regulation of the DNA methyltransferase by the Ras-AP-1 signaling pathway. J Biol Chem 1995;270(4):1595–601.
40. Wu J, Issa JP, Herman J, et al. Expression of an exogenous eukaryotic DNA methyltransferase gene induces transformation of NIH 3T3 cells. Proc Natl Acad Sci U S A 1993;90(19):8891–5.
41. Liang G, Salem CE, Yu MC, et al. DNA methylation differences associated with tumor tissues identified by genome scanning analysis. Genomics 1998;53(3):260–8.
42. Toyota M, Ahuja N, Ohe-Toyota M, et al. CpG island methylator phenotype in colorectal cancer. Proc Natl Acad Sci U S A 1999;96:8681–6.
43. Rhee I, Bachman KE, Park BH, et al. DNMT1 and DNMT3b cooperate to silence genes in human cancer cells. Nature 2002;416(6880):552–6.
44. Sakai T, Toguchida J, Ohtani N, et al. Allele-specific hypermethylation of the retinoblastoma tumor- suppressor gene. Am J Hum Genet 1991;48(5):880–8.
45. Myohanen SK, Baylin SB, Herman JG. Hypermethylation can selectively silence individual p16ink4A alleles in neoplasia. Cancer Res 1998;58(4):591–3.
46. Herman JG, Latif F, Weng Y, et al. Silencing of the VHL tumor-suppressor gene by DNA methylation in renal carcinoma. Proc Natl Acad Sci U S A 1994;91(21):9700–4.
47. Kane MF, Loda M, Gaida GM, et al. Methylation of the hMLH1 promoter correlates with lack of expression of hMLH1 in sporadic colon tumors and mismatch repair- defective human tumor cell lines. Cancer Res 1997;57(5):808–11.
48. Herman JG, Umar A, Polyak K, et al. Incidence and functional consequences of hMLH1 promoter hypermethylation in colorectal carcinoma. Proc Natl Acad Sci U S A 1998;95(12):6870–5.

49. Khorasanizadeh S. The nucleosome. From genomic organization to genomic regulation. Cell 2004;116(2):259–72.
50. Lachner M, Jenuwein T. The many faces of histone lysine methylation. Curr Opin Cell Biol 2002;14(3):286–98.
51. Rice JC, Allis CD. Histone methylation versus histone acetylation: new insights into epigenetic regulation. Curr Opin Cell Biol 2001;13(3):263–73.
52. Haberland M, Montgomery RL, Olson EN. The many roles of histone deacetylases in development and physiology: implications for disease and therapy. Nat Rev Genet 2009;10(1):32–42.
53. Peters AH, Kubicek S, Mechtler K, et al. Partitioning and plasticity of repressive histone methylation states in mammalian chromatin. Mol Cell 2003;12(6): 1577–89.
54. Rice JC, Briggs SD, Ueberheide B, et al. Histone methyltransferases direct different degrees of methylation to define distinct chromatin domains. Mol Cell 2003;12(6):1591–8.
55. Santos-Rosa H, Schneider R, Bannister AJ, et al. Active genes are tri-methylated at K4 of histone H3. Nature 2002;419(6905):407–11.
56. Rougeulle C, Chaumeil J, Sarma K, et al. Differential histone H3 Lys-9 and Lys-27 methylation profiles on the X chromosome. Mol Cell Biol 2004;24(12):5475–84.
57. Pasini D, Bracken AP, Jensen MR, et al. Suz12 is essential for mouse development and for EZH2 histone methyltransferase activity. EMBO J 2004;23: 4061–71.
58. Bernstein BE, Meissner A, Lander ES. The mammalian epigenome. Cell 2007; 128(4):669–81.
59. Goll MG, Bestor TH. Histone modification and replacement in chromatin activation. Genes Dev 2002;16(14):1739–42.
60. Hansen KH, Bracken AP, Pasini D, et al. A model for transmission of the H3K27me3 epigenetic mark. Nat Cell Biol 2008;10(11):1291–300.
61. Mistry AR, Pedersen EW, Solomon E, et al. The molecular pathogenesis of acute promyelocytic leukaemia: implications for the clinical management of the disease. Blood Rev 2003;17(2):71–97.
62. Lehrmann H, Pritchard LL, Harel-Bellan A. Histone acetyltransferases and deacetylases in the control of cell proliferation and differentiation. Adv Cancer Res 2002;86:41–65.
63. Armstrong SA, Golub TR, Korsmeyer SJ. MLL-rearranged leukemias: insights from gene expression profiling. Semin Hematol 2003;40(4):268–73.
64. Du Y, Carling T, Fang W, et al. Hypermethylation in human cancers of the RIZ1 tumor suppressor gene, a member of a histone/protein methyltransferase superfamily. Cancer Res 2001;61(22):8094–9.
65. Varambally S, Dhanasekaran SM, Zhou M, et al. The polycomb group protein EZH2 is involved in progression of prostate cancer. Nature 2002;419(6907): 624–9.
66. Kondo Y, Shen L, Cheng AS, et al. Gene silencing in cancer by histone H3 lysine 27 trimethylation independent of promoter DNA methylation. Nat Genet 2008; 40(6):741–50.
67. Herman JG, Baylin SB. Gene silencing in cancer in association with promoter hypermethylation. N Engl J Med 2003;349(21):2042–54.
68. Ihalainen J, Pakkala S, Savolainen ER, et al. Hypermethylation of the calcitonin gene in the myelodysplastic syndromes. Leukemia 1993;7(2):263–7.
69. Uchida T, Kinoshita T, Nagai H, et al. Hypermethylation of the p15INK4B gene in myelodysplastic syndromes. Blood 1997;90(4):1403–9.

70. Quesnel B, Guillerm G, Vereecque R, et al. Methylation of the p15(INK4b) gene in myelodysplastic syndromes is frequent and acquired during disease progression. Blood 1998;91(8):2985–90.

71. Voso MT, Scardocci A, Guidi F, et al. Aberrant methylation of DAP-kinase in therapy-related acute myeloid leukemia and myelodysplastic syndromes. Blood 2004;103(2):698–700.

72. Johan MF, Bowen DT, Frew ME, et al. Aberrant methylation of the negative regulators RASSFIA, SHP-1 and SOCS-1 in myelodysplastic syndromes and acute myeloid leukaemia. Br J Haematol 2005;129(1):60–5.

73. Iwai M, Kiyoi H, Ozeki K, et al. Expression and methylation status of the FHIT gene in acute myeloid leukemia and myelodysplastic syndrome. Leukemia 2005;19(8):1367–75.

74. Lin J, Yao DM, Qian J, et al. Methylation status of fragile histidine triad (FHIT) gene and its clinical impact on prognosis of patients with myelodysplastic syndrome. Leuk Res 2008;32(10):1541–5.

75. Aggerholm A, Holm MS, Guldberg P, et al. Promoter hypermethylation of p15INK4B, HIC1, CDH1, and ER is frequent in myelodysplastic syndrome and predicts poor prognosis in early-stage patients. Eur J Haematol 2006;76(1):23–32.

76. Grovdal M, Khan R, Aggerholm A, et al. Negative effect of DNA hypermethylation on the outcome of intensive chemotherapy in older patients with high-risk myelodysplastic syndromes and acute myeloid leukemia following myelodysplastic syndrome. Clin Cancer Res 2007;13(23):7107–12.

77. Liu TX, Becker MW, Jelinek J, et al. Chromosome 5q deletion and epigenetic suppression of the gene encoding alpha-catenin (CTNNA1) in myeloid cell transformation. Nat Med 2007;13(1):78–83.

78. Watanabe Y, Kim HS, Castoro RJ, et al. Sensitive and specific detection of early gastric cancer with DNA methylation analysis of gastric washes. Gastroenterology 2009;136(7):2149–58.

79. Boumber YA, Kondo Y, Chen X, et al. RIL, a LIM Gene on 5q31, Is Silenced by Methylation in Cancer and Sensitizes Cancer Cells to Apoptosis. Cancer Res 2007;67(5):1997–2005.

80. Shen L, Kantarjian H, Guo Y, et al. DNA methylation predicts survival and response to therapy in patients with myelodysplastic syndromes. J Clin Oncol 2010;28(4):605–13.

81. Au WY, Fung A, Man C, et al. Aberrant p15 gene promoter methylation in therapy-related myelodysplastic syndrome and acute myeloid leukaemia: clinicopathological and karyotypic associations. Br J Haematol 2003;120(6):1062–5.

82. Christiansen DH, Andersen MK, Pedersen-Bjergaard J. Methylation of p15(INK4B) is common, is associated with deletion of genes on chromosome arm 7q and predicts a poor prognosis in therapy-related myelodysplasia and acute myeloid leukemia. Leukemia 2003;17(9):1813–9.

83. Tien HF, Tang JH, Tsay W, et al. Methylation of the p15(INK4B) gene in myelodysplastic syndrome: it can be detected early at diagnosis or during disease progression and is highly associated with leukaemic transformation. Br J Haematol 2001;112(1):148–54.

84. Aoki E, Uchida T, Ohashi H, et al. Methylation status of the p15INK4B gene in hematopoietic progenitors and peripheral blood cells in myelodysplastic syndromes. Leukemia 2000;14(4):586–93.

85. Rosu-Myles M, Taylor BJ, Wolff L. Loss of the tumor suppressor p15Ink4b enhances myeloid progenitor formation from common myeloid progenitors. Exp Hematol 2007;35(3):394–406.

86. Figueroa ME, Skrabanek L, Li Y, et al. MDS and secondary AML display unique patterns and abundance of aberrant DNA methylation. Blood 2009;114(16): 3448–58.
87. Jiang Y, Dunbar A, Gondek LP, et al. Aberrant DNA methylation is a dominant mechanism in MDS progression to AML. Blood 2009;113(6):1315–25.
88. Gelsi-Boyer V, Trouplin V, Adelaide J, et al. Mutations of polycomb-associated gene ASXL1 in myelodysplastic syndromes and chronic myelomonocytic leukaemia. Br J Haematol 2009;145(6):788–800.
89. Egger G, Liang G, Aparicio A, et al. Epigenetics in human disease and prospects for epigenetic therapy. Nature 2004;429(6990):457–63.
90. Batty N, Malouf GG, Issa JP. Histone deacetylase inhibitors as anti-neoplastic agents. Cancer Lett 2009;280(2):192–200.
91. Qin T, Youssef EM, Jelinek J, et al. Effect of cytarabine and decitabine in combination in human leukemic cell lines. Clin Cancer Res 2007;13(14):4225–32.
92. Kondo Y, Issa JP. Epigenetic changes in colorectal cancer. Cancer Metastasis Rev 2004;23(1–2):29–39.
93. Cameron EE, Bachman KE, Myohanen S, et al. Synergy of demethylation and histone deacetylase inhibition in the re- expression of genes silenced in cancer. Nat Genet 1999;21(1):103–7.
94. Leone G, Teofili L, Voso MT, et al. DNA methylation and demethylating drugs in myelodysplastic syndromes and secondary leukemias. Haematologica 2002; 87(12):1324–41.
95. Santini V, Kantarjian HM, Issa JP. Changes in DNA methylation in neoplasia: pathophysiology and therapeutic implications. Ann Intern Med 2001;134(7): 573–86.
96. Jones PA, Taylor SM. Cellular differentiation, cytidine analogs and DNA methylation. Cell 1980;20(1):85–93.
97. Lubbert M, Wijermans P, Kunzmann R, et al. Cytogenetic responses in high-risk myelodysplastic syndrome following low-dose treatment with the DNA methylation inhibitor 5-aza-2'-deoxycytidine. Br J Haematol 2001;114(2):349–57.
98. Silverman LR, Demakos EP, Peterson BL, et al. Randomized controlled trial of azacitidine in patients with the myelodysplastic syndrome: a study of the cancer and leukemia group B. J Clin Oncol 2002;20(10):2429–40.
99. Kantarjian HM, O'Brien S, Cortes J, et al. Results of decitabine (5-aza-2'deoxycytidine) therapy in 130 patients with chronic myelogenous leukemia. Cancer 2003;98(3):522–8.
100. Marks PA, Miller T, Richon VM. Histone deacetylases. Curr Opin Pharmacol 2003;3(4):344–51.
101. Phiel CJ, Zhang F, Huang EY, et al. Histone deacetylase is a direct target of valproic acid, a potent anticonvulsant, mood stabilizer, and teratogen. J Biol Chem 2001;276(39):36734–41.
102. Ungerstedt JS, Sowa Y, Xu WS, et al. Role of thioredoxin in the response of normal and transformed cells to histone deacetylase inhibitors. Proc Natl Acad Sci U S A 2005;102(3):673–8.
103. Piekarz RL, Robey R, Sandor V, et al. Inhibitor of histone deacetylation, depsipeptide (FR901228), in the treatment of peripheral and cutaneous T-cell lymphoma: a case report. Blood 2001;98(9):2865–8.
104. Garcia-Manero G, Yang H, Bueso-Ramos C, et al. Phase 1 study of the histone deacetylase inhibitor vorinostat (suberoylanilide hydroxamic acid [SAHA]) in patients with advanced leukemias and myelodysplastic syndromes. Blood 2008;111(3):1060–6.

105. Kuendgen A, Strupp C, Aivado M, et al. Treatment of myelodysplastic syndromes with valproic acid alone or in combination with all-trans retinoic acid. Blood 2004;104(5):1266–9.

106. Kubicek S, O'Sullivan RJ, August EM, et al. Reversal of H3K9me2 by a small-molecule inhibitor for the G9a histone methyltransferase. Mol Cell 2007;25(3): 473–81.

107. Tan J, Yang X, Zhuang L, et al. Pharmacologic disruption of Polycomb-repressive complex 2-mediated gene repression selectively induces apoptosis in cancer cells. Genes Dev 2007;21(9):1050–63.

Immunosuppression for Myelodysplastic Syndrome: How Bench to Bedside to Bench Research Led to Success

Elaine M. Sloand, MD*, A.J. Barrett, MD

KEYWORDS

- Immunosuppression • Myelodysplastic syndrome
- Tumor necrosis factor • IFNγ

Laboratory evidence and clinical evidence suggest that some patients with myelodysplastic syndrome (MDS) have immunologically mediated disease. Autoimmune conditions such as Reynaud syndrome, lupus, rheumatoid arthritis, and polymyalgia are more frequent in MDS patients, and activated cytotoxic T cells and elevated levels of tumor necrosis factor alpha (TNF-α) and interferon γ (IFNγ)[1–4] are found in MDS. Cytokine dysregulation and excessive apoptosis are most notable in early MDS,[3–6] where up–regulation of Fas-receptor and Fas-ligand expression are hallmarks of the disease.[7–11]

The concept of using immunosuppressive treatment (IST) for bone marrow (BM) failure originates severe aplastic anemia (SAA) patients.[12] Gluckman and colleagues[13] were the first to show that hematopoietic recovery could occur in SAA following antithymocyte globulin (ATG) treatment alone. As experience and success in IST for SAA accumulated, small numbers of patients with BM failure secondary tp hypoplastic MDS were treated successfully. The response of such patients led to the establishment a clinical trial of IST at the National Institutes of Health in 1994 to evaluate the ability of ATG to improve BM failure in all forms of MDS.[14]

This study showed improvement in 30% of patients with MDS after ATG. Further efforts to identify the profile the characteristics of the IST responder have resulted in better response rates to IST.[15] This article describes the laboratory evidence

---

Hematology Branch, Division of Intramural Research, National Heart, Lung and Blood Institute, Building 10 CRC, 4-5230, 10 Center Drive, Bethesda, MD 20892, USA
* Corresponding author.
E-mail address: sloande@nhlbi.nih.gov

Hematol Oncol Clin N Am 24 (2010) 331–341
doi:10.1016/j.hoc.2010.02.009
0889-8588/10/$ – see front matter. Published by Elsevier Inc.

supporting a role for the immune system in the marrow failure of MDS and clinical trials using IST in these patients.

CYTOKINE DYSREGULATION

TNFα is the cytokine most implicated in the pathophysiology of MDS.[16] TNF is over-expressed in cultured cells from patients with MDS.[17] This cytokine is elevated in marrow biopsies[18] and in plasma.[19] TNF-related apoptosis-inducing ligand (TRAIL)[5] and IFNγ have been reported elevated in peripheral blood lymphocytes from patients with MDS.[17,19] TNF production correlated loosely with disease subtype,[20] being most prominent in patients with low-risk MDS.[21] Some investigators have suggested that the source of TNF, and perhaps other negative regulators, may be macrophages or other cells located within BM stroma.[1,22–24] Both TNF and IFNγ up-regulate Fas expression on the CD34 cell and trigger apoptosis.[25] TRAIL is a member of the TNF family, which controls apoptosis by binding to agonistic receptors 1 and 2 (TRAIL-R1, TRAIL-R2) and decoy receptors 3 and 4 (TRAIL-R3, TRAIL-R4). Although TRAIL is present in negligible amounts in normal marrow, it is constitutively expressed in MDS marrow,[5] where cells are more sensitive to its cytotoxic and inhibitory effects.[5] Interestingly, TRAIL produced apoptosis selectively in cytogenetically abnormal cells, identified by fluorescence situ hybridization markers.[5] These findings were attributed to up-regulation of TRAIL-receptors 1 and 2 on the aneuploid clone and to differential expression (or function) of intracellular inhibitors of apoptosis Fas-associated death domain-like interleukin (IL)-1β-converting enzyme inhibitory protein (FLIP). FLIP is important in controlling apoptosis in normal cells. Isoforms of FLIP, which result from alternative splicing of mRNA, may have either proapoptotic or antiapoptotic properties depending on their length and may regulate apoptosis in normal marrow. In early MDS, when apoptosis is most prominent, the antiapoptotic long isoform of FLIP (FLIP$_L$) is down-regulated.[26]

MODEL FOR IMMUNOLOGICALLY MEDIATED MARROW DESTRUCTION

Early MDS is characterized by an increased apoptosis in marrow cells. It is not clear whether programmed cell death is related to alteration in genetic programming or is a result of an immune attack. Evidence that the ineffective hematopoiesis is immuno-logically mediated comes from experiments showing suppression of hematopoiesis by lymphocytes derived from patients with active disease, but not following successful treatment with ATG.[27] Normally, quiescent lymphocyte populations contain a diverse distribution of thousands of individual clones within 23 T cell receptor (TCR) Vβ fami-lies. During an immune response, expansion of T cell clones specific for the corre-sponding antigen occurs. This expansion may be detected by flow cytometry using antibodies directed against the TCR Vβ subfamilies, or more specifically by spectra-typing or CDR3 length analysis. Like patients with multiple sclerosis,[28] those receiving vaccinations, and patients with infections,[29,30] expanded Vβ subfamilies where they appear to be cytotoxic to hematopoietic cells present in some cases of MDS.[29,30]

The mechanism for immunologically mediated marrow damage in MDS has been defined most clearly in patients presenting with trisomy 8 as a single karyotypic abnor-mality. The authors chose trisomy 8 to investigate, because such patients are likely to respond to IST.[15] Additionally, the dysplastic clone can be identified readily by FISH. Initially, the authors showed that early apoptotic changes appeared to be restricted to the trisomy 8 clone, because flow cytometric-sorted Fas-positive, annexin-positive cells were enriched in, or entirely composed of trisomy 8 cells.[31] T cells from expanded Vβ families selectively killed trisomy 8 cells in vitro, indicating that T cells could target trisomy 8 cells specifically. Consistent with this finding was the observation that depletion of cytotoxic T cells in BM cell improved growth of trisomy 8 colonies. Despite such specificity, it remained a possibility that normal BM cells could be killed as innocent bystanders by TNF and IFN-γ elaborated by activated T cells.[25] Trisomy 8 cells survive despite showing signs of early apoptosis; DNA degradation did not develop, and cell death did not occur.[32] The resistance of trisomy 8 cells to apoptotic cell death might be attributed to up-regulation of c-myc present on chromosome 8, and survivin,[32] which may be responsible for resistance of trisomy 8 cells to T cell attack. Indeed, when these proteins are knocked down or inhibited, trisomy 8 cells generally die in vitro.

It may be hypothesized that CD8+ T cells recognize a neoantigen or an overexpressed self-antigen presented by major histocompatability locus (MHC) class 1 molecules on trisomy 8 cells. The authors searched for candidate antigens by examining microarray data on CD34 cells obtained from MDS patients with trisomy 8 and other cytogenetic abnormalities.[33] Wilms tumor protein 1 (WT-1) was markedly overexpressed in trisomy 8 cells. WT-1 is a zinc finger transcription factor located on chromosome 11p13 and was implicated in the pathogenesis of Wilm tumor. WT1 is expressed at low levels in normal tissues, including kidney, ovary, testis, and spleen, but not in normal BM or peripheral blood (PB). It is overexpressed in various hematological malignancies including leukemia, MDS and paroxysmal nocturnal hemoglobinuria (PNH).[33–40] Cytotoxic T cells recognize a number of epitopes from the WT1 protein.

In MDS, WT1 transcript levels increase with disease progression and correlate with the International Prognostic Scoring System (IPSS) stage.[36] In the authors' studies, WT1 m-RNA and protein were increased in many IPSS-intermediate 1 (int-1) MDS patients, but were highest in patients with trisomy 8. CD8+ T cells from patients who ultimately became IST responders generated TNF-α and IL-2 in response to WT1 peptide stimulation.[41] CD8 cytotoxic T cells, recognizing WT1$_{126}$ peptide, also could be detected by tetramer analysis in HLA-A*0201-positive patients. These findings do not exclude the possibility that other antigens on MDS cells are recognized by the immune system, and that their identification will require further testing of peptide libraries. In this regard, PR1, a peptide derived from myeloid-restricted azurophil granule proteins, can provoke T cell responses in patients with MDS.[42] In summary, therefore, the authors' studies showed that MDS cells could overexpress tumor-specific antigens that are responsible for inducing autologous T cell cytotoxic T cell responses against the MDS lineage. In the case of trisomy 8, however, the MDS target cells are relatively resistant to such T cell-media apoptosis. **Fig. 1** outlines the authors' working model of T cell interactions with trisomy 8 cells that may be extrapolated to other MDS patient responsive to IST.

Patients with trisomy 8 have a high probability of responding to IST. Curiously, the authors found that selective patients may have normal bone marrow cytology despite the persistence of this karyotypic abnormally with trisomy 8 who recover their blood counts after IST to normal marrow morphology yet do not lose the trisomy 8 populations in the marrow. Indeed the percentage of trisomy 8 positive cells by FISH in blood and marrow can actually increase. Despite the increase in karyotypically abnormal cells, these patients remain stable for years and have shown a very low risk of progressing to acute leukemia.[43] These observations reveal unique and unexpected consequences of the interaction of the immune system with MDS. First, in untreated patients, the survival of the trisomy 8 clone despite in the presence of the T cell response suggests that the MDS cells are adapted to survive T cell attack. Experimental data support this idea; trisomy 8 cells show signs of apoptotic induction

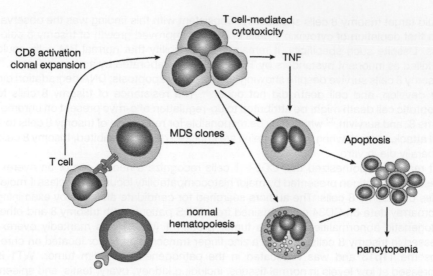

Barrett and Sloand 2008

Fig. 1. Working model for immune dysregulation in MDS.

with increased caspase and BCL-2 but appear to avoid destruction from T cell-mediated apoptosis by up-regulating survivin. This stalled apoptotic process results in "living dead" cells with dysplastic morphology. Second, the recovery of normal morphology in the trisomy 8 cells after IST strongly suggests that morphologic features of dysplasia at least in trisomy 8 disease may represent cellular responses induced by T cell attack. Lastly, and surprisingly, in the absence of T cell attack the expanded trisomy 8 clone can establish normal hematopoiesis, which remains stable for many years.

THE PLACE OF IMMUNOSUPPRESSION IN THE TREATMENT OF MDS

Although BM transplantation is the only curative therapy in MDS, it is important to point out that about half of all deaths are related to cytopenias rather than leukemic progression. Any improvement in hematopoiesis thus may translate into improved survival for this disease.[30,44] Following the considerable success of IST in SAA patients, this treatment was applied with some success first to hypoplastic MDS and then to normo- or hypercellular MDS. About one third of patients had become transfusion independent and enjoyed normal counts for years, but more commonly counts improved but did not revert to normal.[30]

CYCLOSPORINE-BASED TREATMENTS

Many early studies were performed using cyclosporine in low-risk MDS. Jonasova[45] who treated 17 cytopenic patients with refractory anemia (RA) and variable marrow cellularity with cyclosporine (CsA) reported prolonged response in 82% of patients. All responders achieved transfusion independence. A multicenter study in Japan[46] reported responses to CsA in 60% of 50 low-risk patients. Although CSA generally was well tolerated, renal failure occurred in a minority, necessitating stopping the drug. Others have reported no substantial responses to CsA[47] and unacceptable toxicity. Together these findings indicate a potential role for CsA in the treatment of

MDS with careful followup of renal function. It is important to note that responses occurred both in patients with hypocellular and hyper- and normo-cellular marrows.

ATG-BASED REGIMENS

Horse ATG and more recently rabbit ATG (rATG) have been used to treat both aplastic anemia and MDS. Horse ATG rapidly depletes peripheral and lymphoid T cells, but its effect is transient. Rabbit ATG induces more profound and more prolonged immuno-suppression. In vitro data suggest that cocultivation of rATG with normal human peripheral blood mononuclear cells (PBMCs) resulted in marked expansion of functional T regulatory cells by converting CD4+CD25- T cells to CD4+CD25+ T cells.[48] Horse ATG did not expand but rather decreased T regulatory cells.

Formal trials of ATG in MDS first were instituted in 1995.[49] Since then, many other investigators have reported improvement in cytopenias in MDS patients treated with ATG-containing regimens.[50–52] One-hundred-twenty-nine MDS patients were treated with ATG-containing regimens in a trial at the National Institutes of Health (NIH) from 1995 through 2003. Thirty-nine (30%) patients receiving a single course of immuno-suppression responded with significant improvement in cytopenias and transfusion independence.[30] Thirty-one percent (12 of 39) of the responses were complete, resulting in transfusion independence and near-normal blood counts. Factors affecting responses included younger age, low IPSS score, and the presence of HLA DR15. Although responses were equal in patients regardless of cellularity, complete responses were more common in patients with hypocellular MDS. Similar to SAA, the addition of CsA improved the response rate ($P = .048$) and decreased the relapse rate. No controlled trial, however, has yet been performed that compares ATG versus ATG and cyclosporine. Age was a continuous variable, so that the younger the patient, the better was the response to treatment. Median survival of responders was superior to that of responders. Comparison of survival of int-1 MDS less than or equal to 60 years of age treated with IST was superior to that of the historical sample of similar patients treated with supportive care.[30] Multifactorial analysis showed that cellularity did not affect survival or response to therapy. In contrast, Lim and colleagues[53] in the United Kingdom studied a group of 96 patients with MDS, 40 (42%) of whom achieved a hematological response. This group reported that patients with hypocellular BM were most likely to respond and that age did not influence response. The average age of patients in that trial was only 56 years, however, and despite the relation of response to cellularity, 26% of patients with normo- or hypercellular marrows showed improved blood counts.

Trials with younger patients tend to show improved response rates and decreased morbidity associated with the ATG.[54] Geary and colleagues[50] from Manchester, United Kingdom, reported the use of ATG with CsA or oxymetholone in 13 cases of hypoplastic MDS with cytogenetic abnormalities (average age 40). All patients ultimately responded to immunosuppression (with or without androgens), but three eventually relapsed into aplasia. In contrast, Steensma and colleagues[55] from the Mayo Clinic studied a group of older patients (median age 69), finding no responses and considerable toxicity in eight MDS patients (two RA and six refractory anemia with excess blasts) treated with ATG 40 mg/kg/d for 4 days (**Table 1**). At MD Anderson Cancer Center, 32 MDS patients were treated with ATG (40 mg/kg/d intravenously for 4 days plus CsA daily orally for 6 months and methylprednisone 1 mg/kg/intrave-nously before each dose of ATG). Of the 31 evaluable patients, 16% responded; three of these responses were durable remissions (12 to 60+ months). The inclusion of older patients with excess blasts may have accounted for the relatively poorer results

Table 1
Clinical trials of ATG to treat cytopenia in MDS

Center	N	Median Age	% RA	Response n (%)	Response RA (%)	Median Duration (Months)	Response Hypocellular
NIH[65]	129	60	87 (67)	39 (30)	36 (40)	>44	18 (44)
London[52]	30	54.5	13 (65)	10 (50)	8 (62)	15.5	27 (51)
MD Anderson[26,66]	31	59	18 (58)	4 (16)	2 (11)	12–60	NE[a]
Hanover[51]	35	63	24 (68)	12 (34)	10 (42)	>9	2 (50)
Mayo Clinic[55]	8	71	2 (25)	0	0	–	0
Karolinska[54]	20	85		6 (30)	5 (29)	7	2 (50)
Total	253			71 (28%)	61 (41)		

[a] NE data not given.

compared to other studies (see **Table 1**). Of interest is the fact that IST appears to improve nonclonal hematopoiesis. One study from Dusseldorf, Germany[56] examined this phenomenon in 10 female patients with low-risk MDS treated with ALG or ATG. The four responders demonstrated a nonclonal marrow defined by X chromosome inactivation patterns (XCIP), suggesting improved normal progenitor function. It may be hypothesized that this improvement is related to possibly from reduction in bystander damage from TNF and IFNγ.

The comparative effectiveness of hATG versus rATG has not been studied intensively in either MDS or AA. One small study[51] comparing the efficacy of horse ATG (15 mg/kg/d) with rATG (3.75 mg/kg/d) in a cohort of 35 MDS patients treated for 5 days found no significant differences in responses between the two treatments. In patients with RA, overall response rate was 34% and 42% respectively for horse and rabbit ATG. Larger trials will be required to adequately compare these tow treatments.

Patients, who relapse following ATG and receive CsA, generally respond to reinstituting CsA. In the NIH study,[30] there were 13 relapses among the 39 responders. Among the 12 patients with complete responses, four relapsed within the first year, but all responded to reinitiation of immunosuppression. Of these, only two required retreatment with ATG. Three of these patients remain in remission without further treatment at a median follow-up of 6.2 years. Median relapse-free survival was greater than 10.5 years. Of the 40 responders in a European study, 30 (75%) had durable hematological response lasting a median 31.5 months (range: 6 to 92 months).[53] Of the 10 patients with a transient response to ATG therapy, two of three patients subsequently achieved a hematological response following a second course of ATG.

Despite concerns regarding the potential for escape of a malignant clone, IST has not been associated with an increased progression to leukemia.[30] With the notable exception of trisomy 8 (as described previously) samples examined by FISH showed no significant expansion of karyotypically abnormal cells. FISH and cytogenetic analysis of the patient's BM before and following immunosuppression have demonstrated no consistent increase in chromosomal abnormalities indicative of clonal expansion other than in patients with trisomy 8.[43] The trisomy 8 patients remained stable and more likely to respond and maintain their response provided CsA was used as maintenance therapy.[43] Newer immunosuppressive treatment such as alemtuzumab may prove equally or more effective when compared to ATG in patients with MDS.[57]

ANTI-TNF DRUGS

Of all cytokines, TNF-α appears to be the most prominently expressed in MDS. Consequently, many trials have been conducted to evaluate the role of anti-TNF agents as treatment for MDS. Initial trials used thalidomide, which has multiple activities directed against angiogenesis and TNFα production. Response rates were modest, but potentially benefit some MDS patients. Thalidomide has significant toxicity in the elderly population. CC5013 or lenalidomide was developed as an oral analog of thalidomide with a better toxicity profile, notably with fewer neurologic adverse effects, and possibly additional immunomodulatory activities. Its actions however are significantly different than those of thalidomide. Anti-TNF-α monoclonal antibodies,[58–60] soluble TNF-α receptors,[61] and chemical inhibitors of TNF[62–64] have generally been disappointing when used alone.[6]

SUMMARY

Some patients with MDS have an immune-mediated process that compromises hematopoiesis. Improving hematopoiesis in those individuals appears to improve survival. Careful selection of patients to be treated with IST doubtless will improve response rates and eliminate toxicity of those least likely to respond.

REFERENCES

1. Allampallam K, Shetty V, Mundle S, et al. Biological significance of proliferation, apoptosis, cytokines, and monocyte/macrophage cells in bone marrow biopsies of 145 patients with myelodysplastic syndrome. Int J Hematol 2002;75:289–97.
2. Allampallam K, Shetty VT, Raza A. Cytokines and MDS. Cancer Treat Res 2001; 108:93–100.
3. Kitagawa M, Saito I, Kuwata T, et al. Overexpression of tumor necrosis factor (TNF)-alpha and interferon (IFN)-gamma by bone marrow cells from patients with myelodysplastic syndromes. Leukemia 1997;11:2049–54.
4. Koike M, Ishiyama T, Tomoyasu S, et al. Spontaneous cytokine overproduction by peripheral blood mononuclear cells from patients with myelodysplastic syndromes and aplastic anemia. Leuk Res 1995;19:639–44.
5. Zang DY, Goodwin RG, Loken MR, et al. Expression of tumor necrosis factor-related apoptosis-inducing ligand, Apo2L, and its receptors in myelodysplastic syndrome: effects on in vitro hemopoiesis. Blood 2001;98:3058–65.
6. Deeg HJ, Gotlib J, Beckham C, et al. Soluble TNF receptor fusion protein (etanercept) for the treatment of myelodysplastic syndrome: a pilot study. Leukemia 2002;16:162–4.
7. Bouscary D, De Vos J, Guesnu M, et al. Fas/Apo-1 (CD95) expression and apoptosis in patients with myelodysplastic syndromes. Leukemia 1997;11: 839–45.
8. Kitagawa M, Yamaguchi S, Takahashi M, et al. Localization of Fas and Fas ligand in bone marrow cells demonstrating myelodysplasia. Leukemia 1998;12:486–92.
9. Lepelley P, Grardel N, Emy O, et al. Fas/APO-1 (CD95) expression in myelodysplastic syndromes. Leuk Lymphoma 1998;30:307–12.
10. Gupta P, Niehans GA, LeRoy SC, et al. Fas ligand expression in the bone marrow in myelodysplastic syndromes correlates with FAB subtype and anemia, and predicts survival. Leukemia 1999;13:44–53.
11. Claessens YE, Bouscary D, Dupont JM, et al. In vitro proliferation and differentiation of erythroid progenitors from patients with myelodysplastic syndromes: evidence for Fas-dependent apoptosis. Blood 2002;99:1594–601.
12. Mathe G, Schwarzenberg L. Treatment of bone marrow aplasia by mismatched bone marrow transplantation after conditioning with antilymphocyte globulin—long-term results. Transplant Proc 1976;8:595–602.
13. Gluckman E, Devergie A, Poros A, et al. Results of immunosuppression in 170 cases of severe aplastic anaemia. Report of the European Group of bone marrow transplant (EGBMT). Br J Haematol 1982;51:541–50.
14. Molldrem JJ, Jiang YZ, Stetler-Stevenson M, et al. Haematological response of patients with myelodysplastic syndrome to antithymocyte globulin is associated with a loss of lymphocyte-mediated inhibition of CFU-GM and alterations in T cell receptor Vbeta profiles. Br J Haematol 1998;102:1314–22.
15. Sloand EM, Wu CO, Greenberg P, et al. Factors affecting response and survival in patients with myelodysplasia treated with immunosuppressive therapy. J Clin Oncol 2008;26(15):2505–11.
16. Maciejewski JP, Sloand EM, Nunez O, et al. Recombinant humanized anti-IL-2 receptor antibody (daclizumab) produces responses in patients with moderate aplastic anemia. Blood 2003;102:3584–6.

17. Kitagawa M, Takahashi M, Yamaguchi S, et al. Expression of inducible nitric oxide synthase (NOS) in bone marrow cells of myelodysplastic syndromes. Leukemia 1999;13:699–703.
18. Molnar L, Berki T, Hussain A, et al. Detection of TNFα expression in the bone marrow and determination of TNFα production of peripheral blood mononuclear cells in myelodysplastic syndrome. Pathol Oncol Res 2000;6:18–23.
19. Verhoef GE, Schouwer P, Ceuppens JL, et al. Measurement of serum cytokine levels in patients with myelodysplastic syndrome. Leukemia 1992;6:1268–72.
20. Deeg HJ, Appelbaum FR. Hemopoietic stem cell transplantation for myelodysplastic syndrome. Curr Opin Oncol 2000;12:116–20.
21. Stifter G, Heiss S, Gastl G, et al. Over-expression of tumor necrosis factor-alpha in bone marrow biopsies from patients with myelodysplastic syndromes: relationship to anemia and prognosis. Eur J Haematol 2005;75:485–91.
22. Deeg HJ, Beckham C, Loken MR, et al. Negative regulators of hemopoiesis and stroma function in patients with myelodysplastic syndrome. Leuk Lymphoma 2000;37:405–14.
23. Flores-Figueroa E, Gutierrez-Espindola G, Montesinos JJ, et al. In vitro characterization of hematopoietic microenvironment cells from patients with myelodysplastic syndrome. Leuk Res 2002;26:677–86.
24. Tauro S, Hepburn MD, Peddie CM, et al. Functional disturbance of marrow stromal microenvironment in the myelodysplastic syndromes. Leukemia 2002; 16:785–90.
25. Maciejewski J, Selleri C, Anderson S, et al. Fas antigen expression on CD34+ human marrow cells is induced by interferon gamma and tumor necrosis factor alpha and potentiates cytokine-mediated hematopoietic suppression in vitro. Blood 1995;85:3183–90.
26. Benesch M, Platzbecker U, Ward J, et al. Expression of FLIP(Long) and FLIP (Short) in bone marrow mononuclear and CD34+ cells in patients with myelodysplastic syndrome: correlation with apoptosis. Leukemia 2003;17:2460–6.
27. Kochenderfer JN, Kobayashi S, Wieder ED, et al. Loss of T lymphocyte clonal dominance in patients with myelodysplastic syndrome responsive to immunosuppression. Blood 2002;100:3639–45.
28. Zang YC, Hong J, Rivera VM, et al. Human anti-idiotypic T cells induced by TCR peptides corresponding to a common CDR3 sequence motif in myelin basic protein-reactive T cells. Int Immunol 2003;15:1073–80.
29. Melenhorst JJ, Eniafe R, Follmann D, et al. Molecular and flow cytometric characterization of the CD4 and CD8 T cell repertoire in patients with myelodysplastic syndrome. Br J Haematol 2002;119:97–105.
30. Epperson DE, Nakamura R, Saunthararajah Y, et al. Oligoclonal T cell expansion in myelodysplastic syndrome: evidence for an autoimmune process. Leuk Res 2001;25:1075–83.
31. Sloand EM, Kim S, Fuhrer M, et al. Fas-mediated apoptosis is important in regulating cell replication and death in trisomy 8 hematopoietic cells but not in cells with other cytogenetic abnormalities. Blood 2002;100:4427–32.
32. Sloand EM, Pfannes L, Chen G, et al. CD34 cells from patients with trisomy 8 myelodysplastic syndrome (MDS) express early apoptotic markers but avoid programmed cell death by up-regulation of antiapoptotic proteins. Blood 2007; 109:2399–405.
33. Chen G, Zeng W, Miyazato A, et al. Distinctive gene expression profiles of CD34 cells from patients with myelodysplastic syndrome characterized by specific chromosomal abnormalities. Blood 2004;104(13):4210–8.

34. Call KM, Ito CY, Lindberg C, et al. Mapping and characterization of 129 cosmids on human chromosome 11p. Somat Cell Mol Genet 1992;18:463–75.
35. Haber DA, Housman DE. Role of the WT1 gene in Wilms' tumour. Cancer Surv 1992;12:105–17.
36. Cilloni D, Gottardi E, Messa F, et al. Significant correlation between the degree of WT1 expression and the International Prognostic Scoring System score in patients with myelodysplastic syndromes. J Clin Oncol 2003;21:1988–95.
37. Cilloni D, Saglio G. WT1 as a universal marker for minimal residual disease detection and quantification in myeloid leukemias and in myelodysplastic syndrome. Acta Haematol 2004;112:79–84.
38. Cilloni D, Gottardi E, Fava M, et al. Usefulness of quantitative assessment of the WT1 gene transcript as a marker for minimal residual disease detection. Blood 2003;102:773–4.
39. Ellisen LW, Carlesso N, Cheng T, et al. The Wilms tumor suppressor WT1 directs stage-specific quiescence and differentiation of human hematopoietic progenitor cells. EMBO J 2001;20:1897–909.
40. Shichishima T, Okamoto M, Ikeda K, et al. HLA class II haplotype and quantitation of WT1 RNA in Japanese patients with paroxysmal nocturnal hemoglobinuria. Blood 2002;100:22–8.
41. Sloand EM, Rezvani K, Yong A, et al. Cytotoxic CD8 T cell immune responses to Wilms tumor protein (WT-1) characterizes immunosuppression-responsive myelodysplasia (MDS). Blood 2006;108:255.
42. Rezvani K. PR1 vaccination in myeloid malignancies. Expert Rev Vaccines 2008; 7:867–75.
43. Sloand EM, Mainwaring L, Fuhrer M, et al. Preferential suppression of trisomy 8 compared with normal hematopoietic cell growth by autologous lymphocytes in patients with trisomy 8 myelodysplastic syndrome. Blood 2005;106:841–51.
44. Jadersten M, Malcovati L, Dybedal I, et al. Erythropoietin and granulocyte colony-stimulating factor treatment associated with improved survival in myelodysplastic syndrome. J Clin Oncol 2008;26:3607–13.
45. Jonasova A, Neuwirtova R, Cermak J, et al. Cyclosporin A therapy in hypoplastic MDS patients and certain refractory anaemias without hypoplastic bone marrow. Br J Haematol 1998;100:304–9.
46. Shimamoto T, Tohyama K, Okamoto T, et al. Cyclosporin A therapy for patients with myelodysplastic syndrome: multicenter pilot studies in Japan. Leuk Res 2003;27:783–8.
47. Atoyebi W, Bywater L, Rawlings L, et al. Treatment of myelodysplasia with oral cyclosporin. Clin Lab Haematol 2002;24:211–4.
48. Feng X, Kajigaya S, Solomou EE, et al. Rabbit ATG but not horse ATG promotes expansion of functional CD4+CD25highFOXP3+ regulatory T cells in vitro. Blood 2008;111:3675–83.
49. Barrett AJ, Molldrem JJ, Saunthrajarian Y, et al. Prolonged transfusion independence and disease stability in patients with myelodysplastic syndrome (MDS) responding to antithymocyte glogulin (ATG) [abstract]. Blood 1998; 10(Suppl 1):713.
50. Geary CG, Harrison CJ, Philpott NJ, et al. Abnormal cytogenetic clones in patients with aplastic anaemia: response to immunosuppressive therapy. Br J Haematol 1999;104:271–4.
51. Stadler M, Germing U, Kliche KO, et al. A prospective, randomised, phase II study of horse antithymocyte globulin vs rabbit antithymocyte globulin as

immune-modulating therapy in patients with low-risk myelodysplastic syndromes. Leukemia 2004;18:460–5.

52. Killick SB, Mufti G, Cavenagh JD, et al. A pilot study of antithymocyte globulin (ATG) in the treatment of patients with low-risk myelodysplasia. Br J Haematol 2003;120:679–84.

53. Lim ZY, Killick S, Germing U, et al. Low IPSS score and bone marrow hypocellularity in MDS patients predict hematological responses to antithymocyte globulin. Leukemia 2007;21:1436–41.

54. Broliden PA, Dahl IM, Hast R, et al. Antithymocyte globulin and cyclosporine A as combination therapy for low-risk non-sideroblastic myelodysplastic syndromes. Haematologica 2006;91:667–70.

55. Steensma DP, Dispenzieri A, Moore SB, et al. Antithymocyte globulin has limited efficacy and substantial toxicity in unselected anemic patients with myelodysplastic syndrome. Blood 2003;101:2156–8.

56. Aivado M, Rong A, Germing U, et al. Long-term remission after intensive chemotherapy in advanced myelodysplastic syndromes is generally associated with restoration of polyclonal haemopoiesis. Br J Haematol 2000;110:884–6.

57. Sloand EM, Olnes M, Weinstein B, et al. Alemtuzumab treatment of intermediate-1 myelodysplasia patients is associated with sustained improvement in blood counts and cytogenetic remissions. Blood 2009;114:53.

58. Srinivasan R, Geller N, Chakrabarti S, et al. High response rate and improved survival in patients with steroid-refractory acute graft-vs-host disease (SRGVHD) treated with daclizumab with or without infliximab [abstract]. Blood 2002;100:173.

59. Stasi R, Amadori S. Infliximab chimaeric antitumour necrosis factor alpha monoclonal antibody treatment for patients with myelodysplastic syndromes. Br J Haematol 2002;116:334–7.

60. Kobbe G, Schneider P, Rohr U, et al. Treatment of severe steroid refractory acute graft-versus-host disease with infliximab, a chimeric human/mouse anti-TNF-alpha antibody. Bone Marrow Transplant 2001;28:47–9.

61. Maciejewski JP, Risitano AM, Sloand EM, et al. A pilot study of the recombinant soluble human tumour necrosis factor receptor (p75)-Fc fusion protein in patients with myelodysplastic syndrome. Br J Haematol 2002;117:119–26.

62. List A, Kurtin S, Roe DJ, et al. Efficacy of lenalidomide in myelodysplastic syndromes. N Engl J Med 2005;352:549–57.

63. Strupp C, Germing U, Aivado M, et al. Thalidomide for the treatment of patients with myelodysplastic syndromes. Leukemia 2002;16:1–6.

64. Zorat F, Pozzato G. Thalidomide in myelodysplastic syndromes. Biomed Pharmacother 2002;56:20–30.

65. Molldrem JJ, Leifer E, Bahceci E, et al. Antithymocyte globulin for treatment of the bone marrow failure associated with myelodysplastic syndromes. Ann Intern Med 2002;137:156–63.

66. Yazji S, Giles FJ, Tsimberidou AM, et al. Antithymocyte globulin (ATG)-based therapy in patients with myelodysplastic syndromes. Leukemia 2003;17:2101–6.

Innate Immune Signaling in the Myelodysplastic Syndromes

Daniel T. Starczynowski, PhD[a,b,c], Aly Karsan, MD[a,b,c,d,*]

KEYWORDS

- Innate immunity • Myelodysplastic syndromes
- Acute myeloid leukemia • MicroRNAs
- Toll-like receptor • NF-κB

The innate immune system is an evolutionarily conserved defense mechanism against pathogens.[1] Unlike the adaptive immune response, the innate immune system does not recognize every foreign pathogen, but instead recognizes related components shared by many microbes, referred to as "pathogen-associated molecular patterns." Coordinated activation of the innate immune system is achieved by key sentinel cells and a complex sequence of events, including engagement of pathogen-associated molecular patterns responsive receptors, recruitment of phagocytic cells, release of inflammatory mediators, and activation of the complement system resulting in pathogen clearance. The toll-like receptor (TLR) family plays a major role in the initial detection and subsequent elimination of foreign pathogens. This process is achieved through activation of intracellular signaling pathways, such as NF-κB and MAPK, which initiate a coordinated set of responses.

This work was supported by an operating grant to A.K. from the Canadian Institutes of Health Research (MOP 89976).

[a] Genome Sciences Centre, BC Cancer Research Centre, 675 West 10th Avenue, Vancouver, BC V5Z 1L3, Canada

[b] Terry Fox Laboratory, BC Cancer Research Centre, 675 West 10th Avenue, Vancouver, BC V5Z 1L3, Canada

[c] Department of Pathology and Laboratory Medicine, University of British Columbia, 2211 Wesbrook Mall, Vancouver, BC V6T 2B5, Canada

[d] Department of Pathology and Laboratory Medicine, BC Cancer Agency, 600 West 10th Avenue, Vancouver, BC V5Z 4E6, Canada

* Corresponding author. Genome Sciences Centre, BC Cancer Research Centre, 675 West 10th Avenue, Vancouver, BC V5Z 1L3, Canada.
E-mail address: akarsan@bccrc.ca

Hematol Oncol Clin N Am 24 (2010) 343–359
doi:10.1016/j.hoc.2010.02.008
hemonc.theclinics.com

THE INNATE IMMUNE SIGNALING COMPLEX IS ACTIVATED BY FUNCTIONALLY RELATED RECEPTORS

Activation of the innate immunity pathway is the result of the interaction between a ligand (microbial product) and its cognate receptor.[1] The human TLR family comprises 10 members (TLR1–TLR10) involved in the recognition of microbial products, such as lipopolysaccharide (LPS), lipoteichoic acid, peptidoglycan, microbial lipoproteins, and viral nucleic acids (DNA and RNA).[2] The TLRs exhibit homology to the interleukin-1 receptors (IL-1R) and tumor necrosis factor receptors (TNFR). IL-1Rs are a functionally related family of receptors that rely on TRAFs (TNF associated factors) for transmitting intracellular signals.[3] Despite the functional similarities to TLRs, IL-1Rs are not primary sensors of infection but rather secondary sensors that respond to IL-1 from sentinel cells, such as macrophages that have been previously infected.[4] The primary role of IL-1Rs is the production of proinflammatory genes. The TNFR members (eg, TNFR1, LT-βR, Fas, CD40, RANK, EDAR, and LMP) also functionally overlap with innate immune receptors.[3] The main purpose of the TNFR family is to activate genes involved in inflammation and immunoregulatory responses, cell proliferation, viral responses, and growth inhibition. Ligands responsible for activation of TNFR include TNF-α, lymphotoxin (LT), Fas ligand, CD40 ligand, RANK ligand, and EDA.[3] Research on the IL-1R and TNFR family members has revealed mechanistic similarities and related components shared with the TLRs.

COMPONENTS OF THE INNATE IMMUNE SIGNALING SYSTEM

The best-described TLR member, TLR4, is the receptor for LPS. Two pathways diverge downstream of TLR4, the myeloid differentiation primary response gene 88 (MyD88)-dependent and -independent pathways, resulting in the expression of inflammatory cytokines or interferon (IFN)-inducible genes, respectively (**Fig. 1**).[5] The MyD88-dependent pathway mediates a rapid and acute response, whereas the MyD88-independent pathway is responsible for a delayed response. On LPS recognition, a complex is formed on the outer plasma membrane consisting of LPS, TLR4, MD2, and CD14. The LPS-TLR4 interaction is stabilized by MD2 and CD14 coreceptors, which then facilitates intracellular recruitment of protein adaptors required for downstream signaling.[6] MyD88 is a toll–interleukin 1 receptor (TIR)-containing protein adaptor that forms a complex on the corresponding intracellular TIR domain of TLR4. Along with Mal/TIR domain–containing adaptor protein (TIRAP), MyD88 recruits interleukin-1 receptor-associated kinase (IRAK4), which then recruits IRAK1, resulting in subsequent autophosphorylation and disassociation from the TLR4-MyD88 complex. The MyD88-IRAK complex then binds to TRAFs, key effectors of the innate immune signaling complex. The TRAF-containing complex forms the key signaling component, which includes two kinase subunits, IKKα and IKKβ (inhibitor of NF-κB kinase alpha and beta), and a regulatory subunit (IKKγ/NEMO). One of the main TRAF members, TRAF6, is an E3 ligase that self-activates by autoubiquitination and also forms polyubiquitin lysine-63 chains on IKKγ resulting in IKK-mediated activation of NF-κB.[7] Activation of the IKK complex by TRAF6 relies on another complex consisting of TAK1 (transforming growth factor-β activated kinase 1) and TAB1/2 (TAK1 binding protein-1 and -2). Engagement of the TAK1/TAB1/2 complex with TRAF6 not only induces NF-κB, but can also activate specific MAPK pathways (JNK and p38). In contrast, the MyD88-independent pathway forms a TLR4 complex containing TRIF and TRAM adaptor molecules (see **Fig. 1**). As in the MyD88-dependent pathway, TRAF6 plays a key role in downstream activation, but the kinases RIP1 and TBK1 are also necessary for NF-κB and IRF3 activation.[5]

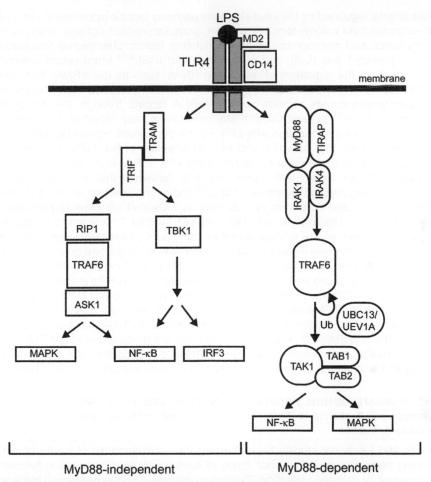

Fig. 1. MyD88-dependent and -independent signaling pathways. LPS is recruited to TLR4 on the outer plasma membrane by association with MD2 and CD14. MyD88 forms a complex on the corresponding intracellular domain of TLR4. Along with Mal/TIRAP, MyD88 recruits IRAK4 and IRAK1, resulting in disassociation from the TLR4/MyD88 complex. The MyD88-IRAK complex then binds to TRAFs. This TRAF-containing complex binds TAK1 and TAB1/2, resulting in the activation of the NF-κB signalasome (IKKα, IKKβ, and IKKγ). TRAF6, an E3 ligase, along with UBC13/UEV1A forms polyubiquitin lysine-63 chains on target proteins including itself. Engagement of the TAK1/TAB1/2 complex with TRAF6 not only induces NF-κB, but can under certain cellular contexts activate the MAPK pathways. In contrast, the MyD88-independent pathway forms a TLR4 complex containing TRIF and TRAM adaptor molecules. TRIF recruits TRAF6, RIP1, and ASK1 to activate MAPK. Alternatively, a TBK1 complex is formed to activate the interferon pathway (IRF). Both pathways can also mediate activation of NF-κB through the MyD88-independent signaling cascade.

GENES REGULATED BY INNATE IMMUNE SIGNALING

Over 1000 protein-coding genes are activated following stimulation of the innate immune system.[8,9] The primary goal of the innate immune system is to generate an immune response by activating the inflammatory cascade. The best characterized genes directly regulated by the innate immune pathway include cytokines (IL-1β, IL-6, TNF-α, granulocyte colony–stimulating factor, granulocyte-macrophage colony–stimulating factor, and macrophage colony–stimulating factor); chemokines (membrane cofactor protein-1 and IL-8); and IFNs (IFN-β and IRG).[9,10] More recent attention has focused on the regulation of noncoding RNAs, such as microRNAs (miRNAs), by the innate immune pathway. miRNAs are 21- to 25-nucleotide noncoding RNAs that posttranscriptionally repress specific mRNA targets through 3′-untranslated region interactions.[11] At least five miRNAs (miRs) have been reported to increase in expression following stimulation with LPS. Four independent groups identified miR-146, miR-147, miR-155, miR-181, and let-7 as effectors of the TLR4 pathway.[12–16] The precise role of these miRs in mediating the LPS-TLR4 response remains to be delineated. Mouse experiments have revealed, however, that miR-155 may be involved in driving myeloid expansion in vivo,[13] and overexpression of miR-147 abrogates a macrophage inflammatory response as indicated by lower expression of TNF-α and IL-6.[15] The roles of miR-146, miR-181, and let-7 have yet to be studied in a similar context, so it is unclear how they contribute to functional innate immune responses. There is some evidence that these miRNAs are important in hematopoiesis and may be involved in differentiation or survival of key immune cells. Knockdown of miR-146 in human or mouse hematopoietic progenitor cells results in increased megakaryopoiesis.[17,18] Ectopic expression of miR-181 in hematopoietic stem and progenitor cells leads to B-lineage differentiation.[19] Some of these miRNAs potentially function as negative-feedback regulators. For instance, miR-146 has been shown to target TRAF6 and IRAK1,[12] and let-7 and miR-181 are predicted to target TLR4.[14,16] It is conceivable that induction of these miRNAs dampens the LPS response by binding and inhibiting multiple components of the innate immune pathway (**Table 1**).

ROLE OF INNATE IMMUNE SIGNALING ON NORMAL HEMATOPOIESIS
Hematopoietic Response to Acute Inflammation and Innate Immune Signaling Activation

Genetic and functional studies have revealed the consequences of innate immune signaling pathways on the distinct steps of hematopoietic differentiation following inflammation or pathogen infection. Extensive discussion and experimental evidence on this topic has been previously reviewed,[1] so only a brief overview is provided. Inflammation and subsequent activation of innate immune signaling results in activation and expansion of mature leukocytes, such as monocytes, dendritic cells, macrophages, and neutrophils, but reduction of B lymphopoiesis in the bone marrow.[20] Similarly in mice, administration of LPS through intravenous injection results in rapid and dynamic effects on myeloid and lymphoid populations in the bone marrow and blood.[13] After LPS injection, expansion of granulocyte-macrophage populations and

Table 1
AML- and MDS-related microRNAs target genes of the innate immune signaling pathway

microRNA	Innate Immunity mRNA Target
miR-145	TIRAP
miR-146	TRAF6, IRAK1
miR-147	TLR4
Let-7a	TLR4
miR-181	TLR2/4/8, NOD2, CARD8

Abbreviations: AML, acute myeloid leukemia; MDS, myelodysplastic syndromes.

reduction in B cells and erythroid precursors are observed in the bone marrow by 72 hours.[13] The inflammatory-mediated imbalance in lymphopoiesis and granulopoiesis is driven by growth factors, chemokines, and cytokines.

Role of Innate Immune Signaling in Hematopoietic Stem and Progenitor Cells

Most work has described the TLRs and the innate immune signaling pathway as critical responders to foreign pathogens in mature myeloid and lymphoid cells. Emerging evidence now suggests that TLR are also important signaling transducers in hematopoietic stem and progenitor cells. Functional TLRs and their coreceptors are expressed on multipotent hematopoietic stem cells.[21] By binding to TLR4, LPS drives hematopoietic stem and progenitor cells to proliferate and differentiate into mature monocytes and macrophages at the expense of lymphoid differentiation in vitro (**Fig. 2**A).[21] Similarly, mice administered LPS show evidence of activated hematopoietic stem cells in the bone marrow and preferential stimulation of macrophage and

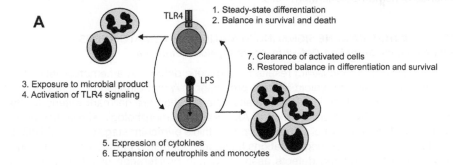

A

TLR4
1. Steady-state differentiation
2. Balance in survival and death

7. Clearance of activated cells
8. Restored balance in differentiation and survival

3. Exposure to microbial product
4. Activation of TLR4 signaling

LPS

5. Expression of cytokines
6. Expansion of neutrophils and monocytes

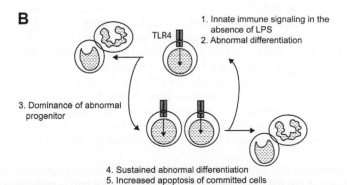

B

TLR4
1. Innate immune signaling in the absence of LPS
2. Abnormal differentiation

3. Dominance of abnormal progenitor

4. Sustained abnormal differentiation
5. Increased apoptosis of committed cells

Fig. 2. Model of acute and constitutive TLR4 signaling in hematopoietic stem/progenitor cells. (A) By binding to TLR4, LPS drives hematopoietic stem/progenitor cells (*gray nucleus*) to proliferate and differentiate into mature monocytes and macrophages (*black nuclei*) at the expense of lymphoid differentiation. Clearance of the pathogen restores normal homeostasis of hematopoietic stem/progenitor cells and mature monocytes and macrophages. (B) Constitutive and unregulated innate immune signaling of hematopoietic stem/progenitor cells (*patterned nucleus*) results in abnormal hematopoietic differentiation and increased cell death of differentiated cells, through autonomous and nonautonomous effects. Prosurvival signals mediated by innate immune pathway maintain and expand the abnormal hematopoietic stem/progenitor. Normal homeostasis of hematopoietic stem/ progenitor cells and mature monocytes and macrophages is disrupted.

monocyte development, whereas B and T lymphoid production is impaired.[13,20] These observations demonstrate a critical role of innate immune signaling in normal hematopoietic stem and progenitor cell differentiation.

The importance of TLR4 signaling in hematopoietic stem cells is further supported by genetic experiments with TAK1, a member of the MAPKKK family and a mediator of TRAF6 signaling (see **Fig. 1**).[22] Under normal physiologic conditions, TAK1 is expressed and activated in hematopoietic stem cells.[22] TAK1 gene-targeted mice show ineffective hematopoiesis leading to pancytopenia. Notably, TAK1-deficient mice display reduced white blood cells, platelets, and nucleated cells in the bone marrow, but hemoglobin levels are unaffected.[22] Detailed examination of the marrow indicates that depletion of TAK1 results in loss of primitive hematopoietic cells in the marrow. The loss of hematopoietic stem and progenitor cells in TAK1-deficient mice is secondary to increased apoptotic signaling, mediated through loss of NF-κB and JNK activation.[22] TAK1 is a key gene of the innate immune pathway responsible for maintenance of hematopoietic stem cells.

ROLE OF INNATE IMMUNE SIGNALING IN MALIGNANT HEMATOPOIESIS
Innate Immune Signaling Defect in Acute Myeloid Leukemia

Acute myeloid leukemia (AML) results from genetic defects in a hematopoietic stem and progenitor cell or myeloid lineage precursor.[23] A combination of increased cell proliferation and a block in hematopoietic differentiation are hallmark criteria for the development of AML. Classification of AML assumes morphologic similarities of the leukemic cells to the normal cell counterpart within a particular stage of myeloid differentiation.[24] Distinct recurring mutations have been identified in AML and are thought to be responsible for the defects associated with proliferation or differentiation of leukemic cells. Balanced translocations, such as t(15;17)/PML-RARA, t(8;21)/AML1-ETO, t(16;16)/CBFB-MY11, t(9;11)/MLLT3-MLL, or other rearrangements of 11q23/MLL are common in de novo AML.[25,26] These alterations, which are now part of the World Health Organization classification of myeloid neoplasias, have been extensively characterized to reveal the roles of the fusion genes in leukemogenesis.[25,26] In addition to genomic alterations, point mutations have also been identified. The most common mutations in AML are ones in the FMS-like tyrosine kinase 3 (FLT3) gene, CEBPA, and NPM1.[26] Internal tandem repeats of FLT3 and overexpression of MN1 are also prognostically important in AML and have been shown to directly contribute to leukemogenesis in mouse models.[27-30] Identification of these alterations in AML patients has improved diagnosis and treatment; however, the heterogeneity of AML and variable survival outcomes suggests that yet undiscovered genes and pathways contribute to AML.

The role of innate immune signaling in AML is becoming increasingly apparent, but the evidence is indirect. IL-1β has been shown to maintain survival and proliferation of AML blasts.[31] Protein levels of TRAF family members are also increased in AML cell lines, but are low or undetectable in normal hematopoietic cells.[32] Consistent with this observation, the downstream pathways regulated by TRAFs, such as NF-κB, are activated in AML blasts but not in normal CD34[+] cells.[33] The importance of NF-κB activation in AML is exemplified by studies using genetic and pharmacologic inhibitors of NF-κB. For example, inhibiting NF-κB signaling suppresses growth of AML blasts and leukemic stem cells.[33]

The contribution of TNFR family members to hematologic malignancies is variable and dependent on the specific receptor. TNFR superfamily members that directly associate with Fas-associated death domain activate the extrinsic apoptotic pathway and have been reported to suppress growth of leukemic cells.[34] In contrast, TNFR members that associate with TNFR1-associated death domain activate prosurvival signaling in parallel with apoptotic pathways, and facilitate leukemic cell growth.[34] One TNFR-family member, CD30 variant, has been identified in a significant proportion (approximately 70%) of AML-M4 and M5.[35] CD30 variant is thought to induce cell growth and differentiation through interactions with TRAF2 or TRAF5 proteins and subsequent activation of NF-κB in AML cell lines.[35] The role of CD40 in AML is more confusing. CD40, which also belongs to the TNFR family, requires TRAFs to propagate signals to NF-κB, STATs, and MAPK.[36] Despite the unresolved role of CD40, it is clear that the ligand for CD40 promotes proliferation, self-renewal, and increased survival potential of AML blasts.[37] Furthermore, circulating levels of CD40 are elevated in AML patients and are associated with poor overall survival.[38]

Individual components of the innate immune pathway have not been as extensively described in AML. Most of the reported research has described components of the MyD88-independent pathway. ASK1, a MAPK member of the MyD88-independent signal, is activated by TRAF6 in response to reactive oxidative species.[39] Knockdown of ASK1 sensitizes AML cells to arsenic trioxide-mediated apoptosis.[40] In contrast, azinomycin epozide induces apoptosis in AML cells through activation of ASK1 and caspase 3.[41] The latter observation supports the original finding that ASK1 induces apoptosis by activating p38.[42] The conflicting data on the role of ASK1 in AML may be resolved by examining ASK1 in a cell-context manner. For example, ASK1 may promote prosurvival pathways in primitive hematopoietic cells, but cell death in committed myeloid progenitors. That the MyD88-independent pathway is responsible for inducing apoptotic pathways is supported by a similar proapoptotic role of RIP1 in myeloid blast cell differentiation.[43]

More recent evidence implicating a key role for innate immune signaling in AML was provided in a miRNA expression study on cytogenetically normal AML patient samples.[44] Only 12 of more than 300 miRNAs examined correlated with overall survival. Five of these miRNAs belong to the miR-181 family. Increased expression of miR-181 family members was associated with decreased risk of death caused by AML.[44] Furthermore, because miRNAs are negative regulators of specific mRNA targets, this study investigated genes and proteins that were inversely correlated with miR-181 expression in the patient samples. It was revealed that genes encoding TLRs (TLR2, TLR4, and TLR8), IL-1β, and various effectors of these pathways (eg, CARD8 and NOD2) were increased in patients with low miR-181 expression.[44] Of these genes, TLR4, IL-1β, and CARD8 are predicted targets of miR-181. It is hypothesized that reduced levels of miR-181 result in increased signaling of the TLR4 or IL1R pathways and contribute to AML progression. In related studies, miR-181 family members have been associated with morphologic subclasses of AML and differentiation of hematopoietic precursors.[45]

Sequential acquisition of genomic alterations, somatic mutations, and deregulation of key signaling pathways contribute to the transformation of a normal hematopoietic stem and progenitor cell to an AML blast. The critical events result in a block in differentiation and increased proliferation of myeloid precursors. According to what is known about signaling pathways downstream of TLRs, deregulation of innate immune signaling likely contributes to resistance to proapoptotic signals and increased survival of AML blasts. At this time, there is no evidence to suggest that innate immune signaling mediates a block in differentiation or promotes self-renewal of primitive hematopoietic stem and precursors resulting in AML.

Innate Immune Signaling Defects in Myelodysplastic Syndromes

The myelodysplastic syndromes (MDS) are a heterogeneous group of clonal hematologic malignancies characterized by peripheral cytopenias, a hypercellular marrow with ineffective hematopoiesis, and a propensity to progress to AML.[46] MDS is thought to arise from a primitive hematopoietic progenitor that has acquired genetic or epigenetic abnormalities.[46] The current World Health Organization classification of MDS comprises eight subtypes, based on biologic, genetic, and morphologic features.[47] Activation of the innate immune system by chronic infection can reproduce hematologic abnormalities resembling MDS, including anemia, neutropenia, thrombocytopenia, and trilineage dysplasia. As examples, chronic infection with *Leishmania* or parvovirus have been reported to induce pancytopenia and dysplastic erythroid and myeloid precursors in the marrow.[48,49] Other evidence that the innate immune system plays a role in MDS comes from the use of immune modulatory drugs for treatment of MDS. The best-known immune modulatory drug, lenalidomide, has been successfully used for treatment of MDS subtypes associated with deletion of chromosome arm 5q.[50] These observations provide indirect evidence that activation of the innate immune pathway may mediate features of MDS.

There are few described mouse models that exhibit features of MDS.[51–58] As evidenced by studies in AML, identification of genetic alterations and the creation of representative mouse model systems may provide insight into the biologic mechanism and potential therapeutic targets for MDS. To further the understanding of the biologic basis of MDS and identify novel therapeutics, efforts to unravel the genetic networks associated with MDS need to be undertaken.

Evidence of Direct Activation of Innate Immune Pathway Genes in MDS

We recently focused on candidate genes and their contribution to 5q syndrome, a common subtype of MDS. 5q syndrome originates in a hematopoietic stem cell and is defined by a heterozygous interstitial deletion of chromosome arm 5q, macrocytic anemia, neutropenia, and thrombocytosis associated with abnormal megakaryocytes.[59] Although deletion of chromosome arm 5q was first reported over 30 years ago, the genes responsible for the clinical manifestation of this disease remained unknown until recently. miRNAs encoded on chromosome 5q were investigated as possible mediators of 5q syndrome. Deletion of chromosome 5q in MDS patients results in loss of at least two functionally related miRNAs (miR-145 and miR-146a).[18] Based on miRNA target prediction algorithms and in vitro validation experiments, TIRAP was identified as a target of miR-145, and TRAF6 was confirmed to be a target of miR-146a (see **Tables 1** and **2**). TIRAP and TRAF6 are two proteins that lie in the MyD88-dependent pathway of innate immune signaling (see **Fig. 1**). Loss of either of these two miRNAs results in depression of innate immune signaling. Expression of TIRAP and TRAF6 proteins is relatively low in primitive hematopoietic cells; however, reduction in miR-145 and miR-146a levels during differentiation results in increased TIRAP and TRAF6 protein, respectively.[18] This suggests that innate immune genes, such as TIRAP and TRAF6, are tightly regulated in hematopoietic stem and progenitor cells. Murine marrow transplant models in which miR-145 and miR-146a are reduced or TRAF6 is overexpressed results in megakaryocytic and platelet defects, and a propensity to develop acute leukemia or marrow failure, through both cell autonomous and nonautonomous mechanisms.[18] Loss of miR-145 and miR-146a does not result in macrocytic anemia, a key clinical finding in 5q- syndrome. Identification of the RPS14 gene in the minimally deleted region of

Table 2		
Mutations that affect innate immune signaling in hematologic malignancies		
Gene	Role in Hematologic Malignancy	Potential Mechanism
miR-145	Deleted in del (5q) MDS/AML, reduced expression in AML	Results in increased TIRAP expression
miR-146a	Deleted in a portion of del (5q) MDS/AML, reduced expression in AML	Results in increased TRAF6 and IRAK1 expression
miR-181	Expression suppressed in AML	Correlates with increased expression of innate immunity genes
c-cbl	Activating mutations in MDS/AML, UPD in MDS	May result in increased TRAF6 signaling
Tel-Syk	Fusion in AML	May result in increased TRAF6 signaling
SOCS-1	Reduced expression because of hypomethylation in MDS and AML	May result in increased TIRAP activation

Abbreviations: AML, acute myeloid leukemia; MDS, myelodysplastic syndromes; UPD, uniparental disomy.

5q- syndrome, however, likely explains the macrocytic anemia.[60–62] The full spectrum of clinical features in 5q syndrome may be explained by the collective loss of miR-145, miR-146a, and RPS14.

The downstream signaling pathways activated by TRAF6 following loss of miR-145 and miR-146a are not completely evaluated in bone marrow cells. Loss of miR-145 and miR-146a, however, results in NF-κB activation in a TRAF6- and TIRAP-dependent manner in fibroblasts.[18] Although NF-κB is implicated in MDS, the mechanism leading to its activation in other MDS subtypes is not clear. Compared with normal CD34+ marrow cells, NF-κB activation is significantly elevated in CD34+ bone marrow cells isolated from low- and high-risk MDS patients, although not in chromic myelomonocytic leukemia.[63,64] A similar increase in NF-κB activity was also documented in MDS cell lines.[64] Blocking NF-κB resulted in apoptosis of MDS and normal CD34+ cells in vitro, suggesting that NF-κB provides survival signals in these cells in part by inducing antiapoptotic genes.[65,66] The contribution of NF-κB to marrow dysplasia has not been extensively studied, although IκBα-deficient mice exhibit dysplastic neutrophils and megakaryocytes.[67] Taken together, myeloid dysplasia and cell survival may be a feature of constitutive NF-κB signaling in MDS (see **Table 2**).

Given that a hallmark of MDS is increased apoptosis of bone marrow precursors and terminally differentiated cells, it is possible that TLRs and TNFR, which have been implicated in inducing apoptosis in other cell types, may similarly mediate cell death and contribute to cytopenias in MDS. TLR2 and TLR4 expression was found to be increased by a TNF-dependent mechanism in CD34+ cells isolated from the marrow of MDS patients, and the level of expression correlated with the extent of apoptosis.[68] TNFR1 was expressed at higher levels in low-risk MDS patients, whereas TNFR2 expression was elevated in high-risk MDS patients. TNFR1 favors cytotoxic signaling, whereas TNFR2 favors cytoprotective signals.[69] The shift from TNFR1 to TNFR2 expression may explain the increase in prosurvival signals found in the marrow of patients with higher-risk MDS.[69] Although TLR and TNFR upregulation is reported in the marrow of MDS patients, it is not clear whether it is the MDS clone or the normal coresident marrow cells that exhibit elevated TLR signaling and are prone to apoptosis.

Gene expression profiling experiments of have also pointed toward a role for activation of innate immune signaling in MDS. In one study, TRAF6 and IRAK1 were overexpressed by greater than 10-fold in CD34$^+$ marrow cells from low- and high-risk MDS patients compared with normal controls.[70] In contrast, TRAF2 is overexpressed only in low-risk MDS and AML, but not in high-risk MDS.[71] By DNA arrays, amplification of the TIRAP locus (chromosome 11q24.2) and the TRAF6 locus (chromosome 11p12) has been reported.[72,73] Whether amplification of the respective loci correlates with increased TIRAP or TRAF6 mRNA expression has not yet been determined. These observations support the finding that loss of miR-145 and miR-146a results in increased protein expression of TIRAP and TRAF6, respectively, in 5q syndrome patients (**Table 3**).

Dysplastic cells in MDS are not exclusively part of the abnormal clone, which suggests that nonautonomous effects contribute to dysplasia. Cytokines that have been shown to be increased in MDS patients include TNFα, IL-1β, IL-6, and IL-3.[74–76] One of the consequences of miR-145 and miR-146 depletion or TRAF6 activation in mouse hematopoietic cells is megakaryocytic and platelet defects caused by nonautonomous effects of IL-6. Circulating IL-6 protein and IL-6 transcripts are elevated in 5q syndrome and approximately 30% of all MDS patients.[74,76,77] IL-6, an NF-κB target gene, is a pleotropic cytokine that stimulates megakaryocyte proliferation, colony formation, and platelet formation.[78] In line with these findings, overexpression of an IL-6 transgene in mouse marrow transplantation experiments produces thrombocytosis, anemia, and transient neutropenia with progression to leukocytosis.[79] The authors found an inverse correlation between IL-6 and miR-145 or miR-146a expression in MDS patient marrow cells, and provide direct evidence that the paracrine effect of TRAF6-induced IL6 elicits some of the features of 5q syndrome. Interestingly, lenalidomide, the main therapy for 5q syndrome, suppresses expression of IL-6.[80]

Evidence of Indirect Activation of Innate Immune Pathway Genes in MDS

Pathways associated with or converging on the innate immune pathway are also deregulated in MDS (see **Table 2**). Missense mutations in c-cbl, which enhance its activity and may explain the clonal dominance in MDS, are identified in approximately 50% of MDS patients with uniparental disomy at chromosome 11q.[81] Contribution of activated c-cbl to MDS may be explained partly through its activation of the MyD88-dependent pathway. c-cbl is recruited along with TRAF6 to form a complex with the intracellular domains of CD40 or TRANCE.[82] Although balanced gene translocations

Table 3		
Innate immune genes implicated in hematologic malignancies		
Innate Immune Gene	**Role in Hematologic Malignancy**	**Potential Mechanism**
TLR4	Overexpressed in MDS	Expands hematopoietic stem cells, survival of abnormal clone
TNFR	Overexpressed in MDS	Prosurvival
TIRAP	Increased protein expression in MDS	Activate NF-κB, prosurvival
TRAF6	Increased protein and mRNA expression in MDS	Activate NF-κB, expand abnormal clones, prosurvival
IRAK1	Overexpressed in MYST3-CREBBP AML	Activate NF-κB
NF-κB	Activated in MDS and AML	Prosurvival

Abbreviations: AML, acute myeloid leukemia; MDS, myelodysplastic syndromes.

are not as common as copy number alterations in MDS, t(9;12)(q22;p12) has been reported in patients with MDS.[83] This fusion involves TEL and Syk, and results in constitutive activation of the Syk tyrosine kinase linked to the PI3K, MAPK, and STAT5 pathways in hematopoietic cells.[84] Whether TEL-Syk expression induces an MDS phenotype in mice has not been investigated; however, TEL-Syk does provide growth factor independent growth in a mouse hematopoietic cell line in vitro.[84] Signaling from Syk has been well studied and requires components of the innate immune pathway. Specifically, IL-1β stimulation formed an IL-1R complex with Syk, TRAF6, and Src in cell lines.[85] Furthermore, TRAF6 is essential for activation of Syk-mediated signaling.[85] It is reasonable to hypothesize that the TEL-Syk fusion identified in MDS patients also requires TRAF6 signaling and contributes to the disease phenotype.

Another example of a common alteration in MDS that may result in deregulation of innate immune signaling is the deletion or epigenetic silencing of suppressor of cytokine signaling (SOCS) proteins.[86,87] SOCS proteins are negative regulators of intracellular signaling, best known for inhibiting JAK kinases.[88] In one study, approximately 30% of MDS patients exhibited hypermethylation of the SOCS-1 locus associated with reduced mRNA expression.[86] Although the consequences of SOCS deletions in other hematologic malignancies has been explored, the role of SOCS hypermethylation in MDS is not known. One possible mechanism may involve TIRAP. SOCS-1 is a negative regulator of TIRAP and blocks activation of downstream pathways by mediating ubiquitination and subsequent degradation of TIRAP.[89]

CLINICAL IMPLICATIONS OF DEREGULATED INNATE IMMUNE SIGNALING IN MDS

Given that innate immune signaling seems to contribute to myeloid hematologic malignancies, it is important to determine whether deregulation of innate immune signaling is associated with adverse outcome, clinical subtypes, or therapeutic response in MDS and AML. The data also suggest that increased expression of TRAF6 and TIRAP or deletion of miR-145/miR-146 in MDS patients who do not have a deletion of chromosome arm 5q presents with similar findings to those with del (5q). The role of other innate immune genes also needs to be evaluated in patients to define the impact of their deregulation on diagnosis and prognosis, and the potential for therapeutic intervention.

To our knowledge, clinically approved drugs that target innate immune system genes are not available, although proteasome inhibitors can block NF-κB activation.[90] Rationale to create such drugs depends on whether experimental knockdown or inhibition of key innate immune genes is beneficial in leukemic model systems. There is some reason to speculate that inhibiting innate immune genes in certain subtypes is beneficial. Although the mechanism is not known, thalidomide analogs can block LPS-induced activation of NF-κB and expression of innate immune-related genes (eg, IL-6, TNFα, and MyD88).[80,91] The therapeutic efficacy of lenalidomide in MDS and other hematologic malignancies[92,93] provides an impetus to design small molecular inhibitors that target innate immune genes.

SUMMARY

Constitutive activation of the innate immune pathway in hematopoietic cells is one likely mechanism leading to abnormal hematopoiesis associated with MDS. Unlike transient activation of the innate immune pathway by acute infection, cell intrinsic defects that cause activation of the innate immune pathway prevent normal homeostasis of differentiation, apoptosis, and proliferation in hematopoietic cells (see

Fig. 2B). Under normal conditions, microbial-mediated activation of TLR4 signaling in hematopoietic cells results in increased expression of cytokines, myeloid-lineage skewing toward neutrophils and monocytes, and eventual elimination of activated cells (see **Fig. 2**B). In contrast, a genetic defect (or chronic exposure to a pathogen) results in constitutive and dysregulated innate immune signaling. Consequently, these cells undergo abnormal hematopoietic differentiation and increased cell death of differentiated cells, through autonomous and nonautonomous effects. Concurrently, prosurvival signals mediated by innate immune pathways maintain and expand the abnormal hematopoietic stem and progenitor cells. Expansion or maintenance of abnormal hematopoietic stem and progenitors allows for subsequent mutations that may promote acute leukemia.

REFERENCES

1. Kimbrell DA, Beutler B. The evolution and genetics of innate immunity. Nat Rev Genet 2001;2(4):256–67.
2. McGettrick AF, O'Neill LA. Toll-like receptors: key activators of leucocytes and regulator of haematopoiesis. Br J Haematol 2007;139(2):185–93.
3. Bradley JR, Pober JS. Tumor necrosis factor receptor-associated factors (TRAFs). Oncogene 2001;20(44):6482–91.
4. Arend WP, Palmer G, Gabay C. IL-1, IL-18, and IL-33 families of cytokines. Immunol Rev 2008;223:20–38.
5. Dauphinee SM, Karsan A. Lipopolysaccharide signaling in endothelial cells. Lab Invest 2006;86(1):9–22.
6. Imler JL, Hoffmann JA. Toll receptors in innate immunity. Trends Cell Biol 2001; 11(7):304–11.
7. Wu H, Arron JR. TRAF6, a molecular bridge spanning adaptive immunity, innate immunity and osteoimmunology. Bioessays 2003;25(11):1096–105.
8. Gao JJ, Diesl V, Wittmann T, et al. Bacterial LPS and CpG DNA differentially induce gene expression profiles in mouse macrophages. J Endotoxin Res 2003;9(4):237–43.
9. Malcolm KC, Arndt PG, Manos EJ, et al. Microarray analysis of lipopolysaccharide-treated human neutrophils. Am J Physiol Lung Cell Mol Physiol 2003; 284(4):L663–70.
10. Hertzog PJ, O'Neill LA, Hamilton JA. The interferon in TLR signaling: more than just antiviral. Trends Immunol 2003;24(10):534–9.
11. Bartel DP. MicroRNAs: genomics, biogenesis, mechanism, and function. Cell 2004;116(2):281–97.
12. Taganov KD, Boldin MP, Chang KJ, et al. NF-kappaB-dependent induction of microRNA miR-146, an inhibitor targeted to signaling proteins of innate immune responses. Proc Natl Acad Sci U S A 2006;103(33):12481–6.
13. O'Connell RM, Rao DS, Chaudhuri AA, et al. Sustained expression of microRNA-155 in hematopoietic stem cells causes a myeloproliferative disorder. J Exp Med 2008;205(3):585–94.
14. Chen XM, Splinter PL, O'Hara SP, et al. A cellular micro-RNA, let-7i, regulates Toll-like receptor 4 expression and contributes to cholangiocyte immune responses against *Cryptosporidium parvum* infection. J Biol Chem 2007;282(39):28929–38.
15. Liu G, Friggeri A, Yang Y, et al. miR-147, a microRNA that is induced upon toll-like receptor stimulation, regulates murine macrophage inflammatory responses. Proc Natl Acad Sci U S A 2009;106(37):15819–24.

16. Androulidaki A, Iliopoulos D, Arranz A, et al. The kinase Akt1 controls macrophage response to lipopolysaccharide by regulating microRNAs. Immunity 2009;31(2):220–31.
17. Labbaye C, Spinello I, Quaranta MT, et al. A three-step pathway comprising PLZF/miR-146a/CXCR4 controls megakaryopoiesis. Nat Cell Biol 2008;10(7): 788–801.
18. Starczynowski DT, Kuchenbauer F, Argiropoulos B, et al. Identification of miR-145 and miR-146a as mediators of the 5q- syndrome phenotype. Nat Med 2010;16: 49–58.
19. Chen CZ, Li L, Lodish HF, et al. MicroRNAs modulate hematopoietic lineage differentiation. Science 2004;303(5654):83–6.
20. Ueda Y, Kondo M, Kelsoe G. Inflammation and the reciprocal production of granulocytes and lymphocytes in bone marrow. J Exp Med 2005;201(11):1771–80.
21. Nagai Y, Garrett KP, Ohta S, et al. Toll-like receptors on hematopoietic progenitor cells stimulate innate immune system replenishment. Immunity 2006;24(6): 801–12.
22. Tang M, Wei X, Guo Y, et al. TAK1 is required for the survival of hematopoietic cells and hepatocytes in mice. J Exp Med 2008;205(7):1611–9.
23. Passegue E, Jamieson CH, Ailles LE, et al. Normal and leukemic hematopoiesis: are leukemias a stem cell disorder or a reacquisition of stem cell characteristics? Proc Natl Acad Sci U S A 2003;100(Suppl 1):11842–9.
24. Vardiman JW. The World Health Organization (WHO) classification of tumors of the hematopoietic and lymphoid tissues: an overview with emphasis on the myeloid neoplasms. Chem Biol Interact 2009 [Epub ahead of print].
25. Alvarez S, Cigudosa JC. Gains, losses and complex karyotypes in myeloid disorders: a light at the end of the tunnel. Hematol Oncol 2005;23(1):18–25.
26. Heerema-McKenney A, Arber DA. Acute myeloid leukemia. Hematol Oncol Clin North Am 2009;23(4):633–54.
27. Heuser M, Argiropoulos B, Kuchenbauer F, et al. MN1 overexpression induces acute myeloid leukemia in mice and predicts ATRA resistance in patients with AML. Blood 2007;110(5):1639–47.
28. Heuser M, Sly LM, Argiropoulos B, et al. Modelling the functional heterogeneity of leukemia stem cells: role of STAT5 in leukemia stem cell self-renewal. Blood 2009; 114:3983–93.
29. Heuser M, Beutel G, Krauter J, et al. High meningioma 1 (MN1) expression as a predictor for poor outcome in acute myeloid leukemia with normal cytogenetics. Blood 2006;108(12):3898–905.
30. Kelly LM, Liu Q, Kutok JL, et al. FLT3 internal tandem duplication mutations associated with human acute myeloid leukemias induce myeloproliferative disease in a murine bone marrow transplant model. Blood 2002;99(1):310–8.
31. Turzanski J, Grundy M, Russell NH, et al. Interleukin-1beta maintains an apoptosis-resistant phenotype in the blast cells of acute myeloid leukaemia via multiple pathways. Leukemia 2004;18(10):1662–70.
32. Zapata JM, Krajewska M, Krajewski S, et al. TNFR-associated factor family protein expression in normal tissues and lymphoid malignancies. J Immunol 2000;165(9):5084–96.
33. Guzman ML, Neering SJ, Upchurch D, et al. Nuclear factor-kappaB is constitutively activated in primitive human acute myelogenous leukemia cells. Blood 2001;98(8):2301–7.
34. Aggarwal BB. Signalling pathways of the TNF superfamily: a double-edged sword. Nat Rev Immunol 2003;3(9):745–56.

35. Horie R, Gattei V, Ito K, et al. Frequent expression of the variant CD30 in human malignant myeloid and lymphoid neoplasms. Am J Pathol 1999;155(6):2029–41.
36. Soni V, Cahir-McFarland E, Kieff E. LMP1 TRAFficking activates growth and survival pathways. Adv Exp Med Biol 2007;597:173–87.
37. Aldinucci D, Poletto D, Nanni P, et al. CD40L induces proliferation, self-renewal, rescue from apoptosis, and production of cytokines by CD40-expressing AML blasts. Exp Hematol 2002;30(11):1283–92.
38. Hock BD, McKenzie JL, Patton NW, et al. Circulating levels and clinical significance of soluble CD40 in patients with hematologic malignancies. Cancer 2006;106(10):2148–57.
39. Hattori K, Naguro I, Runchel C, et al. The roles of ASK family proteins in stress responses and diseases. Cell Commun Signal 2009;7:9.
40. Yan W, Arai A, Aoki M, et al. ASK1 is activated by arsenic trioxide in leukemic cells through accumulation of reactive oxygen species and may play a negative role in induction of apoptosis. Biochem Biophys Res Commun 2007;355(4):1038–44.
41. Casely-Hayford MA, Nicholas SA, Sumbayev VV. Azinomycin epoxide induces activation of apoptosis signal-regulating kinase 1 (ASK1) and caspase 3 in a HIF-1alpha-independent manner in human leukaemia myeloid macrophages. Eur J Pharmacol 2009;602(2-3):262–7.
42. Ichijo H, Nishida E, Irie K, et al. Induction of apoptosis by ASK1, a mammalian MAPKKK that activates SAPK/JNK and p38 signaling pathways. Science 1997; 275(5296):90–4.
43. D'Angelo S, Liebermann D, Hoffman B. The c-myc apoptotic response is not intrinsic to blocking terminal myeloid differentiation. J Cell Physiol 2008;216(1): 120–7.
44. Marcucci G, Radmacher MD, Maharry K, et al. MicroRNA expression in cytogenetically normal acute myeloid leukemia. N Engl J Med 2008;358(18): 1919–28.
45. Debernardi S, Skoulakis S, Molloy G, et al. MicroRNA miR-181a correlates with morphological sub-class of acute myeloid leukaemia and the expression of its target genes in global genome-wide analysis. Leukemia 2007;21(5):912–6.
46. Corey SJ, Minden MD, Barber DL, et al. Myelodysplastic syndromes: the complexity of stem-cell diseases. Nat Rev Cancer 2007;7(2):118–29.
47. Vardiman JW, Thiele J, Arber DA, et al. The 2008 revision of the World Health Organization (WHO) classification of myeloid neoplasms and acute leukemia: rationale and important changes. Blood 2009;114(5):937–51.
48. Kopterides P, Halikias S, Tsavaris N. Visceral leishmaniasis masquerading as myelodysplasia. Am J Hematol 2003;74(3):198–9.
49. Hasle H, Kerndrup G, Jacobsen BB, et al. Chronic parvovirus infection mimicking myelodysplastic syndrome in a child with subclinical immunodeficiency. Am J Pediatr Hematol Oncol 1994;16(4):329–33.
50. List A, Dewald G, Bennett J, et al. Lenalidomide in the myelodysplastic syndrome with chromosome 5q deletion. N Engl J Med 2006;355(14):1456–65.
51. Lin YW, Slape C, Zhang Z, et al. NUP98-HOXD13 transgenic mice develop a highly penetrant, severe myelodysplastic syndrome that progresses to acute leukemia. Blood 2005;106(1):287–95.
52. Chung YJ, Choi CW, Slape C, et al. Transplantation of a myelodysplastic syndrome by a long-term repopulating hematopoietic cell. Proc Natl Acad Sci U S A 2008;105(37):14088–93.
53. Grisendi S, Bernardi R, Rossi M, et al. Role of nucleophosmin in embryonic development and tumorigenesis. Nature 2005;437(7055):147–53.

54. Buonamici S, Li D, Chi Y, et al. EVI1 induces myelodysplastic syndrome in mice. J Clin Invest 2004;114(5):713–9.
55. Moody JL, Xu L, Helgason CD, et al. Anemia, thrombocytopenia, leukocytosis, extramedullary hematopoiesis, and impaired progenitor function in Pten+/-SHIP-/- mice: a novel model of myelodysplasia. Blood 2004;103(12):4503–10.
56. Minella AC, Loeb KR, Knecht A, et al. Cyclin E phosphorylation regulates cell proliferation in hematopoietic and epithelial lineages in vivo. Genes Dev 2008; 22(12):1677–89.
57. Zhou L, Nguyen AN, Sohal D, et al. Inhibition of the TGF-beta receptor I kinase promotes hematopoiesis in MDS. Blood 2008;112(8):3434–43.
58. Peng J, Kitchen SM, West RA, et al. Myeloproliferative defects following targeting of the Drf1 gene encoding the mammalian diaphanous related formin mDia1. Cancer Res 2007;67(16):7565–71.
59. Ebert BL. Deletion 5q in myelodysplastic syndrome: a paradigm for the study of hemizygous deletions in cancer. Leukemia 2009;23(7):1252–6.
60. Ebert BL, Pretz J, Bosco J, et al. Identification of RPS14 as a 5q-syndrome gene by RNA interference screen. Nature 2008;451(7176):335–9.
61. Lehmann S, O'Kelly J, Raynaud S, et al. Common deleted genes in the 5q-syndrome: thrombocytopenia and reduced erythroid colony formation in SPARC null mice. Leukemia 2007;21(9):1931–6.
62. Barlow JL, Drynan LF, Hewett DR, et al. A p53-dependent mechanism underlies macrocytic anemia in a mouse model of human 5q-syndrome. Nat Med 2010;16: 59–66.
63. Kerbauy DM, Lesnikov V, Abbasi N, et al. NF-kappaB and FLIP in arsenic trioxide (ATO)-induced apoptosis in myelodysplastic syndromes (MDSs). Blood 2005; 106(12):3917–25.
64. Fabre C, Carvalho G, Tasdemir E, et al. NF-kappaB inhibition sensitizes to starvation-induced cell death in high-risk myelodysplastic syndrome and acute myeloid leukemia. Oncogene 2007;26(28):4071–83.
65. Pyatt DW, Stillman WS, Yang Y, et al. An essential role for NF-kappaB in human CD34(+) bone marrow cell survival. Blood 1999;93(10):3302–8.
66. Braun T, Carvalho G, Coquelle A, et al. NF-kappaB constitutes a potential therapeutic target in high-risk myelodysplastic syndrome. Blood 2006;107(3): 1156–65.
67. Rupec RA, Jundt F, Rebholz B, et al. Stroma-mediated dysregulation of myelopoiesis in mice lacking I kappa B alpha. Immunity 2005;22(4):479–91.
68. Maratheftis CI, Andreakos E, Moutsopoulos HM, et al. Toll-like receptor-4 is up-regulated in hematopoietic progenitor cells and contributes to increased apoptosis in myelodysplastic syndromes. Clin Cancer Res 2007;13(4):1154–60.
69. Kerbauy DB, Deeg HJ. Apoptosis and antiapoptotic mechanisms in the progression of myelodysplastic syndrome. Exp Hematol 2007;35(11):1739–46.
70. Hofmann WK, de Vos S, Komor M, et al. Characterization of gene expression of CD34+ cells from normal and myelodysplastic bone marrow. Blood 2002; 100(10):3553–60.
71. Sawanobori M, Yamaguchi S, Hasegawa M, et al. Expression of TNF receptors and related signaling molecules in the bone marrow from patients with myelodysplastic syndromes. Leuk Res 2003;27(7):583–91.
72. Starczynowski DT, Vercauteren S, Telenius A, et al. High-resolution whole genome tiling path array CGH analysis of CD34+ cells from patients with low-risk myelodysplastic syndromes reveals cryptic copy number alterations and predicts overall and leukemia-free survival. Blood 2008;112(8):3412–24.

73. Gondek LP, Tiu R, O'Keefe CL, et al. Chromosomal lesions and uniparental disomy detected by SNP arrays in MDS, MDS/MPD, and MDS-derived AML. Blood 2008;111(3):1534–42.

74. Verhoef GE, De Schouwer P, Ceuppens JL, et al. Measurement of serum cytokine levels in patients with myelodysplastic syndromes. Leukemia 1992;6(12): 1268–72.

75. Koike M, Ishiyama T, Tomoyasu S, et al. Spontaneous cytokine overproduction by peripheral blood mononuclear cells from patients with myelodysplastic syndromes and aplastic anemia. Leuk Res 1995;19(9):639–44.

76. Herold M, Schmalzl F, Zwierzina H. Increased serum interleukin 6 levels in patients with myelodysplastic syndromes. Leuk Res 1992;16(6-7):585–8.

77. Hsu HC, Lee YM, Tsai WH, et al. Circulating levels of thrombopoietic and inflammatory cytokines in patients with acute myeloblastic leukemia and myelodysplastic syndrome. Oncology 2002;63(1):64–9.

78. Kishimoto T. Interleukin-6: from basic science to medicine–40 years in immunology. Annu Rev Immunol 2005;23:1–21.

79. Hawley RG, Fong AZ, Burns BF, et al. Transplantable myeloproliferative disease induced in mice by an interleukin 6 retrovirus. J Exp Med 1992;176(4):1149–63.

80. Corral LG, Haslett PA, Muller GW, et al. Differential cytokine modulation and T cell activation by two distinct classes of thalidomide analogues that are potent inhibitors of TNF-alpha. J Immunol 1999;163(1):380–6.

81. Dunbar AJ, Gondek LP, O'Keefe CL, et al. 250K single nucleotide polymorphism array karyotyping identifies acquired uniparental disomy and homozygous mutations, including novel missense substitutions of c-Cbl, in myeloid malignancies. Cancer Res 2008;68(24):10349–57.

82. Arron JR, Vologodskaia M, Wong BR, et al. A positive regulatory role for Cbl family proteins in tumor necrosis factor-related activation-induced cytokine (trance) and CD40L-mediated Akt activation. J Biol Chem 2001;276(32):30011–7.

83. Kuno Y, Abe A, Emi N, et al. Constitutive kinase activation of the TEL-Syk fusion gene in myelodysplastic syndrome with t(9;12)(q22;p12). Blood 2001;97(4): 1050–5.

84. Kanie T, Abe A, Matsuda T, et al. TEL-Syk fusion constitutively activates PI3-K/Akt, MAPK and JAK2-independent STAT5 signal pathways. Leukemia 2004;18(3): 548–55.

85. Yamada T, Fujieda S, Yanagi S, et al. IL-1 induced chemokine production through the association of Syk with TNF receptor-associated factor-6 in nasal fibroblast lines. J Immunol 2001;167(1):283–8.

86. Brakensiek K, Langer F, Schlegelberger B, et al. Hypermethylation of the suppressor of cytokine signalling-1 (SOCS-1) in myelodysplastic syndrome. Br J Haematol 2005;130(2):209–17.

87. Johan MF, Bowen DT, Frew ME, et al. Aberrant methylation of the negative regulators RASSFIA, SHP-1 and SOCS-1 in myelodysplastic syndromes and acute myeloid leukaemia. Br J Haematol 2005;129(1):60–5.

88. Croker BA, Kiu H, Nicholson SE. SOCS regulation of the JAK/STAT signalling pathway. Semin Cell Dev Biol 2008;19(4):414–22.

89. Scott MJ, Liu S, Shapiro RA, et al. Endotoxin uptake in mouse liver is blocked by endotoxin pretreatment through a suppressor of cytokine signaling-1-dependent mechanism. Hepatology 2009;49(5):1695–708.

90. Mitsiades N, Mitsiades CS, Poulaki V, et al. Biologic sequelae of nuclear factor-kappaB blockade in multiple myeloma: therapeutic applications. Blood 2002; 99(11):4079–86.

91. Noman AS, Koide N, Hassan F, et al. Thalidomide inhibits lipopolysaccharide-induced tumor necrosis factor-alpha production via down-regulation of MyD88 expression. Innate Immun 2009;15(1):33–41.

92. Fehniger TA, Byrd JC, Marcucci G, et al. Single-agent lenalidomide induces complete remission of acute myeloid leukemia in patients with isolated trisomy 13. Blood 2009;113(5):1002–5.

93. List A, Kurtin S, Roe DJ, et al. Efficacy of lenalidomide in myelodysplastic syndromes. N Engl J Med 2005;352(6):549–57.

Mouse Models of Myelodysplastic Syndromes

Sarah H. Beachy, PhD, Peter D. Aplan, MD*

KEYWORDS

- Myelodysplastic syndrome • Mouse model • Xenotransplant
- Genetically engineered mice • Hoxa

A wide spectrum of model organisms has been used to investigate the biology of cancer. These model organisms include *Drosophila melanogaster*, *Danio rerio*, *Rattus* (several species), *Mus musculus*, and nonhuman primates. For a variety of reasons, including small body size, high fecundity, well-characterized physiology, and completely sequenced genome, the common laboratory mouse (*M musculus*) has been the model organism of choice for many cancer biologists. Three principal strategies have been used to model cancer in the mouse. Mice have been treated with known mutagenic or carcinogenic agents, most commonly small molecules[1,2] or viruses.[3] In addition, immunodeficient mice have been used in xenotransplant experiments in which primary human malignancies or cell lines are injected into the mouse. Finally, recently developed molecular genetic tools have made possible the generation of genetically engineered mice. All three of these approaches have been used to model myelodysplastic syndrome (MDS) in mice.

Nomenclature for hematopoietic disease in mice has been the topic of considerable debate. The hematopathology subcommittee of the Mouse Models of Human Cancer Consortium has developed a set of guidelines for the uniform description of hematopoietic malignancies in mice.[4] These criteria are presented in **Box 1**. It should be noted that most malignancies fulfilling the criterion for "cytopenia with increased blasts" are classified as acute nonlymphoid leukemias, and not myeloid dysplasia. A mouse that fulfills criteria 1 (cytopenias) and 2B (increased bone marrow [BM] blasts), along with splenomegaly and disseminated disease (as reflected by invasion of parenchymal tissues or >20% circulating blasts) is classified as "acute nonlymphocytic leukemia," not MDS. Dyspoiesis in mice can be difficult to identify. Megaloblastic changes and multinucleate erythroblasts are signs of dysplasia in the erythroid lineage that are

This research was supported by the Intramural Research Program of the National Institutes of Health, National Cancer Institute.

Genetics Branch, Center for Cancer Research, National Cancer Institute, National Institutes of Health, 8901 Wisconsin Avenue, Navy 8 Room 5101, Bethesda, MD 20889–5105, USA

* Corresponding author.

E-mail address: aplanp@mail.nih.gov

Hematol Oncol Clin N Am 24 (2010) 361–375
doi:10.1016/j.hoc.2010.02.002
0889-8588/10/$ – see front matter. Published by Elsevier Inc.

Box 1
Criteria for the diagnosis of myeloid dysplasias in mice

1. At least one of the following findings in peripheral blood

   A. Neutropenia

   B. Thrombocytopenia (in the absence of leukocytosis or erythrocytosis)

   C. Anemia (in the absence of leukocytosis or thrombocytosis)

2. Detection of a maturation defect in nonlymphoid hematopoietic cells manifested by at least one of the following

   A. Dysgranulopoiesis, dyserythropoiesis, or dysplastic megakaryocytes, with or without increased nonlymphoid immature forms or blasts

   B. At least 20% nonlymphoid immature forms or blasts in the bone marrow or spleen

3. Disorder does not meet the criteria for a nonlymphoid leukemia

4. If the disorder complies with

   2A, then the subclassification is a *myelodysplastic syndrome*

   2B, then the subclassification is *cytopenia with increased blasts*

Data from Kogan SC, Ward JM, Anver MR, et al. Bethesda proposals for classification of nonlymphoid hematopoietic neoplasms in mice. Blood 2002;100:238–45.

---

similar in both mice and humans, but ringed sideroblasts are rare in mice. Micromegakaryocytes, large megakaryocytes with unlobated nuclei, and large megakryocytes with bizarre hypersegmentation are signs of megakaryocytic dysplasia in mice. Neutrophil dyspoiesis may be evident in the form of pseudo Pelger-Huët cells with fine nuclear bridging[5] and cells with lobated, as opposed to ring, nuclei.

XENOTRANSPLANTATION

Immunodeficient mouse models bearing human tumor xenografts have been established for the study of solid tumor biology,[4,6,7] and for the study of hematopoietic malignancies and identifications of leukemia-initiating cells.[8–10] Although the xenograft model is an attractive approach for investigating malignant disease, many human tumors are unable to be established in the mouse host. This could be caused by a variety of reasons, including toxicity from ex vivo manipulation of the malignant cells, a lack of necessary growth or survival factors in the tumor microenvironment, or an antitumor immune response generated by the host. Recently, immunodeficient mouse models for the study of leukemia-initiating cells have been subjects of careful scrutiny for the effects of the host immune system on xenografts, specifically sorted primary leukemia cells.[11] In that study, the authors demonstrated that flow cytometric sorting of leukemic cells with a CD38 antibody led to an Fc-mediated clearance of the sorted leukemia cells in vivo. Some of these same challenges may have hindered efforts to establish xenograft models of MDS (perhaps to a further extent).

Several laboratories have attempted to engraft immortal human cell lines established from MDS patients. Until proved otherwise, by recapitulating MDS in a host, these cell lines should not be regarded as MDS cell lines, but rather as acute myeloid leukemia (AML) cell lines that have evolved, in vivo or in vitro, from MDS patients.[12] To provide the growth factors that increase the likelihood of engraftment of F-36P, a cell line derived from a patient with MDS, severe combined immunodeficient (SCID) mice were engineered to express the human forms of granulocyte-macrophage colony–stimulating factor and interleukin-3.[13] Despite the proliferation of F-36P in the transgenic mice, engraftment was only achieved following neutralization of natural killer cells. These mice also developed osteolytic lesions, a rare occurrence in MDS patients.

More recently, the nonobese diabetic (NOD)-SCID mouse has been used in xenograft studies of primary cells from MDS patients, because these mice are defective in complement and natural killer cell activities, in addition to B- and T-cell deficiencies. In one study, hematopoietic cells from seven MDS patients with a 5q deletion were injected into NOD-SCID mice. One of the seven mice showed evidence for low-level (12%) engraftment, and whereas CD45+CD15+ cells contained the 5q deletion, no evidence for clinical disease was found in the recipient mice.[14] Similarly, BM from MDS patients with trisomy 8 was unable to reconstitute lymphoid and myeloid compartments in mice.[15] In a second study, BM from patients with MDS was injected into sublethally irradiated NOD-SCID mice, with or without the delivery of human cytokines.[16] Although subfractions of human CD45+ cells (eg, CD34-CD38+ and T cells) were detected in mice transplanted with MDS BM, decreased percentages of cells from the MDS patients engrafted compared with BM from healthy controls. Additionally, abnormal karyotypes detected in BM from MDS patients (eg, del[5q]) before the transfer of cells to mice were not identified after transplantation, suggesting that most of the human cells that had engrafted were derived from normal bone marrow elements, as opposed to the MDS clone. The authors attribute the lack of observed engraftment of clonal MDS cells to several possibilities, including decreased proliferative potential, adverse microenvironmental conditions, and susceptibility to immune attack.

To evade immune responses, and provide human cytokines in the context of a xenotransplantation assay, Thanopoulou and colleagues[17] designed a study using NOD-SCID mice that lacked β2 microglobulin (β2m$^{-/-}$) and expressed human interleukin-3, granulocyte-macrophage colony–stimulating factor and Steel factor (c-kit ligand). The authors reported that MDS cells from 9 of 11 patients successfully engrafted, and that four of the five samples that had a clonal cytogenetic marker, such as trisomy 8 or del 5q, engrafted the MDS clone. Engraftment level of the MDS clone was typically quite low, however, less than 1% of nucleated cells, and the mice did not develop clinical MDS. Kerbauy and colleagues[18] have recently reported the successful engraftment of human MDS clonal cells using the NOD-SCID-β2m$^{-/-}$ model. The percent of MDS cells in the engrafted mice was small (0.14%–4%), however, and the mice did not develop clinical disease. Taken together, these studies demonstrate that human MDS cells have the capability to engraft in immunodeficient mice, but do not produce clinical disease. The challenge for future work is to improve the engraftment of the MDS clone in sufficient numbers as to generate clinical disease in the engrafted mice.

USE OF GENETICALLY ENGINEERED CELLS

In general, two approaches have been used to generate mouse hematopoietic cells that express (or in the case of putative MDS tumor suppressors genes do not express) genes thought to be relevant for the development of MDS. In the first approach, murine BM nucleated cells are harvested and infected in vitro with a retroviral construct that expresses the gene of interest. The infected BM nucleated cells, including hematopoietic stem and progenitor cells, which now express the gene of interest, are then transplanted into a lethally irradiated, syngeneic host mouse. The second general approach involves modification of the mouse germline, either by pronuclear injection of DNA into fertilized ova to generate transgenic mice, or by homologous recombination of mouse embryonic stem cells, which can then be injected into blastocysts, leading to generation of chimeric mice. Experiments can be designed such that a gene of interest is deleted (knocked out), or so that a gene of interest is introduced (knocked in). In either case, this second general approach leads to mice that have genetically modified germline genomic DNA. More recently, a variety of approaches using conditional promoters (eg, a tetracycline inducible promoter) or tissue-specific transgenes have given investigators the opportunity to control expression in both a temporal and spatial fashion.

Pten/Ship

Because of the influence that Ship (src homology 2- containing 5' phosphoinositol phosphatase) and Pten (phosphatase and tensin homolog) have on the regulation of second messenger PIP3 and the fact that Ship-deficient mice develop a lethal myelo-proliferative condition,[19,20] Pten+/−Ship−/− mice were developed.[21] Although hypothesized that these mice would develop leukemia, instead they displayed features consistent with aberrant hematopoiesis. Pten+/−Ship−/− mice survived only about 5 weeks and during that time, anemia, leukocytosis, and thrombocytopenia were observed. There was no evidence of leukemia; however, extramedullary hematopoiesis in the liver was found. Although increased numbers of neutrophils were present in the peripheral blood, decreases in myeloid progenitors were revealed following methocellulose culture of the BM. The BM from Pten+/−Ship−/− [22] mice failed to reconstitute the peripheral blood of irradiated wild-type mice in a transplantation assay.

Evi1 Overexpression

Transgenic Evi1 mice were developed by Louz and colleagues[23] by using the Sca-1 promoter for expression in hematopoietic stem cells. The expression of Evi1 in the hematopoietic tissues of these mice resulted in a gender-specific response in one of the transgenic lines whereby females remained healthy during an 18-month period in contrast to their male littermates who manifested reduced colony-forming unit erythroid formation. These male mice became severely ill because of impaired erythropoiesis and died within 7 to 11 weeks. Although these mice did not develop MDS or leukemia, the potential for Evi1 to collaborate in tumor formation was demonstrated by the ability of retrovirally infected transgenic Evi1 mice to develop myeloid leukemia more quickly than infected wild-type mice.

Expression of Evi1 in a BM transduction-transplantation model resulted in a progressive pancytopenia, however, which was inevitably fatal by 12 months.[24] On closer examination, necropsy revealed splenomegaly in Evi1-positive mice with an increase in erythroid precursors, iron deposition, and activated caspase-3 compared with spleens from control animals. Similar to clinical MDS, the BM displayed hyperplasia of erythroid cells and megakaryocytes. In contrast to MDS in humans, the Evi1-induced MDS did not transform to leukemia in this study. Before the onset of overt disease, Evi1-positive mice at 4 months had low levels of EpoR and c-Mpl in BM cells, which correlates with the defect in erythropoiesis and platelet generation observed in moribund mice months later. Follow-up studies observed that binding of Evi1 to Gata1 resulted in impaired expression of the EpoR,[25] whereas Evi1 association with PU.1 altered myelopoiesis.[26]

Npm1 Deletion

Npm1 was of interest for study because of its frequent mutation in AML patients (35%), location on chromosome 5q, and ability to regulate tumor suppressor genes [27] One allele of Npm1 was inactivated in mouse embryonic stem cells by homologous recombination that produced a deletion of exons 2 through 7. After generation of chimeric mice and germline transmission, the investigators noted that *Npm1* −/− (*Npm1* knockout) mice were not viable. The *Npm1* −/− mice died between embryonic day E11.5 and E16.5 because of severe anemia and aberrant organogenesis. *Npm1* +/− mice were viable and demonstrated some features that were consistent with MDS.[27] Most mice aged 6 to 18 months presented at least one blood abnormality commonly associated with MDS. *Npm1* +/− mice often demonstrated an elevated mean corpuscular volume and had a wider range of platelet counts, both increased and decreased, than that of wild-type mice; however, the hemoglobin levels did not differ between groups. Approximately two thirds of the *Npm1* +/− mice had morphologic evidence of erythroid or megakaryocytic dysplasia, including binucleated erythroblasts and hypolobated megakaryocytes. In a follow-up study, prolonged (up to 24 months) monitoring of *Npm1* +/− mice revealed an increased incidence of malignancy compared with wild-type mice, including lung and liver tumors, myeloproliferative neoplasms, AML, B-cell lymphoma, and T-cell lymphoma.[28]

Dido1 Deficiency

Dido1 is a gene that was initially identified in a screen for genes whose expression was up-regulated during the initial stages of apoptosis. Homozygous deletion of *Dido1* in mice led to a hematopoietic disease manifested by a variable degree of mild anemia and a variable degree of granulocytosis, in combination with decreased hematopoietic colony formation in vitro.[22] Dysplastic cells in the spleen and BM were reported, but not characterized in detail, and progression to acute leukemia was not noted. The disease was thought to be consistent with a diagnosis of myelodysplastic syndrome/myeloproliferative disease (MDS-MPD) and it was transplantable to recipient mice, indicating that it was cell-autonomous.

NUP98-HOXD13

Over 20[29] chromosomal translocations involving the *NUP98* gene associated with hematopoietic malignancy have been identified.[30,31] Pineault and colleagues[32] described a *NUP98-HOXD13* mouse model in which primary murine BM cells were transduced with a retrovirus carrying a *NUP98-HOXD13* fusion gene, which was initially identified in a patient with MDS.[33] These cells were subsequently transplanted into irradiated recipient mice. Significant decreases in white blood cells were observed in mice expressing the *NUP98-HOXD13* fusion, which was further characterized by a reduction in *B220+* and *CD4+/CD8+* lymphocytes. In contrast, significant increases in myeloid BM cells (*Gr1+/Mac1+*) were identified. Results from colony-forming unit spleen assays with *NUP98-HOXD13*–transduced BM cells indicated a decrease in erythroid precursors (identified by the *Ter119* cell surface marker), an increase in myeloid *Gr1+* cells, and an overall increase in the number of colony-forming unit spleen colonies at day 12. Although some of these mice developed a myeloproliferative disease as early as 4 weeks following transplantation, they did not transition to AML except when mice were engineered to simultaneously express *Meis1*.

In comparison, *NUP98-HOXD13* (*NHD13*) transgenic mice that used Vav 1 regulatory elements to direct expression of the *NHD13* transgene in hematopoietic tissues developed anemia, neutropenia, and lymphopenia at 4 to 7 months.[5] These mice also had a variable degree of thrombocytopenia and macrocytosis; however, these differences were not statistically significant. Despite the peripheral blood cytopenias, these mice had hypercellular or normocellular BMs, indicating ineffective hematopoiesis. Morphologically, the *NHD13* mice showed dysplasia in the form of binucleate erythroblasts, megaloblastosis, pseudo Pelger-Huët cells, and micromegakaroyctes. Similar to the progression pattern observed in patients with MDS, approximately half of the *NHD13* mice with MDS developed an acute leukemia, typically at 10 to 14 months of age. A variety of leukemic phenotypes were identified, most commonly AML. Some animals developed pre–T-lymphoblastic leukemia-lymphoma (pre–T-LBL), however, which is rarely seen in secondary leukemia that evolves from patients with MDS. Although the development of pre–T-LBL was somewhat surprising, it was not completely unexpected given that *NUP98* fusion genes have been associated with both T-cell and myeloid malignancies.[34] Of note, although the initial studies of the *NHD13* fusion used *FVB/N* mice, the entire study was subsequently repeated with *C57Bl/6* mice. The results were remarkably similar in terms of peripheral blood cytopenias, dysplastic morphology, and progression to acute leukemia, demonstrating that the effect of the transgene was not mouse strain-dependent.[5] There are both similarities and differences between the transgenic and retroviral transduction-transplantation models. Both lead to anemia, lymphopenia, and neutropenia initially; however, the retrovirally transduced model quickly transforms to a myeloproliferative disease, whereas the transgenic mice transform more slowly, usually to an AML. The differences between the transgenic and retroviral transduction models could be caused by differences in mouse strain, ex vivo manipulation of cells, effects from BM reconstitution, or differential susceptibility of the BM stem and progenitor cells by the *NUP98-HOXD13* retrovirus.

SALL4 Overexpression

SALL4B is a zinc finger transcription factor expressed early during embryonic development, and is involved in the transcriptional regulation of *Oct4* and *Nanog*.[35] *SALL4B* was constitutively expressed in mouse tissues under the control of the cytomegalovirus promoter.[36] These mice developed some classic features of MDS within a few months of life, including peripheral blood leukopenia and dysplasia, and a mild anemia. BM from these mice was hypercellular and showed an increased number of Mac1+/Gr1+ cells, and increased apoptosis when compared with wild-type counterparts. Half of the transgenic mice transformed to AML by an average of 14.5 months of age and the disease was transplantable. In addition to the hematopoietic abnormalities, most of the transgenic mice were also diagnosed with polycystic kidneys and a minority was identified as having cerebral spinal fluid accumulation in the brain that affected motor function.

BCL-2 and NRAS

To study the process of MDS transformation to AML, overexpression of an inducible *BCL-2* transgene along with simultaneous expression of an *NRAS* mutant (*NrasD12*) were selected for examination in a mouse model.[37] In collaboration with the increased proliferative effects attributed to mutant *NRAS*, it was predicted that a complementary mutation, induced by overexpression of antiapoptotic *BCL-2*, would induce MDS or AML. The authors found that mice that expressed *BCL-2* and mutant *NRAS* developed a mild leukocytosis and thrombocytopenia, without anemia. The mice also displayed hepatosplenomegaly, dysplastic neutrophils, and increased BM blasts (mean of 15%). Serial transplantations of the *lin^{neg}* but not the *lin^{pos}* cells from mice with MDS into immunodeficient mice were successful.

RUNX1 Mutations

Watanabe-Okochi and colleagues[38] infected mouse BM with retroviral constructs that encoded one of two different *RUNX1* (also know as *AML1*) gene mutations that were initially identified in patients with MDS or AML. The D171N mutation is a missense mutation involving the runt homology domain, and the AML1-S291fsX300 mutation is a frameshift mutation that results in truncation of the C-terminal region of the AML1 protein. Most mice that expressed the D171N *RUNX1* mutation developed MDS with an increased red blood cell mean corpuscular volume, dysplasia, anemia, leukopenia, and progression to AML **(Table 1)**.[38] Of note, a fraction of the *RUNX1*-D171N mice had integrations of the retroviral vector used to express the *RUNX1* mutant at the *Evi1* locus, and transplantation of BM cells coinfected with *RUNX1*-D171N and *Evi1* reduced the latency of the disease to 3 to 5 months. This study provides support for the cooperation of *RUNX1* mutants and *Evi1* for inducing MDS with progression to AML.

Arid4a Deficiency

ARID4A and ARID4B (also known as "RBBP1" and "RBBP1L1") are proteins that contain an AT-rich interaction domain (ARID). ARID4A, but not ARID4B, interacts with RB and recruits histone deacetylases to E2F-dependent promoters.[39] Arid4a deficient (*Arid4a*−/−) mice were identified by a gene trap mutagenesis screen.[40] Young (2–5 month old) *Arid4a*−/− mice developed lymphopenia, neutropenia, thrombocytopenia, and a mild anemia, with a normocellular BM.[41] The peripheral blood cytopenias described previously became progressively more severe, with a marked increase in monocytes, as the mice aged. These changes were accompanied by BM fibrosis with increased reticulin fibers and hepatosplenomegaly secondary to a compensatory extramedullary hematopoiesis. These features are reminiscent of a chronic myelomonocytic leukemia (CMML) that has evolved from a MDS/MPD. In 12% of the mice, the disease transformed to a frank AML, with high peripheral blood white blood cell, at ages between 12 and 22 months. BM from the *Arid4a*−/− mice had decreased levels of several *Hoxb* cluster genes (*Hoxb3*, *5*, *6*, and *8*) that are normally expressed in BM, but levels of *Hoxa7*, *Hoxa9*, and *Meis1*, which are up-regulated in some MDS cases in mice and patients (see previously), were normal.[41] Although mice that had deleted both *Arid4a* and *Arid4b* were not viable (*Arid4a*−/− *Arid4b*−/−), *Arid4a* −/− *Arid4b*+/− developed AML with a higher frequency (83%) at an early age (7–15 months).

DNA Polymerase Gamma (Polg) Mutations

Although controversial because of the inexorable accumulation of mitochondrial DNA mutations with age,[42,43] some studies have suggested that MDS patients have an increased frequency of mitochondrial DNA mutations.[44–46] DNA polymerase gamma (Polg), a protein that is encoded by the nuclear genome, is responsible for replication of mitochondrial DNA. Polg has two enzymatic activities: a C-terminal polymerase and an N-terminal "proofreading" exonuclease. Mice with targeted instability of the mitochondrial genome were produced by selective elimination of the N-terminal proofreading activity through gene-targeted creation of a missense mutation (*Polg* D257A); the mutant allele is designated *Polg*[A].[47] Homozygous mutant mice (designated *Polg*[A/A]) show an increase in the frequency of mitochondrial DNA mutations and exhibit features of premature aging, including hair loss, thymic involution, testicular atrophy, and loss of intestinal crypts. In addition, the mice showed a progressive, fatal severe megaloblastic anemia and impaired lymphopoiesis, but there was no evidence for transformation to acute leukemia.[48] Of note given the loss of intestinal crypts in the *Polg*[A/A] mice, the megaloblastic anemia was demonstrated to be caused by mitochondrial defects in the hematopoietic compartment, as opposed to malabsorption, by transplantation of *Polg* [A/A] cells in wild-type recipient mice.

Clinical Implications of Modeling MDS in Mice

Mouse models are developed to study, in detail, questions that cannot easily (or are impossible to) be addressed in the clinic. A useful animal model for MDS would

Table 1
Summary of genetically engineered mouse models for MDS

Genes	Technique	Findings	Reference
Pten/Ship	Pten haploinsufficient Ship knockout	Leukocytosis, neutrophilia, anemia, thrombocytopenia, hepatosplenomegaly, extramedullary hematopoiesis. Lethal by 5 weeks of age, no leukemia.	21
Evi1	Retroviral transduction	Anemia, thrombocytopenia, variable leukopenia, hypercellular BM, BM dysplasia, uniformly fatal (14 mo), no leukemia.	24
Npm1	Npm1 haploinsufficient	No anemia, variable thrombocytosis or thrombocytopenia, BM dysplasia and hypercellularity. Lung, liver tumors, AML, lymphoma at advanced age.	27,28
Dido	Knockout	Variable anemia, variable leukocytosis, variable splenomegaly, BM dysplasia. Survival 55% at 26 mo, no leukemia.	22
NUP98-HOXD13	Transgenic (Vav promoter)	Anemia, macrocytosis, leukopenia, variable thrombocytopenia, hypercellular-normocellular BM, dysplasia. Survival 5% at 14 mo, 60% leukemic transformation (AML and ALL).	5,49-51
SALL4B	Transgenic (CMV promoter)	Mild anemia, mild neutropenia, variable thrombocytosis, BM dysplasia and hypercellularity. Survival 12% at 24 mo, 50% leukemic transformation (AML).	36
BCL2/NRASD12	Transgenic(tTA, MRP8 promoters)	No anemia, mild leukocytosis, mild thrombocytopenia, BM dysplasia, hepatosplenomegaly, survival and leukemia not reported.	37
RUNX1	Retroviral transduction (S291fs)	Anemia, macrocytosis, leukopenia, thrombocytopenia, hypercellular-normocellular BM, dysplasia. Survival 10% at 14 mo, 60% leukemic transformation.	38
Arid4a	Knockout	Mild anemia, leukopenia, lymphopenia, thrombocytopenia, hypercellular-normocellular BM with fibrosis. 12% AML at 12-22 mo.	41
Polg	Knock-in of mutant (Polg$^{A/A}$)	Anemia, lymphopenia, BM dysplasia, mitochondrial dysfunction. Lethal by 16 mo because of severe megaloblastic anemia.	48

Abbreviations: ALL, acute lymphocytic leukemia; AML, acute myeloid leukemia; BM, bone marrow.

accurately represent genetic aberrations in patients, provide similar microenvironmental conditions for reproducing hematopoietic phenotypes (eg, impaired differentiation and increased apoptosis), recapitulate patient symptoms and responses to existing treatment regimens, and progress to AML with similar kinetics and features as seen in the clinic. Although a model that satisfies all of these criteria may not exist, cancer biologists have several different models to choose from, and can select an available animal model, being cognizant of its caveats. Once an MDS model is developed and validated, it can be used to advance the understanding of the molecular biology of the disease and provide a platform for cultivation of new therapeutic approaches. This section focuses on mice with NUP98-HOX fusions, because there have been a number of follow-up studies[34,49–54] performed with these mice beyond the initial description, providing examples for the types of additional studies that are possible with these animal models.

Although rare, many of the NUP98 translocations, including NUP98-TOP1, NUP98-DDX10, and NUP98-HOX fusions, have been seen in patients with MDS, especially younger patients.[33,55–59] Furthermore, the NUP98-HOXA9 and NUP98-HOXD13 translocations both lead to overexpression of HOXA9 in mice; marked (10-fold–1000-fold greater than normal BM or CD34+ cells) overexpression of HOXA9 is a common finding in patients with AML[60] and MDS.[61] NHD13 mice develop a variety of leukemias including myeloid, erythroid, megakaryocytic, and undifferentiated; however, although unexpected, about 15% to 25% of NHD13 mice developed pre–T- or pre–B-LBLs.[5,34] This is in contrast to reports of human MDS transformation to lymphoid leukemias, which are rare.[62–65] Despite this difference between MDS patients and mouse models of the disease, 60% of NHD13 mice developed acute leukemias and 20% died because of severe MDS, statistics that are similar with patient progression.[34]

Additional studies based on the NHD13 translocation have sought to describe the implications of this mutation and to understand its mechanistic role in MDS. The NHD13 protein can inhibit maturation of the K562 cell line, suggesting that NHD13 expression plays a role in hematopoietic precursors by impairing their differentiation.[5] To study the impaired differentiation attributed to the NHD13 protein, colony-forming cell assays were performed with BM from the NHD13 transgenic mice. Although the number of colonies formed by plating whole BM from wild-type and NHD13 mice were similar, 10-fold fewer total colonies were observed from the NHD13 lin[neg] BM population (which contains the stem and progenitor cells) than from the wild-type lin[neg] BM cells.[50] Lin[neg] cells from NHD13 mouse BM also showed dramatic increases in apoptosis following treatment with hematopoietic cytokines that promote survival and differentiation of wild-type murine hematopoietic stem and progenitor cells. Moreover, most of the surviving NHD13 cells were undifferentiated lin[neg] cells. Taken together, these findings indicate that the NHD13 fusion impairs differentiation of hematopoietic stem and progenitor cells and predisposes these cells to apoptotic death; these findings are reminiscent of the maturation arrest and increased apoptosis seen in patients with MDS.

Subsequent studies in the lymphoid system of NHD13 mice revealed impaired B-lymphocyte differentiation at the pro-B to pre-B transition and impaired differentiation of T lymphocytes during the transition from double negative (DN) DN2 to DN3 thymocytes.[49] Hoxa7, Hoxa9, and Hoxa10 were overexpressed in the thymus of NHD13 mice compared with that of wild-type mice, an association that has previously been observed with impaired thymocyte differentiation.

Additional studies have identified a long-term repopulating MDS-initiating cell by demonstration of successful engraftment of lin[neg] NHD13-expressing BM cells into primary and secondary lethally irradiated wild-type recipients. Importantly, mice that received the *NHD13* BM developed signs and symptoms of MDS, including peripheral blood cytopenias caused by ineffective hematopoiesis, morphologic dysplasia, and transformation to acute leukemia.[51] These studies also demonstrated that, in a competitive repopulation assay, the *NHD13* BM cells were able to out-compete normal wild-type BM cells, even when a 10-fold excess of wild-type BM was transplanted. Finally, limiting dilution experiments identified the frequency of the MDS-initiating cell to be similar to the frequency of hematopoietic stem cells from wild-type mice (approximately 1 per 20,000).

In addition to elucidating the role of *NHD13* in MDS, its contribution to the development of leukemia is also of interest. In the context of the recently developed two-class mutation hypothesis for AML,[66] the *NUP98-HOX* fusions can be classified as Type II, or differentiation-impairing, mutations.[52,67] Infection of primary BM cells by replication-competent retroviral particles predisposes mice to develop leukemia through a process known as "retroviral insertional mutagenesis."[68] This happens because of integration of the retrovirus, with the retroviral LTR serving as a powerful promoter-enhancer, near to cellular proto-oncogenes. Activation of two or more collaborative proto-oncogenes leads to leukemia or lymphoma in the infected mice. When *NHD13* mice were infected with the MOL4070LTR retrovirus, the time from MDS to leukemic transformation was shortened by 6 months, providing further support that a second event is needed in collaboration with the *NHD13* fusion for progression to leukemia.[53] Potential collaborators with *NHD13* identified by retroviral insertional mutagenesis include *Meis1*, *Mn1*, *Gata2*, *miR29a*, and *miR29b1*.[53]

To identify spontaneous mutations that might collaborate with *NHD13* as the MDS converts to an AML, genes frequently mutated in human AML were resequenced in leukemic tissue from *NHD13* mice that had developed AML. In *NHD13* mice with AML, 32% of mice assessed were found to have a *Nras* or *Kras* mutation of codon 12.[54] Interestingly, no codon 13 or 61 mutations were found, although a codon 61 *Nras* mutation was identified in a *NHD13* mouse with a pre–T-LBL. One mouse was found to have a mutation in *Cbl*, specifically an exon 8 deletion. These results, along with the lack of mutations observed in *Npm1* and *Runx1* (both classified as Type II, or differentiation-blocking mutations), are again consistent with *NHD13* being a Type II mutation. Given that *KIT* mutations are most commonly found in patients with core-binding factor translocations, it may not have been surprising that *Kit* mutations were not identified in the *NHD13* AMLs, because the *NHD13* fusion does not seem to affect the core-binding factor pathways. It was curious that no *Flt3* mutations were identified, however, because *Flt3* mutations are commonly associated with lesions (eg, fusions of the *MLL* gene) that up-regulate *HOXA* cluster genes.[54]

In addition to verifying that mutations (eg, *Runx1* point mutations or *NUP-HOX* gene fusions) found in MDS patients are important in the disease process, mouse models provide a platform that can be used for preclinical testing. In addition to testing small molecules, singly or in combination, these animal models can be used to study the mechanisms by which allogeneic hematopoietic stem cell transplant is curative for patients with MDS. Hematopoietic stem cell transplant is the only known definitive treatment for MDS patients, and is thought to be effective by a combination of myeloablative radiochemotherapy and adoptive immunotherapy leading to a graft-versus-tumor effect. Inbred strains of mice with complete or partial major histocompatibility complex mismatches afford the ability to test the relative contributions of these two effects. In addition, these animal models may also be useful for examining possible autoimmune contributions to MDS initiation as proposed when immunosuppressive therapy resulted in positive responses in certain patient subsets.[69–71]

SUMMARY

Despite the challenges encountered in the long-term growth and proliferation of primary MDS cells in vitro and in vivo, modeling the disease in mice has recently met with some success. Additional studies are needed to characterize more fully the genetic lesions that lead to MDS, and which complementary mutations lead to leukemic transformation of the MDS clone. This information, along with insight into the fundamental basis for the impaired differentiation and apoptosis associated with MDS, may be extracted from many of the models discussed in this article. It is hoped that studies using the recently described animal models discussed will be useful in developing new therapeutic approaches for patients with MDS in the near future.

ACKNOWLEDGMENTS

The authors thank Tim Graubert, Martin Carroll, James Thompson, Li Chai, Chris Slape, Ying Wei Lin, and members of the Aplan laboratory at the Genetics Branch, National Cancer Institute, for helpful discussions.

REFERENCES

1. Funk RK, Maxwell TJ, Izumi M, et al. Quantitative trait loci associated with susceptibility to therapy-related acute murine promyelocytic leukemia in hCG-PML/RARA transgenic mice. Blood 2008;112:1434.
2. Fenske TS, McMahon C, Edwin D, et al. Identification of candidate alkylator-induced cancer susceptibility genes by whole genome scanning in mice. Cancer Res 2006;66:5029.
3. Suzuki T, Shen H, Akagi K, et al. New genes involved in cancer identified by retroviral tagging. Nat Genet 2002;32:166.
4. Naka T, Sugamura K, Hylander BL, et al. Effects of tumor necrosis factor-related apoptosis-inducing ligand alone and in combination with chemotherapeutic agents on patients' colon tumors grown in SCID mice. Cancer Res 2002;62:5800.
5. Lin YW, Slape C, Zhang Z, et al. NUP98-HOXD13 transgenic mice develop a highly penetrant, severe myelodysplastic syndrome that progresses to acute leukemia. Blood 2005;106:287.
6. Xu Y, Silver DF, Yang NP, et al. Characterization of human ovarian carcinomas in a SCID mouse model. Gynecol Oncol 1999;72:161.
7. Sakakibara T, Xu Y, Bumpers HL, et al. Growth and metastasis of surgical specimens of human breast carcinomas in SCID mice. Cancer J Sci Am 1996;2:291.
8. Bonnet D, Dick JE. Human acute myeloid leukemia is organized as a hierarchy that originates from a primitive hematopoietic cell. Nat Med 1997;3:730.
9. Wang JC, Lapidot T, Cashman JD, et al. High level engraftment of NOD/SCID mice by primitive normal and leukemic hematopoietic cells from patients with chronic myeloid leukemia in chronic phase. Blood 1998;91:2406.
10. Lapidot T, Sirard C, Vormoor J, et al. A cell initiating human acute myeloid leukaemia after transplantation into SCID mice. Nature 1994;367:645.
11. Taussig DC, Miraki-Moud F, Anjos-Afonso F, et al. Anti-CD38 antibody-mediated clearance of human repopulating cells masks the heterogeneity of leukemia-initiating cells. Blood 2008;112:568.

12. Steube KG, Gignac SM, Hu ZB, et al. In vitro culture studies of childhood myelo-dysplastic syndrome: establishment of the cell line MUTZ-1. Leuk Lymphoma 1997;25:345.

13. Kim DK, Kojima M, Fukushima T, et al. Engraftment of human myelodysplastic syndrome derived cell line in transgenic severe combined immunodeficient (TG-SCID) mice expressing human GM-CSF and IL-3. Eur J Haematol 1998;61:93.

14. Nilsson L, Astrand-Grundstrom I, Arvidsson I, et al. Isolation and characterization of hematopoietic progenitor/stem cells in 5q-deleted myelodysplastic syndromes: evidence for involvement at the hematopoietic stem cell level. Blood 2000;96:2012.

15. Nilsson L, Astrand-Grundstrom I, Anderson K, et al. Involvement and functional impairment of the CD34(+)CD38(-)Thy-1(+) hematopoietic stem cell pool in myelodysplastic syndromes with trisomy 8. Blood 2002;100:259.

16. Benito AI, Bryant E, Loken MR, et al. NOD/SCID mice transplanted with marrow from patients with myelodysplastic syndrome (MDS) show long-term propagation of normal but not clonal human precursors. Leuk Res 2003;27:425.

17. Thanopoulou E, Cashman J, Kakagianne T, et al. Engraftment of NOD/SCID-beta2 microglobulin null mice with multilineage neoplastic cells from patients with myelodysplastic syndrome. Blood 2004;103:4285.

18. Kerbauy DM, Lesnikov V, Torok-Storb B, et al. Engraftment of distinct clonal MDS-derived hematopoietic precursors in NOD/SCID-beta2-microglobulin-deficient mice after intramedullary transplantation of hematopoietic and stromal cells. Blood 2004;104:2202.

19. Helgason CD, Damen JE, Rosten P, et al. Targeted disruption of SHIP leads to hemopoietic perturbations, lung pathology, and a shortened life span. Genes Dev 1998;12:1610.

20. Liu Q, Sasaki T, Kozieradzki I, et al. SHIP is a negative regulator of growth factor receptor-mediated PKB/Akt activation and myeloid cell survival. Genes Dev 1999;13:786.

21. Moody JL, Xu L, Helgason CD, et al. Anemia, thrombocytopenia, leukocytosis, extramedullary hematopoiesis, and impaired progenitor function in Pten+/-SHIP-/- mice: a novel model of myelodysplasia. Blood 2004;103:4503.

22. Futterer A, Campanero MR, Leonardo E, et al. Dido gene expression alterations are implicated in the induction of hematological myeloid neoplasms. J Clin Invest 2005;115:2351.

23. Louz D, van den Broek M, Verbakel S, et al. Erythroid defects and increased retro-virally-induced tumor formation in Evi1 transgenic mice. Leukemia 2000;14:1876.

24. Buonamici S, Li D, Chi Y, et al. EVI1 induces myelodysplastic syndrome in mice. J Clin Invest 2004;114:713.

25. Laricchia-Robbio L, Fazzina R, Li D, et al. Point mutations in two EVI1 Zn fingers abolish EVI1-GATA1 interaction and allow erythroid differentiation of murine bone marrow cells. Mol Cell Biol 2006;26:7658.

26. Laricchia-Robbio L, Premanand K, Rinaldi CR, et al. EVI1 Impairs myelopoiesis by deregulation of PU.1 function. Cancer Res 2009;69:1633.

27. Grisendi S, Bernardi R, Rossi M, et al. Role of nucleophosmin in embryonic development and tumorigenesis. Nature 2005;437:147.

28. Sportoletti P, Grisendi S, Majid SM, et al. Npm1 is a haploinsufficient suppressor of myeloid and lymphoid malignancies in the mouse. Blood 2008;111:3859.

29. Tosic N, Stojiljkovic M, Colovic N, et al. Acute myeloid leukemia with NUP98-HOXC13 fusion and FLT3 internal tandem duplication mutation: case report and literature review. Cancer Genet Cytogenet 2009;193:98.

30. Moore MA, Chung KY, Plasilova M, et al. NUP98 dysregulation in myeloid leuke-mogenesis. Ann N Y Acad Sci 2007;1106:114.
31. Slape C, Aplan PD. The role of NUP98 gene fusions in hematologic malignancy. Leuk Lymphoma 2004;45:1341.
32. Pineault N, Buske C, Feuring-Buske M, et al. Induction of acute myeloid leukemia in mice by the human leukemia-specific fusion gene NUP98-HOXD13 in concert with Meis1. Blood 2003;101:4529.
33. Raza-Egilmez SZ, Jani-Sait SN, Grossi M, et al. NUP98-HOXD13 gene fusion in therapy-related acute myelogenous leukemia. Cancer Res 1998;58:4269.
34. Slape C, Lin YW, Hartung H, et al. NUP98-HOX translocations lead to myelodys-plastic syndrome in mice and men. J Natl Cancer Inst Monographs 2008;64.
35. Yang J, Chai L, Fowles TC, et al. Genome-wide analysis reveals Sall4 to be a major regulator of pluripotency in murine-embryonic stem cells. Proc Natl Acad Sci U S A 2008;105:19756.
36. Ma Y, Cui W, Yang J, et al. SALL4, a novel oncogene, is constitutively expressed in human acute myeloid leukemia (AML) and induces AML in transgenic mice. Blood 2006;108:2726.
37. Omidvar N, Kogan S, Beurlet S, et al. BCL-2 and mutant NRAS interact physically and functionally in a mouse model of progressive myelodysplasia. Cancer Res 2007;67:11657.
38. Watanabe-Okochi N, Kitaura J, Ono R, et al. AML1 mutations induced MDS and MDS/AML in a mouse BMT model. Blood 2008;111:4297.
39. Lai A, Kennedy BK, Barbie DA, et al. RBP1 recruits the mSIN3-histone deacety-lase complex to the pocket of retinoblastoma tumor suppressor family proteins found in limited discrete regions of the nucleus at growth arrest. Mol Cell Biol 2001;21:2918.
40. Wu MY, Tsai TF, Beaudet AL. Deficiency of Rbbp1/Arid4a and Rbbp1l1/Arid4b alters epigenetic modifications and suppresses an imprinting defect in the PWS/AS domain. Genes Dev 2006;20:2859.
41. Wu MY, Eldin KW, Beaudet AL. Identification of chromatin remodeling genes Arid4a and Arid4b as leukemia suppressor genes. J Natl Cancer Inst 2008;100:1247.
42. Shin MG, Kajigaya S, Levin BC, et al. Mitochondrial DNA mutations in patients with myelodysplastic syndromes. Blood 2003;101:3118.
43. Shin MG, Kajigaya S, McCoy JP Jr, et al. Marked mitochondrial DNA sequence heterogeneity in single CD34+ cell clones from normal adult bone marrow. Blood 2004;103:553.
44. Gattermann N, Wulfert M, Junge B, et al. Ineffective hematopoiesis linked with a mitochondrial tRNA mutation (G3242A) in a patient with myelodysplastic syndrome. Blood 2004;103:1499.
45. Wulfert M, Kupper AC, Tapprich C, et al. Analysis of mitochondrial DNA in 104 patients with myelodysplastic syndromes. Exp Hematol 2008;36:577.
46. Yao YG, Ogasawara Y, Kajigaya S, et al. Mitochondrial DNA sequence variation in single cells from leukemia patients. Blood 2007;109:756.
47. Kujoth GC, Hiona A, Pugh TD, et al. Mitochondrial DNA mutations, oxidative stress, and apoptosis in mammalian aging. Science 2005;309:481.
48. Chen ML, Logan TD, Hochberg ML, et al. Erythroid dysplasia, megaloblastic anemia, and impaired lymphopoiesis arising from mitochondrial dysfunction. Blood 2009;114:4045.
49. Choi CW, Chung YJ, Slape C, et al. A NUP98-HOXD13 fusion gene impairs differ-entiation of B and T lymphocytes and leads to expansion of thymocytes with partial TCRB gene rearrangement. J Immunol 2009;183:6227.

50. Choi CW, Chung YJ, Slape C, et al. Impaired differentiation and apoptosis of hematopoietic precursors in a mouse model of myelodysplastic syndrome. Haematologica 2008;93:1394.
51. Chung YJ, Choi CW, Slape C, et al. Transplantation of a myelodysplastic syndrome by a long-term repopulating hematopoietic cell. Proc Natl Acad Sci U S A 2008;105:14088.
52. Slape C, Chung YJ, Soloway PD, et al. Mouse embryonic stem cells that express a NUP98-HOXD13 fusion protein are impaired in their ability to differentiate and can be complemented by BCR-ABL. Leukemia 2007;21:1239.
53. Slape C, Hartung H, Lin YW, et al. Retroviral insertional mutagenesis identifies genes that collaborate with NUP98-HOXD13 during leukemic transformation. Cancer Res 2007;67:5148.
54. Slape C, Liu LY, Beachy S, et al. Leukemic transformation in mice expressing a NUP98-HOXD13 transgene is accompanied by spontaneous mutations in Nras, Kras, and Cbl. Blood 2008;112:2017.
55. Ahuja HG, Felix CA, Aplan PD. The t(11;20)(p15;q11) chromosomal translocation associated with therapy-related myelodysplastic syndrome results in an NUP98-TOP1 fusion. Blood 1999;94:3258.
56. Brown J, Jawad M, Twigg SR, et al. A cryptic t(5;11)(q35;p15.5) in 2 children with acute myeloid leukemia with apparently normal karyotypes, identified by a multiplex fluorescence in situ hybridization telomere assay. Blood 2002;99:2526.
57. Ikeda T, Ikeda K, Sasaki K, et al. The inv(11)(p15q22) chromosome translocation of therapy-related myelodysplasia with NUP98-DDX10 and DDX10-NUP98 fusion transcripts. Int J Hematol 1999;69:160.
58. Jaju RJ, Fidler C, Haas OA, et al. A novel gene, NSD1, is fused to NUP98 in the t(5;11)(q35;p15.5) in de novo childhood acute myeloid leukemia. Blood 2001;98: 1264.
59. Romana SP, Radford-Weiss I, Ben Abdelali R, et al. NUP98 rearrangements in hematopoietic malignancies: a study of the Groupe Francophone de Cytogenetique Hematologique. Leukemia 2006;20:696.
60. Palmqvist L, Pineault N, Wasslavik C, et al. Candidate genes for expansion and transformation of hematopoietic stem cells by NUP98-HOX fusion genes. PLoS one 2007;2:e768.
61. Chen G, Zeng W, Miyazato A, et al. Distinctive gene expression profiles of CD34 cells from patients with myelodysplastic syndrome characterized by specific chromosomal abnormalities. Blood 2004;104:4210.
62. Disperati P, Ichim CV, Tkachuk D, et al. Progression of myelodysplasia to acute lymphoblastic leukaemia: implications for disease biology. Leuk Res 2006;30:233.
63. Sato N, Nakazato T, Kizaki M, et al. Transformation of myelodysplastic syndrome to acute lymphoblastic leukemia: a case report and review of the literature. Int J Hematol 2004;79:147.
64. San Miguel JF, Hernandez JM, Gonzalez-Sarmiento R, et al. Acute leukemia after a primary myelodysplastic syndrome: immunophenotypic, genotypic, and clinical characteristics. Blood 1991;78:768.
65. Bonati A, Delia D, Starcich R. Progression of a myelodysplastic syndrome to pre-B acute lymphoblastic leukaemia with unusual phenotype. Br J Haematol 1986; 64:487.
66. Gilliland DG, Tallman MS. Focus on acute leukemias. Cancer Cell 2002;1:417.
67. Dash AB, Williams IR, Kutok JL, et al. A murine model of CML blast crisis induced by cooperation between BCR/ABL and NUP98/HOXA9. Proc Natl Acad Sci U S A 2002;99:7622.

68. Touw IP, Erkeland SJ. Retroviral insertion mutagenesis in mice as a comparative oncogenomics tool to identify disease genes in human leukemia. Mol Ther 2007; 15:13.
69. Broliden PA, Dahl IM, Hast R, et al. Antithymocyte globulin and cyclosporine A as combination therapy for low-risk non-sideroblastic myelodysplastic syndromes. Haematologica 2006;91:667.
70. Yazji S, Giles FJ, Tsimberidou AM, et al. Antithymocyte globulin (ATG)-based therapy in patients with myelodysplastic syndromes. Leukemia 2003;17:2101.
71. Kochenderfer JN, Kobayashi S, Wieder ED, et al. Loss of T-lymphocyte clonal dominance in patients with myelodysplastic syndrome responsive to immunosup-pression. Blood 2002;100:3639.

Lenalidomide for Treatment of Myelodysplastic Syndromes: Current Status and Future Directions

Rami S. Komrokji, MD*, Alan F. List, MD

KEYWORDS

- Lenalidomide • Myelodysplastic syndromes • Deletion 5q

Myelodysplastic syndromes (MDS) are a spectrum of hematopoietic stem cell malignancies characterized pathologically by the presence of cytologic dysplasia and clinically by bone marrow failure with persistent and progressive variant cytopenias.[1] More than 90% of patients diagnosed with MDS will have anemia during their disease course, and 30% to 50% of patients will be transfusion-dependent, more so in higher risk patients.[2,3] Red blood cell (RBC) transfusion dependency is an independent adverse prognostic factor in MDS.[4,5]

Anemia is predominantly the result of ineffective erythropoeisis.[6] Accelerated apoptosis is the hallmark of early disease, while up-regulation of survival signals, proliferation, and clonal evolution are features of higher-risk disease.[7] Impaired clonogenic growth of primitive erythroid progenitors and impaired erythropoietin receptor signaling are major causes of anemia.[6] Inflammatory cytokines amplify apoptosis of hematopoietic progenitors and the inherent defective erythroid maturation.[6] Immunologic derangements can contribute to anemia also.

In the past, options for treating anemia were limited to the use of erythroid stimulating factors (ESAs) and RBC transfusions. Unfortunately, only 20% to 40% of patients will respond to ESAs alone or ESA combined with granulocyte colony-stimulating factor (G-CSF).[8] In the past 5 years, three drugs were approved for the treatment of MDS. Lenalidomide, a second-generation, immunomodulatory drug (IMiD), was approved by the US Food and Drug Administration (FDA) in December 2005 for

Department of Malignant Hematology, H. Lee Moffitt Cancer Center and Research Institute, University of South Florida, FOB-3rd Floor, 12902 Magnolia Drive, Tampa, FL 33612, USA
* Corresponding author.
E-mail address: rami.komrokji@moffitt.org

Hematol Oncol Clin N Am 24 (2010) 377–388
doi:10.1016/j.hoc.2010.02.013
0889-8588/10/$ – see front matter © 2010 Elsevier Inc. All rights reserved.

hemonc.theclinics.com

treatment of transfusion-dependent anemia in patients with lower–risk MDS with interstitial deletion of a segment of the long arm of chromosome 5 (del[5q]). This article summarizes the relevant data that led to the FDA approval of lenalidomide in patients with del(5q), discusses the role of lenalidomide in the treatment of anemia in non-del(5q) patients, highlights some of the new insights into the mechanism of action and resistance, and finally discusses current and future strategies of using lenalidomide in the treatment of MDS.

THE RATIONALE FOR LENALIDOMIDE IN MDS

Thalidomide paved the road for the use of lenalidomide for the treatment of MDS. The story of thalidomide's evolution into an established anticancer agent is well known, including both its triumph and tragedy.[9]

IMiDs exert a variety of biologic effects, including their action to modify ligand-induced receptor signals that include inflammatory cytokine generation, antiangiogenic effects, immune and cell adhesion response, and direct antiproliferative effects.[10] All those effects make the use of IMiDs appealing for treating MDS patients.

In MDS, stromal abnormalities and immune changes lead to production of inflammatory and hematopoietic inhibitory cytokines, such as tumor necrosis factor (TNF)-α. IMiDs exert different cytokine modulation effects based on the type of cell and stimulus. IMiDs decrease TNF-α production from monocytes after lipopolysaccharide or microbial stimulation, while they potentiate TNF-α production through T cell costimulation to enhance immune response. Lenalidomide is a 100- to 50,000-fold more potent inhibitor of monocyte TNF-α production than thalidomide.[11–13]

Angiogenesis is thought to contribute to the progression of MDS to higher-risk disease. IMiDs' angiogenic properties derive in part from suppression of vascular endothelial growth factor (VEGF) production and VEGF cellular response. IMiDs decrease microvessel density and inhibit new vessel growth in rat models, and this has been evidenced from correlative studies in clinical trials.[14–17]

Different immune alterations have been described in MDS.[18,19] In lymphoid cells, lenalidomide facilitates and potentiates T cell costimulation in response to antigen activation to enhance CD8 + and NK cell-mediated cytotoxicity. It also restores the balance between CD-4 + T helper Th1 and Th2 cells.[20–22]

Thalidomide was the first IMiD tested in MDS. Overall, hematologic improvement rates approximated 20% and mainly were restricted to the erythroid lineage. The erythroid responses, however, were robust and often longstanding.[23] The toxicity of long-term use of thalidomide, namely neuropathy, precluded further development, and lenalidomide, based on its more favorable activity/toxicity profile, emerged as the next IMiD for clinical development.

EFFICACY OF LENALIDOMIDE IN MDS

Lenalidomide's activity and safety in the treatment of MDS patients was established in three consecutive clinical studies.[24–26]

The MDS-001 study was the exploratory single-institution phase 1/2 study.[24] This trial enrolled 43 patients with MDS who had either symptomatic anemia or were transfusion-dependent (defined as need for 4 U of RBC within 8 weeks before enrollment). All patients had failed treatment with recombinant erythropoietin (EPO) (77%) or had low probability of response to an ESA based an endogenous serum EPO level and heavy transfusion burden (23%). The study excluded patients with neutropenia less than 500/mm^3 or platelets less than 10,000 mm^3. Most patients (77%) had refractory anemia (RA) or RA with ringed sideroblasts (RARS), and 88% were low-to-intermediate-1 (int-1) risk scores according to the International Prognostic Scoring System (IPSS). Two thirds of the patients were transfusion-dependent, and 30% failed treatment with thalidomide. An abnormal karyotype was present in 43% of patients, and 12 patients had a del(5q) abnormality. The overall hematologic response rate was 56%. Twenty-one patients (49%) achieved a major erythroid response. Among transfusion-dependent patients, 63% achieved transfusion independence. The most important finding was the significant relation between cytogenetics and hematologic response, where 83% of patients with a del(5q) abnormality had an erythroid response, compared with 57% of those with a normal karyotype and 12% of those with other cytogenetic abnormalities ($P = .007$). Among 20 patients with an abnormal karyotype, 11 patients achieved a cytogenetic response. Out of the 12 patients with del(5q) abnormality, 10 (83%) had a cytogenetic response, and 9 (75%) had a complete cytogenetic response.

Correlative biologic studies confirmed much of the proposed rationale for the use of lenalidomide in MDS. Bone marrow concentrations of proapoptotic cytokines decreased significantly in responders to lenalidomide; erythroid maturation also increased with a significant reduction in microvessel density in responder patients, particularly in patients with del(5q) abnormality.[17] The biomarker studies also supported a karyotype-specific mechanism of action, where reduction in microvessel density was greatest in patients with del(5q), while reduction in proliferative index was greater in non-del(5q) erythroid responders (**Fig. 1**).

LENALIDOMIDE IN LOWER-RISK MDS WITH DEL(5Q)

The MDS-003 study (**Table 1**) was the pivotal study for the FDA approval of lenalidomide for lower-risk MDS patients with del(5q) abnormality.[25] The study design and eligibility criteria were similar to the MDS-001 study; however, eligibility was limited to patients with a del(5q) abnormality. The study enrolled 148 patients. Treatment consisted of lenalidomide 10 mg daily for 21 days every 28-day cycle. Shortly after the study activation, the schedule was amended to a continuous schedule given the apparent faster time to response observed with this schedule in the MDS-001 study. Sixty-four percent of the patients had the French American British subtypes RA or RARS, and most were low or int-1 IPSS. Two thirds of the patients had isolated del(5q), but only 26% overall had the 5q syndrome. Most patients were treated previously with an ESA (73%) and were heavily transfusion-dependent (71%, 2 U or more).

The overall transfusion response rate was 76% (112 patients). Ninety-nine patients (67%) achieved transfusion independence, and 13 patients (9%) had more than a 50% reduction in transfusion. The median time to response was short (4.6 weeks), and the median rise in Hgb compared with baseline was 5.4 g/dL. The duration of response was durable, lasting more than 2 years, even longer for patients with isolated del(5q). Forty-nine patients (77%) with isolated 5q achieved a cytogenetic response after 24 weeks of treatment, including 45% with a complete cytogenetic response. In patients with del(5q) and one additional abnormality, 67% had a cytogenetic response and 40% having a complete response. The cytogenetic response rate was 50% in patients with a complex karyotype. In del(5q) MDS patients, development of a treatment-induced cytopenia in the first 8 weeks on lenalidomide treatment (at least 50% decrease in platelets or at least 75% decrease in neutrophil count) was associated with a higher rate of hematologic response and cytogenetic response, indicating that early cytopenias may be a surrogate marker for suppression of the del(5q) clone.[27]

Among the patients with del(5q) treated on MDS-001 and MDS-003, cytogenetic response strongly correlated with extended survival (hazard ratio [HR], 5.295;

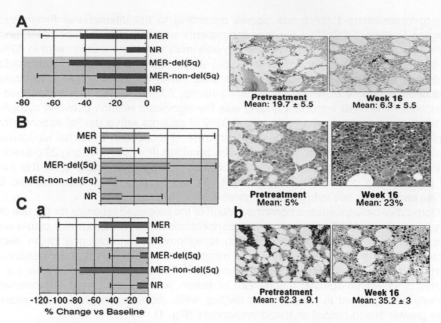

Fig. 1. (*A*) Change in bone marrow microvessel density (MVD) according to erythroid response and cytogenetic category. (*B*) Change in apoptotic index according to erythroid response and cytogenetic category. Apoptosis was assessed by detection of the p85 fragment of poly (ADP-ribose) polymerase (PARP) in trephine biopsy specimens. (*C*) Change in marrow proliferation index according to erythroid response and cytogenetic category. Proliferation index was assessed by immunohistochemical staining of trephine biopsy specimens for the Ki67 proliferation. *Abbreviations:* MER, major erythroid response; NR, no response. (*Modified from* List AF, Baker AF, Green S, et al. Lenalidomide: targeted anemia therapy for myelodysplastic syndromes. Cancer Control 2006;13:4–11; with permission.)

$P<.001$). Kaplan-Meier estimates of overall survival from the start of lenalidomide treatment showed that cytogenetic responders had a significant survival advantage compared with nonresponders (NR) (median, not reached vs 28 months; $P<.0001$). The 10-year survival estimate for cytogenetic responders was 78% compared with 4% in the NR cohort. The 10-year estimated risk for leukemia progression was 15% in responding patients compared with 67% in the NR group ($P = .010$).[28]

In a small cohort of European patients (n = 22) enrolled on MDS-003 progression to acute mycloid leukemia (AML) was reported in 8 patients (two patients with del(5q) syndrome, four with refractory cytopemia with multi lineage dysplasia, 2 with refractory anemia with excess blasts). Progression to AML was accompanied by development of complex karyotype clonal evolution in seven of those patients.[29] It is not clear if lenalidomide increases chromosomal instability or if this reflects the natural course of the disease. More recent data suggest that the median overall survival for patients with untreated del(5q) may be shorter than what originally was estimated. The median overall survival was 3 years in a prospective analysis of German patients with del(5q) before introduction of lenalidomide.[30]

LENALIDOMIDE FOR LOWER-RISK MDS WITHOUT DEL(5Q)

The MDS-002 (**Table 2**) clinical trial was similar in design to MDS-003 but examined the role of lenalidomide in MDS patients lacking a del(5q).[26] Two-hundred fourteen

Table 1 MDS 003 clinical study summary	
Number of patients	148
Median age	71 years
Baseline characteristics	IPSS risk category—number (%) Low 55 (37) Intermediate—1 65 (44) Intermediate—2 or high 8 (5) Unclassified 20 (14) Karyotype—number (%) Isolated 5 out of every 110 (74) 5q + additional abn 37 (25)
Responses	Overall erythroid response 112 (76%) Transfusion independency (TI) 99 (67%) ≥50% transfusion reduction 13 (9%) TI frequency by karyotype complexity Isolated del(5q) 79 (72%) Del(5q) + 1 additional 12 (48%) Complex (>30) 8 (67%) Overall cytogenetic response 62/85 (73%) Complete response 38/85 (45%) Median Hgb increase 5.4 g/dL
Time to response	Median time to response 4.6 weeks Median duration of response 115 weeks
Hematological toxicity (number of patients [%])	Grade 3 or 4 Neutropenia 81 (55) Thrombocytopenia 65 (44) Anemia 10 (7)

patients were enrolled. Most patients were low or int-1 IPSS risk (79%). The median age of patients was 72 years. The overall transfusion response to lenalidomide was 43% according to International Working Group (IWG) 2000 criteria, where 56 (26%) patients achieved transfusion independence, and 37 (17%) patients had a reduction in transfusions of at least 50%. According to the new IWG 2006 response criteria, 33% achieved hematological improvement. The median hemoglobin increase was 3.2 g/dL. The median time to response was 4.8 weeks, and the median duration of response was 41 weeks. Overall, cytogenetic responses were infrequent, occurring in only19% of patients. Similarly, development of cytopenia on treatment in the non-del(5q) population did not correlate with hematologic response.[27]

The hematological improvement rate observed in non-del(5q) MDS patients treated with lenalidomide is clinically relevant and similar to other available options including ESA and hypomethylating agents. Strategies to improve those responses, however, will be clearly of great benefit to the patients. One strategy is identifying patients who will have better chances of response. No clinical predictors of response have been described, where contrary to del(5q) therapy, related thrombocytopenia and neutropenia did not correlate with hematological improvement. Ebert and his colleagues[31] reported an erythroid differentiation signature using gene profiling as a biomarker that could predict response. The signature was developed using a training set of 16 samples of patients with non-del(5q) from MDS-002 and validated in 26 other samples. Decreased expression of erythroid specific genes was noted in responders. Many of these genes are targets of the erythropoietin-specific transcriptional factors,

Table 2 MDS 002 clinical study summary	
Number of patients	214
Median age	72 years
IPSS risk category—number (%)	Low—92 (43) Intermediate—1 76 (36) Intermediate—2 or high—8 (5) Unclassified—38 (18)
Response	Hematological responses: Overall erythroid response 93 (43%) Transfusion independence (TI) 56 (26%) ≥50% transfusion reduction 37 (17%) TI by IPSS risk Low—31 (34%) Intermediate—1 23 (30%) High risk—0 Median Hgb increase 3.2 g/dL
Time to response	Median time to response 4.8 weeks Median duration of response 41 weeks
Hematological toxicity (number of patients [%])	Grade 3 or 4 Neutropenia 25% Thrombocytopenia 20%

GATA-1 and STAT-5. This observation confirms the suggested mechanism of action in non-del(5q) of promoting erythroid signaling, which will be discussed later.

The other strategy to be pursued in attempt to improve outcome is combination strategies. An example of this is combining lenalidomide with ESA, which is currently subject of a phase 3 intergroup study (E2905) based on promising single-institution results demonstrating response to the combination after monotherapy with lenalidomide and ESA failed previously.[32] Based on preclinical observations showing that lenalidomide significantly potentiated erythropoietin receptor signaling, a pilot pharmacokinetic study was conducted. Patients with low and int-1 risk MDS that had failed prior treatment with an ESA were treated with lenalidomide for 16 weeks, after which epoetin alpha 40,000 U/week was added for an additional 8-week course if no response was seen with lenalidomide monotherapy.[32] Forty patients were treated with lenalidomide, and 19 patients who did not respond to monotherapy were treated with the combination. The major erythroid response was 33% with lenalidomide alone and 16% in patients who received the combination therapy. Median serum erythropoietin concentration at baseline was more than 10-fold higher in monotherapy responders compared with nonresponders, while a low endogenous serum erythropoietin level before combination therapy was associated with response to the combination.

LENALIDOMIDE FOR HIGH-RISK MDS

The success of lenalidomide in lower-risk del(5q) MDS raised interest in its possible application in patients with higher-risk disease with this cytogenetic abnormality. The Groupe Franchophone des MDS treated 46 del(5q) patients with int-2 or high-risk MDS with lenalidomide at a dose of 10 mg for 21days every 28 days. Most patients had additional cytogenetic abnormalities.[33] Treatment was associated with significant hematological toxicity, and 80% of patients required hospitalization owing to cytopenia complications. Five (12%) patients achieved complete remission, and two (5%)

patients had a marrow complete remission. The overall cytogenetic response was 19%, and a corresponding hematological response rate of 26% with transfusion independence was achieved in 24%.

Studies exploring role of lenalidomide for higher-risk disease are ongoing. Promising preliminary results of combing azacitidine with lenalidomide were reported. Among 17 evaluable patients in the phase 1 trial, 12 patients achieved a response, including 7 complete remissions and 5 additional patients with hematologic improvements. Dose-intensive lenalidomide for treating AML patients with del5(q) abnormalities is the subject of South West Oncology Group study. A phase 1 study of sequential standard 3 + 7 induction chemotherapy followed by lenalidomide is also ongoing.

ADVERSE EVENTS AND TOXICITY OF LENALIDOMIDE IN MDS

In general, lenalidomide usually is well tolerated. The most common adverse events are neutropenia thrombocytopenia, rash, diarrhea, muscle cramps, and pruritus. Other rare adverse effects are hypothyroidism and hypogonadism.[34,35]

Myelosuppression (neutropenia and thrombocytopenia) is the most common adverse event observed in clinical trials.[24–26] In del(5q) MDS patients treated in the MDS-003 study, more than half (55%) experienced neutropenia, and 44% experienced thrombocytopenia (World Health Organization [WHO] grade 3 or 4). Most of those events occurred in the first 8 weeks of treatment (62%). Dose reductions or interruptions for adverse events were needed in 84% of patients in the del(5q) group. The median time to first dose reduction was 22 days. In non-del(5q) patients, neutropenia and thrombocytopenia were encountered less commonly; however, they remained among the most common toxicities observed.[26]

Dry skin, rash, and pruritus are common, and itching of the scalp is reported frequently in the first week of lenalidomide treatment. Antihistamines offer some relief, and in more severe cases, a short course of low-dose corticosteroids can be used. Diarrhea is more difficult to treat, and in chronic cases, temporary interruption of lenalidomide might be necessary. Hypothyroidism has been reported in about 7% of patients and is almost exclusively autoimmune in nature.[34,35]

Patients with renal insufficiency were excluded from MDS clinical studies. The risk of toxicity is expected to be greater in patients with known renal impairment. In those patients, it is prudent to adjust the dosage based on creatinine clearance.[36] The incidence of venous thromboembolic events (VTE) in MDS patients treated with lenalidomide monotherapy is generally low; VTE was observed in 3% of del(5q) patients in MDS-003 and 1% of patients non-del(5q) disease in MDS-002.[34,35]

CURRENT UNDERSTANDING OF THE MECHANISM OF ACTION

As discussed previously, correlative biologic studies in the MDS-001 trial suggested different mechanism of action in del(5q) patients. The clinical experience emphasized a karyotype-specific dual mechanism of action for the drug, where in del(5q), lenalidomide suppresses the clone, evidenced by the concordance between cytogenetic and hematologic responses and by the initial myelosuppression that correlates with response. On the other hand, in non-del(5q) MDS, lenalidomide generally promotes effective erythropoiesis within the existing clone (Fig. 2).

The commonly deleted region (CDR) on chromosome 5 in del(5q) MDS involves a 1.5 Mb interstitial segment that extends between 5q31 and 5q32. The CDR contains 44 genes.[37] Until recently, the specific genes in the CDR that might contribute to the del(5q) phenotype were not known. Ebert and colleagues demonstrated that reduced expression of the RPS14 gene as a result of haploinsufficiency is critical to the MDS

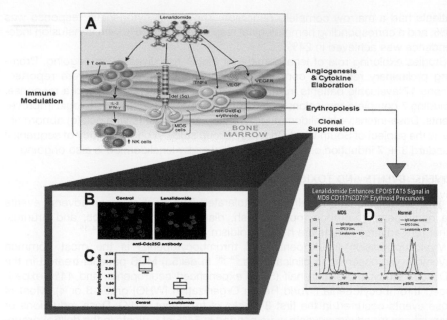

Fig. 2. Mechanism of action of lenalidomide in MDS. Part A summarizes lenalidomide effect including antiangiogenic activity, immunomodulatory effect, and cytokine inhibitory effect. (*Data from* Sekeres Mikkael A, List A. Immunomodulation in myelodysplastic syndromes. Best Practice & Research Clinical Haematology 2006;19(4):757–67.) In part B, lenalidomide increases Cdc25C cytoplasmic sequestration; U937 cells were treated with or without lenalidomide at the concentration of 1 _M for 3 hours. Cytospins were prepared and stained with anti-Cdc25C primary antibody, AlexaFlour-594 secondary, and DAPI (original magnification, 400×). In C, Quantitative analysis of nuclear/cytoplasmic ratio of Cdc25C for lenalidomide-treated cells is significantly lower compared with that of the control (*P*<.0001). (B and C *modified from* Wei S, Chen X, Rocha K, et al. A critical role for phosphatase haplodeficiency in the selective suppression of deletion 5q MDS by lenalidomide. Proc Natl Acad Sci U S A 2009;106:12974–9; with permission.) Part D demonstrates that lenalidomide enhances EPO/STAT5 signaling in non-del(5q)MDS.

phenotype observed in patients with del(5q). The RPS14 protein is an integral component of the ribosomal subunit (40s), which is essential for cleavage of the18SE/18S rRNA molecule. Using a functional RNA interference screen for each of the 41 genes in the CDR, only knock down of the RPS14 gene yielded a phenotype similar to the del(5q) deletion characterized by impaired erythroid differentiation and survival while preserving megakaryocytopoiesis.[38] Interestingly, mutational inactivation of RPS19, another gene involved in ribosomal biogenesis, is implicated in the pathogenesis of another hypoplastic anemia, Diamond-Blackfan anemia, establishing the linkage between congenital and acquired bone marrow failure syndromes.[39–41] Impaired ribosome biogenesis results in the release of L11, regardless of a 60S protein component, which binds to the E3 ubiquitin ligase MDM2, resulting in stabilization of p53 with cell cycle arrest and apoptotic cell death.[42] Although haploinsufficiency of RPS 14 explains the MDS phenotype observed in patients with del(5q), it is not the target for lenalidomide, nor does it explain the differential mechanism of drug action.

Lenalidomide selectively inhibits the growth of del(5q) erythroblasts in vitro and induces expression of the SPARC gene encoded in the CDR region in both MDS patients with del(5q) and normal marrow donors. The only differentially regulated gene in lenalidomide-treated MDS erythroblasts was activin A.[43] Wei and colleagues demonstrated that haploinsufficiency of two dual-specificity phosphatase cell cycle regulators encoded within the CDR can explain the differential lenalidomide effect in del(5q). First, they showed that lenalidomide selectively induced apoptosis in del(5q) myeloblasts and caused preferential cell cycle arrest at the G2 checkpoint. The cell division cycle 25 C (Cdc25C) and the protein phosphatase 2A (PP2A) are important cell cycle regulators, dephosphorylation of Cdc25C, are critical cell cycle regulators enabling mitotic entry. Cdc25C normally is dephosphorylated by PP2A to promote 14–3-3 disassembly and its nuclear translocation. Expression of Cdc25C and PP2A mRNA was significantly lower in del(5q) specimens commensurate with haplodeficiency. Lenalidomide directly inhibits Cdc25C and indirectly inhibits PP2A, increasing cytoplasmic sequestration of Cdc25C. Dual knock-down by small interfering (si) RNA in primary bone marrow cells from MDS patients with a normal karyotype promoted lenalidomide-specific apoptosis.[44] Resistance to lenalidomide in del(5q) patients can be related to overexpression of Cdc25C and PP2A at the time of treatment failure with consequent restoration of wild-type P53 mutation[45] Inhibiting Cdc25c may overcome resistance to lenalidomide or improve responses in non-del(5q) patients.

The mechanism of action is different in non-del(5q). Lenalidomide restores and promotes effective erythropoiesis with no direct cytotoxic effect.[46] Also, lenalidomide promotes erythropoiesis and fetal hemoglobin production in human CD34 cells.[47] Lenalidomide relieves repression of ligand-dependent activation of the EPO-receptor/STAT-5 pathway (signal transduction and activator of transcription). This is supported by gene expression profiling studies from patients treated with lenalidomide, showing that the profound underexpression of genes involved in erythroid differentiation in drug-responsive individuals is caused by transcriptional targets of the erythropoietin-responsive transcription factors, STAT5 and GATA-1.[31] In vitro, lenalidomide delays erythroid maturation by increasing erythropoietin-responsive immature progenitors and inducing hemoglobin-F transcription.[47]

The translational research using lenalidomide in treating MDS is a remarkable example where bench observations provided a rational for testing the agent in MDS, with clinical results that led to laboratory investigations delineating insight as to the mechanism of action.

PRACTICAL RECOMMENDATIONS FOR USING LENALIDOMIDE

Lenalidomide is currently the therapy of choice for patients with lower-risk MDS with del(5q) who are transfusion-dependent after a trial of an ESA or who have a poor ESA response profile. Patients should have adequate platelets and neutrophil counts. The starting dose is 10 mg orally daily if creatinine clearance is more than 50 mL/min. Weekly observation of peripheral blood counts is warranted in the first 8 weeks. Almost two thirds of patients will require dose reduction or interruption after 3 weeks of initiating therapy. Dose interruption on average lasts 3 weeks followed by resumption of treatment at a reduced dose of 5 mg/d, and if necessary again, to a 5 mg orally every other day. Growth factors should be used judiciously for prolonged neutropenia or in setting of febrile neutropenia. After the initial 8 weeks of treatment, blood counts and kidney function should be monitored monthly or as clinically indicated.

In lower-risk non-del(5q) patients with anemia and adequate platelet and neutrophil counts, lenalidomide may be considered after failure of primary treatment with an ESA or hypomethylating agent. The same dosage and monitoring recommendations should be applied but with expectations for less severe myelosuppression. If no response is observed within 4 months, lenalidomide should be discontinued given that 90% of responses occur within this treatment window.

SUMMARY

Lenalidomide is active agent for the treatment of anemia in lower-risk MDS patients. The rates of response and transfusion independence are comparable to other treatment options in non-del(5q) patients and are clearly superior for patients with del(5q) MDS. Myelosuppression is the most frequent adverse event that requires close observation and dose adjustment/interruption. Treatment-related cytopenia correlates with response only in del(5q) patients. The difference in clinically observed response rates and treatment-related cytopenias derives from the karyotype-specific mechanism of action. Future directions include further understanding of the mechanism of resistance in patients with del(5q), translating the biologic predictive markers into a readily available clinical tool to better select non-del(5q) patients, improve response rates with combination strategies, and address the role of lenalidomide in higher-risk MDS.

REFERENCES

1. Bennett JM, Komrokji RS. The myelodysplastic syndromes: diagnosis, molecular biology and risk assessment. Hematology 2005;10(Suppl 1):258–69.
2. Bennett JM, List AF. Disparities in criteria for initiating chelation therapy for iron overload in patients with myelodysplastic syndromes (MDS). ASH Annual Meeting Abstracts 2005;106(11):2535.
3. Bennett JM. Consensus statement on iron overload in myelodysplastic syndromes. Am J Hematol 2008;83(11):858–61.
4. Malcovati L, Germing U, Kuendgen A, et al. Time-dependent prognostic scoring system for predicting survival and leukemic evolution in myelodysplastic syndromes. J Clin Oncol 2007;25(23):3503–10.
5. Malcovati L, Della Porta MG, Cazzola M. Predicting survival and leukemic evolution in patients with myelodysplastic syndrome. Haematologica 2006;91(12):1588–90.
6. Melchert M, List AF. Management of RBC-transfusion dependence. Hematology 2007;2007(1):398–404.
7. Bennett JM, Komrokji R, Kouides P. The myelodysplastic syndromes. In: Abeloff MD, Armitage JO, Niederhuber JE, editors. Clincial oncology. New York: Churchill Livingstone; 2004. p. 2849–81.
8. Hellstrom-Lindberg E. Efficacy of erythropoietin in the myelodysplastic syndromes: a meta-analysis of 205 patients from 17 studies. Br J Haematol 1995;89(1):67–71.
9. Melchert M, List A. The thalidomide saga. Int J Biochem Cell Biol 2007;39:1489–99.
10. Bartlett JB, Dredge K, Dalgleish AG. The evolution of thalidomide and its IMiD derivatives as anticancer agents. Nat Rev Cancer 2004;4(4):314–22.
11. Muller GW, Corral LG, Shire MG, et al. Structural modifications of thalidomide produce analogs with enhanced tumor necrosis factor inhibitory activity. J Med Chem 1996;39(17):3238–40.
12. Muller GW, Chen R, Huang SY, et al. Amino-substituted thalidomide analogs: potent inhibitors of TNF-alpha production. Bioorg Med Chem Lett 1999;9(11):1625–30.

13. Marriott JB, Clarke IA, Dredge K, et al. Thalidomide and its analogues have distinct and opposing effects on TNF-alpha and TNFR2 during co-stimulation of both CD4(+) and CD8(+) T cells. Clin Exp Immunol 2002;130(1):75–84.
14. D'amato RJ, Loughnan MS, Flynn E, et al. Thalidomide is an inhibitor of angiogenesis. Proc Natl Acad Sci U S A 1994;91(9):4082–5.
15. Gupta D, Treon SP, Shima Y, et al. Adherence of multiple myeloma cells to bone marrow stromal cells upregulates vascular endothelial growth factor secretion: therapeutic applications. Leukemia 2001;15(12):1950–61.
16. Dredge K, Horsfall R, Robinson SP, et al. Orally administered lenalidomide (CC-5013) is antiangiogenic in vivo and inhibits endothelial cell migration and Akt phosphorylation in vitro. Microvasc Res 2005;69(1–2):56–63.
17. List AF, Baker AF, Green S, et al. Lenalidomide: targeted anemia therapy for myelodysplastic syndromes. Cancer Control 2006;13(Suppl):4–11.
18. Epling-Burnette PK, List AF. Advancements in the molecular pathogenesis of myelodysplastic syndrome. Curr Opin Hematol 2009;16(2):70–6.
19. Epling-Burnette PK, Painter JS, Rollison DE, et al. Prevalence and clinical association of clonal T cell expansions in myelodysplastic syndrome. Leukemia 2007;21(4):659–67.
20. Mchugh SM, Rifkin IR, Deighton J, et al. The immunosuppressive drug thalidomide induces T helper cell type 2 (Th2) and concomitantly inhibits Th1 cytokine production in mitogen- and antigen-stimulated human peripheral blood mononuclear cell cultures. Clin Exp Immunol 1995;99(2):160–7.
21. Dredge K, Marriott JB, Todryk SM, et al. Protective antitumor immunity induced by a costimulatory thalidomide analog in conjunction with whole tumor cell vaccination is mediated by increased Th1-type immunity. J Immunol 2002;168(10):4914–9.
22. Davies FE, Raje N, Hideshima T, et al. Thalidomide and immunomodulatory derivatives augment natural killer cell cytotoxicity in multiple myeloma. Blood 2001;98(1):210–6.
23. Musto P. Thalidomide therapy for myelodysplastic syndromes: current status and future perspectives. Leuk Res 2004;28(4):325–32.
24. List A, Kurtin S, Roe DJ, et al. Efficacy of lenalidomide in myelodysplastic syndromes. N Engl J Med 2005;352(6):549–57.
25. List A, Dewald G, Bennett J, et al. Lenalidomide in the myelodysplastic syndrome with chromosome 5q deletion. N Engl J Med 2006;355(14):1456–65.
26. Raza A, Reeves JA, Feldman EJ, et al. Phase 2 study of lenalidomide in transfusion-dependent, low-risk, and intermediate-1 risk myelodysplastic syndromes with karyotypes other than deletion 5q. Blood 2008;111(1):86–93.
27. Sekeres MA, Maciejewski JP, Giagounidis AAN, et al. Relationship of treatment-related cytopenias and response to lenalidomide in patients with lower-risk myelodysplastic syndromes. J Clin Oncol 2008;26(36):5943–9.
28. List A, Wride K, Dewald G, et al. Cytogenetic response to lenalidomide is associated with improved survival in patients with chromosome 5q deletion. Leuk Res 2007;31(Suppl 1):s38.
29. Gohring G, Giagounidis A, Aul C, et al. Long-term cytogenetic follow-up of MDS patients with 5q- treated within the MDS-003 (CC-5013-MDS-003) study: evolution to complex clones and progression to AML. ASH Annual Meeting Abstracts 2008;112(11):1647.
30. Germing U, Strupp C, Kuendgen A, et al. Prospective validation of the WHO proposals for the classification of myelodysplastic syndromes. Haematologica 2006;91(12):1596–604.

31. Ebert BL, Galili N, Tamayo P, et al. An erythroid differentiation signature predicts response to lenalidomide in myelodysplastic syndrome. PLoS Med 2008;5(2): e35.

32. List AF, Lancet JE, Melchert M, et al. Two-stage pharmacokinetic & efficacy study of lenalidomide alone or combined with recombinant erythropoietin (EPO) in lower risk MDS EPO-failures [PK-002]. ASH Annual Meeting Abstracts 2007; 110(11):4626.

33. Burcheri S, Prebet T, Beyne-Rauzy O, et al. Lenalidomide (LEN) in INT 2 and high risk MDS with DEL 5q. Interim results of a phase II trial by the GFM. ASH Annual Meeting Abstracts 2007;110(11):820.

34. Komrokji R, Giagounidis A, List A. Lenalidomide therapy in MDS. In: Steensma DP, editor. Myelodysplastic syndromes: pathobiology and clinical management. 2nd edition. London: Informa Health Care; 2008. p. 457–83.

35. Giagounidis A, Fenaux P, Mufti GJ, et al. Practical recommendations on the use of lenalidomide in the management of myelodysplastic syndromes. Ann Hematol 2008;87(5):345–52.

36. Chen N, Lau H, Kong L, et al. Pharmacokinetics of lenalidomide in subjects with various degrees of renal impairment and in subjects on hemodialysis. J Clin Pharmacol 2007;47(12):1466–75.

37. Giagounidis AA, Germing U, Wainscoat JS, et al. The 5q syndrome. Hematology 2004;9(4):271–7.

38. Ebert BL, Pretz J, Bosco J, et al. Identification of RPS14 as the 5qsyndrome gene by RNA interference screen. ASH Annual Meeting Abstracts 2007;110(11):1.

39. Boultwood J, Pellagatti A, Cattan H, et al. Gene expression profiling of CD34+ cells in patients with the 5q- syndrome. Br J Haematol 2007;139(4):578–89.

40. Liu TX, Becker MW, Jelinek J, et al. Chromosome 5q deletion and epigenetic suppression of the gene encoding alpha-catenin (CTNNA1) in myeloid cell transformation. Nat Med 2007;13(1):78–83.

41. Joslin JM, Fernald AA, Tennant TR, et al. Haploinsufficiency of EGR1, a candidate gene in the del(5q), leads to the development of myeloid disorders. Blood 2007; 110(2):719–26.

42. Ferreira-Cerca S, Hurt E. Cell biology: arrest by ribosome. Nature 2009; 459(7243):46–7.

43. Pellagatti A, Jadersten M, Forsblom AM, et al. Lenalidomide inhibits the malignant clone and up-regulates the SPARC gene mapping to the commonly deleted region in 5q- syndrome patients. Proc Natl Acad Sci U S A 2007;104(27): 11406–11.

44. Wei S, Chen X, Rocha K, et al. A critical role for phosphatase haplodeficiency in the selective suppression of deletion 5q MDS by lenalidomide. Proc Natl Acad Sci U S A 2009;106(31):12974–9.

45. List AF, Rocha K, Zhang L, et al. Secondary resistance to lenalidomide in del(5q) MDS is associated with CDC25C and PP2A overexpression blood. ASH Annual Meeting Abstracts 2009;114:292.

46. Hoefsloot LH, Van Amelsvoort MP, Broeders LC, et al. Erythropoietin-induced activation of STAT5 is impaired in the myelodysplastic syndrome. Blood 1997; 89(5):1690–700.

47. Moutouh-De Parseval LA, Verhelle D, Glezer E, et al. Pomalidomide and lenalidomide regulate erythropoiesis and fetal hemoglobin production in human CD34+ cells. J Clin Invest 2008;118(1):248–58.

Practical Recommendations for Hypomethylating Agent Therapy of Patients With Myelodysplastic Syndromes

David P. Steensma, MD[a,b,*], Richard M. Stone, MD[a,b]

KEYWORDS

- Myelodysplastic syndromes • Azacitidine • Decitabine
- Hypomethylating agents • Drug therapy

The U S Food and Drug Administration (FDA) approved azacitidine for treatment of patients with myelodysplastic syndromes (MDS) in May 2004, and the FDA subsequently granted regulatory approval to decitabine for MDS in May 2006. The European Medicines Agency (EMEA) formally approved azacitidine for treatment of MDS and acute myeloid leukemia (AML) in March 2009, and either azacitidine or decitabine is now available in most countries in the developed world. As a class of drugs, hypomethylating agents are now second only to erythropoiesis-stimulating agents in the frequency with which they are prescribed for patients with MDS outside of clinical trials.[1,2]

Despite widespread clinical use of azacitidine and decitabine, several important practical questions remain with respect to these agents, including uncertainty about optimal patient and drug selection, dose and schedule for administration, and management of adverse events such as treatment-emergent cytopenias.[3] Ideally, such questions would be addressed individually in well-designed clinical trials. However, the multiplicity of issues, the ready commercial availability of the drugs, and the great interest in trials of newer agents mean that it is unlikely future clinical trials will be initiated to resolve all of these areas of uncertainty. In addition, the

[a] Department of Hematologic Malignancies, Dana-Farber Cancer Institute, 44 Binney Street, Suite D1B30, Boston, MA 02115, USA
[b] Harvard Medical School, Boston, MA, USA
* Corresponding author. Department of Hematologic Malignancies, Dana-Farber Cancer Institute, 44 Binney Street, Suite D1B30, Boston, MA 02115.
E-mail address: david_steensma@dfci.harvard.edu

Hematol Oncol Clin N Am 24 (2010) 389–406
doi:10.1016/j.hoc.2010.02.012
0889-8588/10/$ – see front matter © 2010 Elsevier Inc. All rights reserved.

relatively short duration of the remaining patent life and marketing exclusivity for both azacitidine and decitabine in the United States likely will limit the industry funding available for such postmarketing studies.

This article discusses the authors' current approach treating patients with MDS using hypomethylating agents. This approach is based on both published data and the authors' own clinical experience, and comments should be interpreted in light of the fact that lack of definitive study results does not obviate the need to make decisions in the clinic.

BACKGROUND

Azacitidine and decitabine are both potent inhibitors of DNA methyltransferases, a family of enzymes that have been highly conserved throughout evolution and are expressed in all tissues, and which are responsible for initiation and maintenance of 5' methylation of cytosine nucleosides and associated gene silencing.[4–6] Inhibition of DNA methyltransferases can result in hypomethylation of CpG dinucleotides in gene promoters and consequent reactivation of previously silenced genes.[7] If some of these newly activated genes encode tumor suppressors or promoters of healthy cell differentiation, the consequences of reactivation of expression could be beneficial in MDS, since clonal hematopoiesis and impaired differentiation are central MDS-associated pathobiological features.[8–10]

In addition to these epigenetic effects, both azacitidine and decitabine also have cytotoxic activity similar to the nucleoside analog cytarabine, as manifested by formation of γ-H2AX foci, a marker of double-stranded DNA breakage.[11,12] The relative contribution of epigenetic mechanisms versus cytotoxicity to the clinical activity of the hypomethylating agents is currently unknown. A more detailed discussion of the biologic mechanisms of hypomethylating agents and their future prospects in neoplasia can be found (See the article by Jean-Pierre Issa elsewhere in this issue for further explanation of this topic.).

Clinical trial experience with either of the hypomethylating agents demonstrates complete responses in 9% to 37% of patients (using International Working Group 2000 criteria[13]), reduction in marrow blast burden without full hematological recovery in a similar proportion of patients, and hematological improvement in 20% to 48% of patients (overall objective response rates 30% to 73%) (**Table 1**).[14–20] In addition, about one third of patients with an abnormal karyotype experience complete cytogenetic remission during treatment with azacitidine or decitabine, indicating the potential for hypomethylating agent therapy to modify the natural history of MDS.[17–19] Indeed, for patients with International Prognostic Scoring System (IPSS) intermediate-2 and high-risk MDS, the AZA-001 randomized trial demonstrated a 9-month overall benefit in median survival (ie, 24 months versus 15 months) for patients treated with azacitidine, compared with those who received supportive care alone.[15] In contrast, a European randomized study with decitabine in higher-risk patients, GMDSSG/EORTC 06011, observed a modest 0.3-year improvement in median progression-free survival with decitabine treatment compared with supportive care, but failed to show improved overall survival.[20]

Current clinical trial efforts in MDS focus on improving response rates and response duration by combining hypomethylating agents with other biologically active agents, such as histone deacetylase inhibitors, for which there is in vitro evidence of synergy.[21] A review of combination therapy is beyond the scope of the present discussion, but the initial results and prospects for histone deacetylase inhibitors in MDS are discussed in more detail in this issue (See the article by David P. Steensma elsewhere in this issue for further explanation of this topic.).

WHICH PATIENTS ARE MOST APPROPRIATE TO TREAT
WITH A HYPOMETHYLATING AGENT?

In view of the demonstrated improvement in survival[15] with azacitidine treatment of patients who have IPSS intermediate-2 or high risk MDS, individuals with higher-risk MDS are excellent candidates for hypomethylating agent therapy. Patients with 20% to 30% marrow blasts—currently classified as AML by the World Health Organization, but formerly classified as MDS subtype refractory anemia with excess blasts in transformation (RAEB-T)—also were included in the AZA-001 trial, and this group also experienced a survival benefit with azacitidine compared with supportive care.

It is not yet known whether a similar survival benefit will be accrued for lower-risk patients with MDS who receive azacitidine; nor is it known whether decitabine, when optimally administered, has an impact on survival comparable to azacitidine. When hypomethylating agent clinical trials have included lower-risk MDS patients, such as the CALGB 9221 azacitidine trial or the D-0007 decitabine registration study, the lower-risk patients have experienced similar overall hematopoietic response rates as were seen in higher-risk patients.[22,23]

The lower-risk patients who have the most compelling indication for hypomethylating agent treatment are those patients who are transfusion-dependent, and for whom hematopoietic growth factors such as recombinant erythropoietin have failed. Reported red cell transfusion independence rates have ranged from 23% to 56% in transfusion-requiring patients treated with hypomethylating agents (see **Table 1**).[14–20] Reduction of transfusion needs improves patient convenience, and also may delay or prevent the development of transfusion-related iron overload. There is considerable controversy at present, however, with respect to the actual clinical importance of iron overload in MDS relative to the other risks patients face, such as infection, bleeding, and disease progression.[24–26]

Given the potential risks associated with hypomethylating agent treatment and relative paucity of active treatments in MDS generally, it seems prudent to withhold therapy from asymptomatic and minimally symptomatic patients with lower-risk disease, especially those who do not yet require transfusions. It is not yet known whether early treatment is better than late treatment in MDS. In hypomethylating agent trials enrolling patients with higher-risk disease, patients who were within 1 year of diagnosis had modestly higher response rates than those who had their disease for longer than 1 year, but it is not clear that a higher likelihood of response with earlier treatment also applies to lower-risk disease.[19]

Another circumstance in which treatment with a hypomethylating agent may be appropriate is for patients with MDS who are candidates for allogeneic stem cell transplantation.[27] Azacitidine or decitabine may stabilize disease for a few months while stem cell transplantation is coordinated and insurance approval is obtained, or, for patients who lack a sibling donor, while a search for an unrelated donor is ongoing. Because the median age of patients with MDS is 65 to 70 years, most patients with MDS who undergo stem cell transplantation receive reduced-intensity conditioning (RIC), in which the principle method of eliminating neoplastic cells is via a graft-versus-leukemia immunologic effect.[28] Because patients who proceed to RIC stem cell transplant with less than 5% marrow blasts do better than those with higher marrow blast proportion,[29] cytoreduction of patients with excess marrow blasts before conditioning also could represent an appropriate use of hypomethylating agents, although this hypothesis has not been tested formally. Although it also is not known whether it is beneficial to treat patients who already have less than 5% blasts before transplantation, the delays inherent in organizing an allogeneic

Table 1
Major clinical trial results with hypomethylating agents in MDS

Trial	CALGB 9221	AZA-001	US Oncology	D-0007	ICD03-180 (MD Anderson)	DACO-020 (ADOPT)	GMDSSG/ EORTC 06011
First author and year of primary publication	Silverman 2002, 2006[14,32,a]	Fenaux 2009[15]	Lyons 2009[16]	Kantarjian 2006[17]	Kantarjian 2007[18]	Steensma 2009[19]	Wijermans 2008[20]
Number of patients enrolled	191	358	151	170	95	99	233
Number treated with hypomethylating agent	150[b]	179	151	89	95	99	119
Study type	Phase III (US registration)	Phase 3 (US registration)	Phase 2 (randomized)	Phase 3 (US registration)	Phase 2 (randomized)	Phase 2 (singlearm)	Phase 3
Drug regimen	Azacitidine SC 75 mg/m^2 daily × 7 d; total dose 525 mg/m^2	Azacitidine SC 75 mg/m^2 daily × 7 d; total dose 525 mg/m^2	Azacitidine SC over 5–10 d (3 arms) sparing weekends; total doses 375–525 mg/m^2	Decitabine IV 15 mg/m^2 every 8 h × 9 doses; total dose 135 mg/m^2	Decitabine IV or SC over 5 or 10 d (3 arms); total dose 100 mg/m^2	Decitabine IV 20 mg/m^2 daily × 5 d; total dose 100 mg/m^2	Decitabine IV 15 mg/m^2 every 8 h × 9 doses; total dose 135 mg/m^2
Proportion with IPSS INT-2 or high-risk disease	46%	87%	IPSS not assessed	70%	66%	46%	93%

Proportion with de novo MDS	80%	100%	100%	87%	70%	89%	88%
Median treatment cycles administered	>4	9	6	3	7	5	4
CR rate (IWG 2000) in azacitidine- or decitabine-randomized group (where applicable)	9%	17%	NR	9%	37%	15%	13%
Overall improvement rate (CR + PR + HI)	48%	49%	>48%	30%	73%	43%	34%
Cytogenetic CR rate	NR	NR	NR	35%	35%	33%	NR
Proportion of RBC transfusion dependent patients who became transfusion-free	45%	45%	56%	23%	NR	33%	32%

Abbreviations: CR, complete response; HI, hematological improvement; IPSS, International Prognostic Scoring System; IV, intravenous; IWG, International Working Group on Clinical Trial Response Criteria in Myelodysplastic Syndromes; MDS, myelodysplastic syndromes; NR, not reported; PR, partial response; RBC, red blood cell; SC, subcutaneous.

[a] Ref.[32] also includes data from earlier CALGB azacitidine trials (8421 and 8921).

[b] Ninety-nine patients were randomized to receive azacitidine; 51 additional patients initially randomized to supportive care later crossed over to receive azacitidine.

transplant procedure make pretransplant hypomethylating therapy reasonable in this group, with the goal of temporary disease stabilization rather than cytoreduction.

Some physicians also use hypomethylating agents in patients without evidence of active disease—for example, to try to prevent relapse after induction chemotherapy in patients who experienced leukemic progression of MDS, or after stem cell transplantation. There are at present no data to support such an approach, and the authors feel that treatment of patients without active disease only should be considered in the context of a clinical trial.

ONCE A DECISION HAS BEEN MADE TO ADMINISTER A HYPOMETHYLATING AGENT, WHICH DRUG SHOULD BE CHOSEN?

In 2009, the National Comprehensive Cancer Network (NCCN) changed its MDS treatment guidelines (http://www.nccn.org) to recommend azacitidine as the preferred therapy for patients with higher-risk MDS, with decitabine an alternative. The NCCN made this change because of the survival advantage observed with azacitidine in the AZA-001 trial, and the unknown effect of decitabine on survival in MDS. The GMDSSG/EORTC 06011 decitabine survival study failed to show a survival benefit for reasons unrelated to the choice of hypomethylating agent. The reason for this may be because a decitabine regimen with suboptimal pharmacokinetics was used (ie, the 3-day inpatient regimen used in the D-0007 US registration trial[17] and earlier phase 2 trials in Europe,[30] instead of the widely used 5-day outpatient regimen developed at M.D. Anderson Cancer Center in Houston[18]). It is also possible that the trial was negative because many patients received a short duration of decitabine therapy (median four cycles of treatment in GMDSSG/EORTC 06011, with 40% of patients receiving two cycles or less, compared with a median of nine cycles in AZA-001), or because salvage chemotherapy was administered to more than 20% of patients who had been randomized to receive supportive care.[20] Still, the trial's negative result means that there are no studies demonstrating an overall survival benefit in MDS with decitabine treatment. The patent life and marketing exclusivity issues and other logistical considerations mentioned previously mean that it likely never will be known whether there is actually a survival benefit with decitabine in higher-risk MDS, so a preference for azacitidine seems appropriate, at least for patients who would have qualified for the AZA-001 trial.

Given the survival data with azacitidine, is there ever a reason to use decitabine? Leaving aside the fact that many clinicians have developed a comfort level with one agent or another because of local usage patterns, the highest complete response rate reported to date with a hypomethylating agent in MDS (37%, using IWG 2000 criteria) was observed in the single-institution MD Anderson study employing the 5-day 20 mg/m²/d intravenous decitabine regimen.[18] This encouraging complete response rate continues to drive decitabine use. Idiosyncrasies of patient selection or trial design may be a factor in these results. A multicenter study[19] of the same 5-day decitabine regimen showed a lower complete response rate (15%) compared with the single-center study, only slightly better than that reported with the 3-day decitabine regimen (9% to 13%).[17,20]

It has been the authors' impression that the intensity of therapy is greater with the commonly used 5-day decitabine regimen, compared with the 7-day 75 mg/m²/d azacitidine regimen (ie, these two outpatient regimens are not dose-equivalent). For instance, the rate of febrile neutropenia was higher in the ID03-0180[18] (14% of patients were hospitalized per treatment course, with 66% of patients hospitalized overall) and DACO-020 (alternative dosing for outpatient therapy [ADOPT])[19] (17% febrile neutropenia rate) 5-day decitabine trials, compared with CALGB 9221 or AZA-001 7-day azacitidine trials,[31] in which there was no significant difference in the rate of febrile neutropenia between patients treated with azacitidine or those who received supportive care alone.[31,32] In addition, the rate of response to decitabine seems to be somewhat more rapid: 82% of patients who would ultimately respond to decitabine in DACO-020 (ADOPT) had experienced an initial response by the end of two cycles,[19] compared with 75% of responders showing improvement by cycle 4 of azacitidine in CALGB 9221,[32] and 81% showing improvement after six cycles of azacitidine in AZA-001.[33] Comparing across studies, however, is somewhat perilous, because enrolled populations may have differed. An azacitidine versus decitabine head-to-head trial is planned, which should answer some questions about relative pace of response and frequency of adverse effects, although the planned study will be too small to assess survival endpoints using noninferiority methods.[34]

For the time being, the authors tend to prefer 7-day azacitidine in patients who would have been eligible for AZA-001 and for frailer patients, and 5-day decitabine in patients who appear to have more rapidly progressive disease. The authors discuss both agents with each patient, and consider patient preferences. They still use the older 3-day inpatient decitabine regimen studied in D-0007 and GMDSSG/EORTC 06011, but only rarely (eg, if the authors want to initiate a hypomethylating agent while the patient needs to be in the hospital for some other reason, or if patients prefer hospitalization to treatment in the outpatient clinic for logistical reasons).

If one hypomethylating agent has failed the patient, is there any reason to try the other? Despite the chemical similarity of azacitidine (5-azacitidine) and decitabine (5-aza-2'-deoxycitidine), which differ from one another only in a single hydroxyl group on the sugar moiety, there are biologic reasons why a patient might respond to one compound and not the other. Cellular metabolism of azacitidine and decitabine is similar, but not identical. Upon entry to the cell via cell surface equilibrative nucleoside transporters (ENTs), azacitidine is phosphorylated to 5-azacytidine monophosphate by uridine–cytidine kinase, whereas decitabine is phosphorylated by deoxycytidine kinase (the rate-limiting step in intracellular drug activation.)[35] Low expression of deoxycytidine kinase correlates with decitabine resistance in neoplastic cell lines, but would not be expected to have an effect on azacitidine metabolism.[36] In cell lines, sensitivity to decitabine correlates better with sensitivity to cytarabine than with sensitivity to azacitidine.[36] In addition, the global pattern of hypomethylation induced in vitro by azacitidine is distinct from that induced by decitabine.[37] These data suggest that there may be some patients who are destined to respond better to one hypomethylating agent than the other, and that some day it may be possible to obtain a gene expression signature before treatment to select the most appropriate agent. This approach, however, needs to be validated formally.

There is only one small published series describing the results of decitabine therapy for patients who were intolerant of, or had failed, azacitidine.[38] In this report of 14 patients, 3 patients achieved complete remission, and 1 patient experienced hematological improvement.

WHAT ARE THE OPTIMAL DOSE, SCHEDULE, AND ROUTE OF ADMINISTRATION FOR HYPOMETHYLATING AGENT TREATMENT?

Because the positive AZA-001 survival study employed azacitidine administered subcutaneously over 7 consecutive days at a dose of 75 mg/m^2/d, repeated every 28 days (total dose per cycle 525 mg/m^2), this dose and schedule should be considered the standard of care for patients with higher-risk MDS. The chief practical obstacle to administration of azacitidine according to this schedule is the need for weekend treatment, because many chemotherapy infusion centers are only open 5 or 6 days per week. Several weekend-sparing azacitidine administration schedules have been tested,[16] with hematological improvement rates similar to that seen with the 7-day schedule, but these schedules were not directly compared with the 7-day schedule. Additionally, it is not known whether these regimens yield a comparable survival benefit. Therefore, the authors feel that whenever possible, the 7-day regimen should be chosen.

The pharmacokinetics of intravenous azacitidine are almost identical to those of subcutaneous azacitidine,[39] but there are scant published clinical data with intravenous azacitidine: only a single phase 2 study of 22 evaluable patients, which employed 5 consecutive days of a 20-minute intravenous infusion of 75 mg/m^2 azacitidine and observed a 27% response rate.[40] Despite the limited published response data, intravenous azacitidine is a reasonable alternative for patients who suffer injection site reactions with subcutaneous administration, and a supplemental New Drug Application for intravenous azacitidine was approved by the FDA in January 2007. An oral preparation of azacitidine is in development, but is not yet approved. Early trials of oral azacitidine were limited by rapid catabolism of the compound in aqueous environments, but the development of a film-coated formulation improved stability.[41] However, there remains considerable interpatient variation in the absorption and bioavailability of oral azacitidine, and this may be an obstacle to successful development of the compound.[42]

The initial FDA approval of decitabine, based on the D-0007 US registration trial[17] and early experience with decitabine in higher-risk patients with MDS in Europe,[30] was for a schedule of intravenous administration of nine doses, given once every 8 hours over 3 days, 15 mg/m^2/dose (total 135 mg/m^2 per course). In July 2009, the FDA accepted a supplemental application for the 5-day course of outpatient intravenous decitabine, 20 mg/m^2/d over 1 hour (total 100 mg/m^2 per course), based on the results of the MD Anderson ID03-0180 and multicenter DACO-020 (ADOPT) trials.[18,19] Almost all decitabine in the United States (>90%) currently is administered using the 5-day outpatient regimen, because of the increased convenience of outpatient administration and higher complete response rates reported with this regimen compared with the 3-day inpatient regimen. as mentioned previously, however, the authors still use the older 3-day inpatient decitabine if the patient needs to be in the hospital for some other reason, such as treatment of thrombocytopenia-related bleeding or neutropenia-associated infection, or for logistical reasons. The 3-day regimen can be completed more quickly and facilitates earlier hospital dismissal. Subsequent cycles might be given in the outpatient clinic using the 5-day schedule.

Subcutaneous administration of decitabine has been reported in patients with disorders other than MDS, such as sickle cell anemia (to augment γ-globin production and increase fetal hemoglobin levels) and primary myelofibrosis.[43,44] Subcutaneous administration of decitabine, however, has not been tested systematically in MDS, and at present there is no good reason to do it. Just as for azacitidine, an oral formulation of decitabine is in development, but clinical results have not yet been reported, and this compound is not approved by the FDA.[45]

Although both azacitidine and decitabine typically are readministered once every 28 days, many clinicians delay retreatment when treatment-emergent grade 4 cytopenias or active infections remain present and it is time to proceed with the next cycle. It is not clear how critical it is to stay on schedule with hypomethylating agents, or whether dose delays are permissible.

IS ANTIMICROBIAL PROPHYLAXIS INDICATED DURING HYPOMETHYLATING AGENT THERAPY?

Infection is the most frequent serious adverse event that occurs in patients undergoing therapy with hypomethylating agents. Because infection is also the most common cause of death for patients with MDS who are not undergoing treatment,[46] and febrile episodes occur in patients receiving only supportive care at an average rate of approximately 1 episode per 250 days during the first year after diagnosis,[47] it is usually not possible to distinguish treatment-related infection from infection caused by the underlying disease. Pooled data from the CALGB 8421, 8921, and 9221 azacitidine trials suggested that febrile neutropenia is not significantly more common in patients treated with the usual 7-day subcutaneous azacitidine regimen, compared with those patients receiving only supportive care.[32] Nevertheless, treatment-emergent severe neutropenia in patients undergoing therapy must pose some risks, and the likelihood of an infection-related death appears to be highest in the first two cycles of treatment, before treatment-induced clonal evolution has had a chance to occur, with subsequent restoration of normal hematopoiesis in those fortunate patients who achieve a complete response.[19]

Clinicians vary widely in their use of antimicrobial prophylaxis during hypomethylating agent therapy. Some clinicians offer no prophylaxis, and treat infections expectantly; others employ antibacterial prophylaxis, antifungal prophylaxis, antiviral prophylaxis, or some combination of these three. There are no randomized trials comparing the various potential antimicrobial prophylactic strategies in patients with MDS undergoing azacitidine or decitabine treatment, so the data on which to base decisions are derived from other settings.

The rate of febrile neutropenia in the D-0007 trial decitabine arm was 23%, compared with 4% for the supportive care control group.[17] In the DACO-020 (ADOPT) single-arm study, the rate of febrile neutropenia was 17%; most febrile episodes occurred in the first two cycles, and 5 of 11 deaths on study were thought to be caused by infection.[19] Antibiotic prophylaxis was not mandated in the DACO-020 (ADOPT) trial and was used according to local protocols. In contrast, the 3-month mortality was only 7% in the MD Anderson Cancer Center ID03-180 study that used the same decitabine regimen as DACO-020 (ADOPT), and in that study levofloxacin antibacterial prophylaxis was employed universally. Fluoroquinolone prophylaxis is well established in the setting of stem cell transplantation and induction chemotherapy for leukemia, but the rates of mucosal barrier disruption are higher in those settings than with hypomethylating agent treatment of MDS. Additionally, grade 4 neutropenia is universal with high-dose chemotherapy.[48–50]

Invasive fungal infections are uncommon during hypomethylating agent therapy, and adverse effects of newer triazole antifungals, such as transaminase elevation, are relatively frequent. Nevertheless, because posaconazole has been demonstrated to reduce invasive fungal infections and improve overall survival in randomized trials of patients with AML or MDS undergoing intensive chemotherapy,[51] and voriconazole also reduces invasive fungal infections in the same setting (trials of voriconazole with survival endpoint were terminated prematurely because of ethical concerns with placebo randomization after the posaconazole data became available[52]), some clinicians prescribe voriconazole or posaconazole to patients undergoing hypomethylating treatment also. Posaconazole primary prophylaxis in patients with AML or MDS undergoing intensive chemotherapy is supported by formal recommendations by infectious disease expert groups.[53] Fluconazole is useful in the setting of Candida infections, but has no anti-Aspergillus activity, and posaconazole has been shown to be superior to both itraconazole and fluconazole in primary prophylaxis against invasive fungal infections in patients with AML or MDS.[51]

Drug–drug interactions are common with triazoles. Notably, drug–drug interaction studies have not been performed with azacitidine or decitabine, but neither hypomethylating agent appears to be extensively metabolized by the cytochrome P450 system, which commonly mediates such interactions.

Acyclovir and its prodrug valacyclovir are the agents most commonly used for antiviral prophylaxis in patients with MDS who are undergoing disease-modifying treatment. In part, this is because randomized, placebo-controlled trials in the 1990s showed some benefit from acyclovir in terms of delaying the onset of fever and reducing the number of nonfungal oral infections outside the soft palate in herpes simplex virus (HSV)-seropositive patients undergoing remission induction chemotherapy for AML.[54] Acyclovir has no effect on mortality in patients receiving chemotherapy for hematological malignancies.[55] Valacyclovir is not as well studied in AML, and there are no systematic studies with either acyclovir or valacyclovir in MDS. The incidence of mouth ulcers caused by HSV in patients with MDS undergoing hypomethylating agent therapy is unknown, but is likely to be less than in patients undergoing AML remission induction therapy, because of the shorter duration of neutropenia. For this reason, many clinicians do not choose to employ antiviral prophylaxis routinely in patients receiving azacitidine or decitabine.

In the authors' clinical decisions about antimicrobial prophylaxis, they take into account the patient's prior history of infections and duration and degree of pretreatment neutropenia.[56] The first author treats all patients initiating hypomethylating therapy with prophylactic oral levofloxacin, at least for the first two cycles of therapy when the infection risk is the greatest. The second author does not use antibiotic prophylaxis routinely because of the theoretical risk of engendering infections with quinolone-resistant organisms. The authors do not use antifungals as primary prophylaxis in patients with MDS, but they do use these agents as secondary prophylaxis in patients with a history of invasive fungal infection, and also begin voriconazole or posaconazole at the first sign of pulmonary infiltrates or other signs or possible invasive fungal infection. The authors use prophylactic acyclovir or valacyclovir only in patients with a history of HSV-associated mouth ulcers.

HOW SHOULD CYTOPENIAS AND OTHER TREATMENT-ASSOCIATED ADVERSE EVENTS BE MANAGED?
Gastrointestinal Adverse Events

When gastrointestinal adverse events such as nausea, vomiting, or diarrhea develop in association with hypomethylating agent therapy, the symptoms are usually mild, and they respond well to the usual antiemetics (eg, prochlorperazine, metoclopramide, or serotonin 5-HT3 receptor antagonists) and hypomotility drugs (eg, loperamide or diphenoxylate-atropine). Most hematologists and oncologists are very comfortable with managing such chemotherapy-associated symptoms, so they will not be discussed further here.

Oral Ulcers and Mucositis

Severe mucositis is rare with hypomethylating agents, but in the authors' experience, aphthous-like mouth ulcers occasionally occur, especially with decitabine. Stomatitis and tongue ulcers were reported in 12% and 7% of patients in the D-0007 study, respectively, compared with rates of 6% and 2% in those patients treated with supportive care. A stomatitis rate of 7.7% was noted in the prescribing information for azacitidine. Antimicrobial mouth rinses seem to be of little help in preventing these ulcers, although once established, it is possible that antibacterial rinses or other compounds might speed healing. This issue is poorly studied in hematological malignancies other than acute leukemia and after stem cell transplantation.[57] Topical viscous lidocaine is effective local pain control, although there is systemic absorption with repeated use, so that patients should be cautioned against excess.[58] Various agents have been found to prevent or speed healing of mucositis in patients undergoing therapy for cancer, as summarized by a recent Cochrane Collaboration systemic review,[59] but none have been tested formally in patients with MDS. In the setting of mucositis caused by chemotherapy or radiotherapy, acyclovir improves healing when HSV-1 is present, but has little effect if swabs for HSV-1 are negative[60]; acyclovir also has not been studied in MDS.

Cytopenias

The most common treatment-emergent adverse event with hypomethylating agents is the development of cytopenias, or a worsening in the degree of existing cytopenias. For instance, in the AZA-001 azacitidine trial, grade 3 or 4 neutropenia was reported in 91% of patients, while grade 3 or 4 thrombocytopenia was present in 85%. In the D-0007 decitabine registration trial, grade 3 or 4 neutropenia was present in 87% of decitabine-treated patients compared with 50% receiving supportive care, while grade 3 or 4 thrombocytopenia was present in 85% in decitabine-treated patients, compared with 43% of those receiving supportive care alone.[15,17] There is no consensus on the best way to deal with cytopenias induced by hypomethylating agents. Potential strategies include dose delay, dose reduction, administration of hematopoietic growth factors, or just simply riding it out.

Those who argue in favor of dose reduction point out that it is not clear that there is a threshold dose for the clinical effects of hypomethylating agents, but that cytopenias do appear to be dose-dependent. Modulation of gene expression can occur at very low doses of hypomethylating agents (eg, in patients with sickle cell disease, successful induction of γ-globin expression was accomplished by use of just 0.2 mg/kg of decitabine, administered subcutaneously one to three times per week in two cycles of 6-week duration).[43] A dose reduction might occur at treatment initiation if the patient already has severe cytopenias, or in later cycles if cytopenias prove to be problematic.

In contrast, other clinicians argue that cytopenias are often not an adverse event so much as they are a marker of clonal evolution, just as cytopenias associated with lenalidomide therapy predict a higher likelihood of complete cytogenetic response.[61] The MD Anderson group always uses full doses and stays on schedule for at least the first three cycles of hypomethylating therapy, administering the drug every 4 weeks regardless of cytopenias. The authors tend to follow this approach whenever possible, although active infection and other emergent problems sometimes mandate delay. Dose delay can allow recovery of blood counts, but lengthy dose delay also can allow re-emergence of a neoplastic clone, especially if the interval between doses is longer than 8 weeks.

The prescribing information for decitabine recommends dose delay and reduction in subsequent cycles if recovery to a platelet count of $\geq 50 \times 10^9$/L and absolute neutrophil count $\geq 1 \times 10^9$/L do not occur by week 6 after initial therapy. It also recommends performing a bone marrow aspirate to assess for disease progression if recovery has not occurred by week 8. The prescribing information for azacitidine recommends a more complex dose adjustment and dose delay algorithm, based on marrow cellularity, baseline counts, and degree of drop of white count and platelet count in each cycle (**Table 2**). This algorithm appears to be based on expert opinion rather than data. Moreover, these recommendations are unwieldy and could be considered impractical.

The use of G-CSF or GM-CSF has not been studied formally in patients undergoing hypomethylating agent therapy. In patients receiving azacitidine, however, a randomized study of the novel thrombopoietin receptor agonist romiplostim indicated that concomitant weekly subcutaneous administration of romiplostim improved platelet nadir and reduced platelet transfusion needs.[62] There are as yet no data with the orally administered thrombopoietin agonist eltrombopag in MDS, either as a single agent or in combination with hypomethylating agents.

Injection Site Reactions

When azacitidine is administered subcutaneously, injection site reactions (erythema and pain) are common. In the AZA-001 trial, injection site redness was reported by 43% of patients, and other injection site reactions were reported by 29% of patients.[15,31] In a small case series, application of evening primrose oil (*Oenothera biennis*) topically at the injection site after injection ameliorated this complication.[63] This approach, however, has not been subjected to formal clinical trials. Other commonly used but not formally tested approaches include warm compresses, antihistamines, and nonsteroidal anti-inflammatory drugs. Of course, if skin symptoms are severe, switching to intravenous azacitidine will eliminate them, but there are fewer data with intravenous azacitidine than with subcutaneous azacitidine.[40]

Table 2			
Azacitidine dosage adjustment based on hematology laboratory values			
Nadir Counts[a]			**% Dose in the Next Course**
ANC ($\times 10^9$/L)		**Platelets ($\times 10^9$/L)**	
<0.5		<25	50%
0.5–1.5		25–50	67%
>1.5		>50	100%
WBC or Platelet Nadir (% Decrease in Counts from Baseline)[b]	**Bone Marrow Biopsy Cellularity at the Time of Nadir (%)**		
	30–60	**15–30**	**<15**
	% Decrease in Dose in the Next Course		
50%–75%	100%	50%	33%
>75%	75%	50%	33%

If a nadir as defined in the table above has occurred, the next course of treatment should be given 28 days after the start of the preceding course, provided that both the WBC and the platelet counts are >25% above the nadir and rising. If a >25% increase above the nadir is not seen by day 28, counts should be reassessed every 7 days. If a 25% increase is not seen by day 42, then the patient should be treated with 50% of the scheduled dose.

[a] For patients with baseline (start of treatment) WBC count $\geq 3.0 \times 10^9$/L, absolute neutrophil count (ANC) $\geq 1.5 \times 10^9$/L, and platelets $\geq 75.0 \times 10^9$/L, adjust the dose as follows, based on nadir counts for any given cycle.

[b] For patients whose baseline counts are WBC <3.0 $\times 10^9$/L, ANC <1.5 $\times 10^9$/L, or platelets <75 $\times 10^9$/L, dose adjustments should be based on nadir counts and bone marrow biopsy cellularity at the time of the nadir as noted below, unless there is clear improvement in differentiation (percentage of mature granulocytes is higher, and ANC is higher than at onset of that course) at the time of the next cycle, in which case the dose of the current treatment should be continued.

From Vidaza prescribing information, November 2009.

Fatigue

The most common symptom reported by patients with MDS is debilitating fatigue, regardless of whether they are receiving treatment.[2] Fatigue also has been reported commonly as an adverse event in clinical trials of hypomethylating agents, although in this setting it can be difficult to disentangle fatigue related to the underlying disease from treatment-associated fatigue. In general, fatigue is an especially challenging symptom to address. It seems reasonable to encourage patients to remain as active as possible physically. Some clinicians have employed modafinil, a novel centrally acting wakefulness-inducing agent that does not appear to be habit forming, with encouraging results in MDS and cancer-related fatigue.[64] This agent is approved in the United States for narcolepsy and shift work-associated sleep disorders, so it is usually not reimbursed by insurance companies when used off-label in other settings such as cancer-associated fatigue. Additionally, there is a strong potential for a placebo effect, and controlled trials will be necessary before modafinil can be recommended for MDS-associated fatigue. Methylphenidate also is employed by some clinicians to treat fatigue, as it is much less costly than modafinil, but signs and symptoms of central nervous system overstimulation can be problematic.

HOW LONG SHOULD HYPOMETHYLATING AGENT THERAPY BE CONTINUED, BOTH IN THE PRESENCE AND IN THE ABSENCE OF RESPONSE?

In patients who are fortunate enough to achieve an objective response during therapy with a hypomethylating agent, some of the same questions arise regarding maintenance therapy as arise when treating patients with follicular non-Hodgkin lymphoma. Azacitidine and decitabine do not appear to be curative; continued therapy is necessary to maintain a response, and resistance eventually emerges. As a result, some clinicians argue in favor of continuing therapy indefinitely, to minimize the risk of emergence of a resistant clone. Others argue that because azacitidine and decitabine are palliative rather than curative, and the mechanism of acquired resistance to hypomethylating agents is not known, once the best response is achieved, it is acceptable to allow patients to take a break from therapy and then re-treat at the time of relapse. Although continued treatment has not been compared with retreatment at the time of relapse, at least one study indicates that retreatment after relapse is associated with lower likelihood of response (although it is true that emergence of resistance might have occurred in nonresponders in this study, even with continued treatment).[65] Because azacitidine and decitabine are not a major burden on quality of life (indeed, in the CALGB 9221, azacitidine treatment was associated with improved quality of life, compared with supportive care alone),[66] the authors tend to continue to treat responding patients until the time of disease progression, as long as they tolerate the drug.

Although no one would argue for continuing hypomethylating agent therapy in a patient with MDS who has progressive disease despite that therapy, some investigators have stated that therapy should be continued indefinitely in those patients who tolerate the hypomethylating drug acceptably, even in the absence of measurable response.[33] This suggestion is based on a post-hoc analysis of the AZA-001 trial that indicated that a complete response was not necessary for patients to derive a survival benefit. Patients whose best response was a partial response, hematological improvement, or even stable disease had a reduced hazard ratio for death, compared with the whole cohort of patients treated with supportive care alone.[67] It is not clear, however, whether azacitidine was responsible for the stable disease in all of these patients; for some, their disease likely would have remained stable without any intervention. With a potentially lethal condition such as MDS, stability of disease is a necessary (but not sufficient) condition for long-term survival, regardless of what treatment is being administered, so it is not surprising that those who have stable disease have better outcomes than those who have progressive disease.

In practice, it is often difficult to convince patients to receive a therapy indefinitely in the absence of measurable benefit, and many patients are not persuaded by the argument that their disease might be worse if they were not taking the drug. Once a patient has completed a four- to six-cycle trial with azacitidine or decitabine without a response, if another effective therapy or an attractive clinical trial is available, the authors generally discontinue the hypomethylating agent and try something else. If a response is observed, however, the authors continue treating the patient with the hypomethylating agent until either disease progression, or the patient no longer can tolerate therapy.

Because response to hypomethylating agents can be delayed, it is important not to give up too soon when administering these drugs. The azacitidine package insert recommends a trial of at least four to six cycles to allow adequate time for a response, and the decitabine prescribing information recommends a trial of at least four cycles. The authors follow these suggestions.

SUMMARY

The hypomethylating agents azacitidine and decitabine have been an important addition to the therapeutic armamentarium for patients with MDS. Although many of the practical decisions described previously must be made in the absence of high-quality data, the benefit that these agents offer to appropriately selected patients makes their use worthwhile, and the responses are often quite satisfying.

REFERENCES

1. Sekeres MA, Schoonen WM, Kantarjian H, et al. Characteristics of US patients with myelodysplastic syndromes: results of six cross-sectional physician surveys. J Natl Cancer Inst 2008;100:1542–51.
2. Steensma DP, Heptinstall KV, Johnson VM, et al. Common troublesome symptoms and their impact on quality of life in patients with myelodysplastic syndromes (MDS): results of a large internet-based survey. Leuk Res 2008;32: 691–8.
3. Silverman LR, Mufti GJ. Methylation inhibitor therapy in the treatment of myelodysplastic syndrome. Nat Clin Pract Oncol 2005;2(Suppl 1):S12–23.
4. Garcia-Manero G. Modifying the epigenome as a therapeutic strategy in myelodysplasia. Hematology Am Soc Hematol Educ Program 2007;405–11.
5. Garcia-Manero G. Demethylating agents in myeloid malignancies. Curr Opin Oncol 2008;20:705–10.
6. Jones PA, Taylor SM, Wilson VL. Inhibition of DNA methylation by 5-azacytidine. Recent Results Cancer Res 1983;84:202–11.
7. Vesely J. Mode of action and effects of 5-azacytidine and of its derivatives in eukaryotic cells. Pharmacol Ther 1985;28:227–35.
8. Boultwood J, Wainscoat JS. Clonality in the myelodysplastic syndromes. Int J Hematol 2001;73:411–5.
9. Jones PA, Baylin SB. The fundamental role of epigenetic events in cancer. Nat Rev Genet 2002;3:415–28.
10. Kuendgen A, Lubbert M. Current status of epigenetic treatment in myelodysplastic syndromes. Ann Hematol 2008;87:601–11.

11. Oka M, Meacham AM, Hamazaki T, et al. De novo DNA methyltransferases Dnmt3a and Dnmt3b primarily mediate the cytotoxic effect of 5-aza-2'-deoxycytidine. Oncogene 2005;24:3091–9.
12. Palii SS, Van Emburgh BO, Sankpal UT, et al. DNA methylation inhibitor 5-Aza-2'-deoxycytidine induces reversible genome-wide DNA damage that is distinctly influenced by DNA methyltransferases 1 and 3B. Mol Cell Biol 2008;28:752–71.
13. Cheson BD, Bennett JM, Kantarjian H, et al. Report of an international working group to standardize response criteria for myelodysplastic syndromes. Blood 2000;96:3671–4.
14. Silverman LR, Demakos EP, Peterson BL, et al. Randomized controlled trial of azacitidine in patients with the myelodysplastic syndrome: a study of the cancer and leukemia group B. J Clin Oncol 2002;20:2429–40.
15. Fenaux P, Mufti GJ, Hellstrom-Lindberg E, et al. Efficacy of azacitidine compared with that of conventional care regimens in the treatment of higher-risk myelodysplastic syndromes: a randomised, open-label, phase III study. Lancet Oncol 2009;10:223–32.
16. Lyons RM, Cosgriff TM, Modi SS, et al. Hematologic response to three alternative dosing schedules of azacitidine in patients with myelodysplastic syndromes. J Clin Oncol 2009;27:1850–6.
17. Kantarjian H, Issa JP, Rosenfeld CS, et al. Decitabine improves patient outcomes in myelodysplastic syndromes: results of a phase III randomized study. Cancer 2006;106:1794–803.
18. Kantarjian H, Oki Y, Garcia-Manero G, et al. Results of a randomized study of 3 schedules of low-dose decitabine in higher-risk myelodysplastic syndrome and chronic myelomonocytic leukemia. Blood 2007;109:52–7.
19. Steensma DP, Baer MR, Slack JL, et al. Multicenter study of decitabine administered daily for 5 days every 4 weeks to adults with myelodysplastic syndromes: the alternative dosing for outpatient treatment (ADOPT) trial. J Clin Oncol 2009; 27:3842–8.
20. Wijermans P, Suciu S, Baila L, et al. Low dose decitabine versus best supportive care in elderly patients with intermediate or high risk mds not eligible for intensive chemotherapy: final results of the randomized Phase III study (06011) of the EORTC Leukemia and German MDS Study Groups. ASH Annual Meeting Abstracts 2008;112:226.
21. Santini V, Gozzini A, Ferrari G. Histone deacetylase inhibitors: molecular and biological activity as a premise to clinical application. Curr Drug Metab 2007;8:383–93.
22. Lyons RM. Clinical roundtable monograph. Choosing an appropriate therapy for lower-risk MDS in the community setting. Clin Adv Hematol Oncol 2009;7:S5–7.
23. Stone R, Sekeres M, Garcia-Manero G, et al. Recent advances in low- and intermediate-1-risk myelodysplastic syndrome: developing a consensus for optimal therapy. Clin Adv Hematol Oncol 2008;6:1–15.
24. Steensma DP. Myelodysplasia paranoia: iron as the new radon. Leuk Res 2009; 33:1158–63.
25. Tefferi A, Stone RM. Iron chelation therapy in myelodysplastic syndrome - Cui bono? Leukemia 2009;23:1373.
26. Stone R. Elevated serum ferritin in patients with a myelodysplastic syndrome: how much of a problem? Am J Hematol 2008;83:609–10.
27. Kindwall-Keller T, Isola LM. The evolution of hematopoietic SCT in myelodysplastic syndrome. Bone Marrow Transplant 2009;43:597–609.
28. Deeg HJ. Optimization of transplant regimens for patients with Myelodysplastic Syndrome (MDS). Hematology Am Soc Hematol Educ Program 2005;167–73.

29. Benesch M, Deeg HJ. Hemopoietic cell transplantation for myelodysplastic syndromes. Curr Hematol Rep 2003;2:209–16.
30. Wijermans P, Lubbert M, Verhoef G, et al. Low-dose 5-aza-2′-deoxycytidine, a DNA hypomethylating agent, for the treatment of high-risk myelodysplastic syndrome: a multicenter phase II study in elderly patients. J Clin Oncol 2000; 18:956–62.
31. Santini V, Fenaux P, Mufti GJ, et al. Management and supportive care measures of adverse events (AEs) in higher-risk MDS patients (Pts) treated with azacitidine (AZA). ASH Annual Meeting Abstracts 2008;112:1653.
32. Silverman LR, McKenzie DR, Peterson BL, et al. Further analysis of trials with azacitidine in patients with myelodysplastic syndrome: studies 8421, 8921, and 9221 by the Cancer and Leukemia Group B. J Clin Oncol 2006;24:3895–903.
33. Silverman LR, Fenaux P, Mufti GJ, et al. The effects of continued azacitidine (AZA) treatment cycles on response in higher-risk patients (pts) with myelodysplastic syndromes (MDS). ASH Annual Meeting Abstracts 2008;112:227.
34. Anonymous. First head-to-head study comparing Dacogen(R) (decitabine for injection) And Vidaza(R) (azacitidine) in patients with myelodysplastic syndromes: eisai press release. Available at: http://www.medicalnewstoday.com/articles/131641.php. December 3, 2008. Accessed October 31, 2009.
35. Kaminskas E, Farrell A, Abraham S, et al. Approval summary: azacitidine for treatment of myelodysplastic syndrome subtypes. Clin Cancer Res 2005;11:3604–8.
36. Qin T, Jelinek J, Si J, et al. Mechanisms of resistance to 5-aza-2′-deoxycytidine in human cancer cell lines. Blood 2009;113:659–67.
37. Flotho C, Claus R, Batz C, et al. The DNA methyltransferase inhibitors azacitidine, decitabine, and zebularine exert differential effects on cancer gene expression in acute myeloid leukemia cells. Leukemia 2009;23:1019–28.
38. Borthakur G, Ahdab SE, Ravandi F, et al. Activity of decitabine in patients with myelodysplastic syndrome previously treated with azacitidine. Leuk Lymphoma 2008;49:690–5.
39. Marcucci G, Silverman L, Eller M, et al. Bioavailability of azacitidine subcutaneous versus intravenous in patients with the myelodysplastic syndromes. J Clin Pharmacol 2005;45:597–602.
40. Martin MG, Walgren RA, Procknow E, et al. A phase II study of 5-day intravenous azacitidine in patients with myelodysplastic syndromes. Am J Hematol 2009;84: 560–4.
41. Garcia-Manero G, Stoltz ML, Ward MR, et al. A pilot pharmacokinetic study of oral azacitidine. Leukemia 2008;22:1680–4.
42. Skikne BS, Ward MR, Nasser A, et al. A phase I, open-label, dose-escalation study to evaluate the safety, pharmacokinetics, and pharmacodynamics of oral azacitidine in subjects with myelodysplastic syndromes (MDS) or acute myelogenous leukemia (AML) [abstract]. J Clin Oncol 2008;26.
43. Saunthararajah Y, Hillery CA, Lavelle D, et al. Effects of 5-aza-2′-deoxycytidine on fetal hemoglobin levels, red cell adhesion, and hematopoietic differentiation in patients with sickle cell disease. Blood 2003;102:3865–70.
44. Odenike OM, Godwin JE, Van Besien K, et al. Phase II trial of low dose, subcutaneous decitabine in myelofibrosis. ASH Annual Meeting Abstracts 2008;112:2809.
45. Lavelle D, Chin J, Vaitkus K, et al. Oral decitabine reactivates expression of the methylated gamma-globin gene in Papio anubis. Am J Hematol 2007;82:981–5.
46. Pomeroy C, Oken MM, Rydell RE, et al. Infection in the myelodysplastic syndromes. Am J Med 1991;90:338–44.

47. Oguma S, Yoshida Y, Uchino H, et al. Infection in myelodysplastic syndromes before evolution into acute non-lymphoblastic leukemia. Int J Hematol 1994;60:129–36.

48. Moon S, Williams S, Cullen M. Role of prophylactic antibiotics in the prevention of infections after chemotherapy: a literature review. Support Cancer Ther 2006;3:207–16.

49. Cullen M, Baijal S. Prevention of febrile neutropenia: use of prophylactic antibiotics. Br J Cancer 2009;101(Suppl 1):S11–4.

50. Lo N, Cullen M. Antibiotic prophylaxis in chemotherapy-induced neutropenia: time to reconsider. Hematol Oncol 2006;24:120–5.

51. Cornely OA, Maertens J, Winston DJ, et al. Posaconazole vs. fluconazole or itraconazole prophylaxis in patients with neutropenia. N Engl J Med 2007;356:348–59.

52. Vehreschild JJ, Bohme A, Buchheidt D, et al. A double-blind trial on prophylactic voriconazole (VRC) or placebo during induction chemotherapy for acute myelogenous leukaemia (AML). J Infect 2007;55:445–9.

53. Cornely OA, Bohme A, Buchheidt D, et al. Primary prophylaxis of invasive fungal infections in patients with hematologic malignancies. Recommendations of the Infectious Diseases Working Party of the German Society for Haematology and Oncology. Haematologica 2009;94:113–22.

54. Bergmann OJ, Mogensen SC, Ellermann-Eriksen S, et al. Acyclovir prophylaxis and fever during remission-induction therapy of patients with acute myeloid leukemia: a randomized, double-blind, placebo-controlled trial. J Clin Oncol 1997;15:2269–74.

55. Yahav D, Gafter-Gvili A, Muchtar E, et al. Antiviral prophylaxis in haematological patients: Systematic review and meta-analysis. Eur J Cancer 2009;45:3131–48.

56. Angarone M, Ison MG. Prevention and early treatment of opportunistic viral infections in patients with leukemia and allogeneic stem cell transplantation recipients. J Natl Compr Canc Netw 2008;6:191–201.

57. Alvarado Y, Bellm LA, Giles FJ. Oral mucositis: time for more studies. Hematology 2002;7:281–9.

58. Elad S, Cohen G, Zylber-Katz E, et al. Systemic absorption of lidocaine after topical application for the treatment of oral mucositis in bone marrow transplantation patients. J Oral Pathol Med 1999;28:170–2.

59. Worthington HV, Clarkson JE, Eden OB. Interventions for preventing oral mucositis for patients with cancer receiving treatment. Cochrane Database Syst Rev 2007;(4):CD000978.

60. Nicolatou-Galitis O, Athanassiadou P, Kouloulias V, et al. Herpes simplex virus-1 (HSV-1) infection in radiation-induced oral mucositis. Support Care Cancer 2006; 14:753–62.

61. Sekeres MA, Maciejewski JP, Giagounidis AA, et al. Relationship of treatment-related cytopenias and response to lenalidomide in patients with lower-risk myelodysplastic syndromes. J Clin Oncol 2008;26:5943–9.

62. Kantarjian H, Giles F, Greenberg P, et al. Effect of romiplostim in patients (pts) with low or intermediate risk myelodysplastic syndrome (MDS) receiving azacytidine. ASH Annual Meeting Abstracts 2008;112:224.

63. Platzbecker U, Aul C, Ehninger G, et al. Reduction of 5-azacitidine induced skin reactions in MDS patients with evening primrose oil. Ann Hematol 2009. [Epub ahead of print].

64. Cooper MR, Bird HM, Steinberg M. Efficacy and safety of modafinil in the treatment of cancer-related fatigue. Ann Pharmacother 2009;43:721–5.

65. Ruter B, Wijermans PW, Lubbert M. Superiority of prolonged low-dose azanucleoside administration? Results of 5-aza-2′-deoxycytidine retreatment in high-risk myelodysplasia patients. Cancer 2006;106:1744–50.

66. Kornblith AB, Herndon JE 2nd, Silverman LR, et al. Impact of azacytidine on the quality of life of patients with myelodysplastic syndrome treated in a randomized phase III trial: a Cancer and Leukemia Group B study. J Clin Oncol 2002;20: 2441–52.

67. List AF, Fenaux P, Mufti GJ, et al. Effect of azacitidine (AZA) on overall survival in higher-risk myelodysplastic syndromes (MDS) without complete remission [abstract]. J Clin Oncol 2008. [Epub ahead of print].

Hematopoietic Stem Cell Transplantation for MDS

Matthias Bartenstein, MD[a], H. Joachim Deeg, MD[a,b],*

KEYWORDS

- Transplantation for MDS • Conditioning intensity
- Cytogenetics and relapse

The myelodysplastic syndromes (MDS) comprise a heterogeneous group of clonal bone marrow diseases characterized by ineffective production of normal mature blood cells and peripheral blood cytopenias.[1] Generally required for the diagnosis are dysplastic changes in blood and marrow cells. In approximately one third of patients, MDS will eventually evolve to acute myeloid leukemia (AML).[2] A detailed description of the disease characteristics, including the cellular and molecular biology of MDS, is provided elsewhere in this issue.

Infections caused by neutropenia and neutrophil dysfunction represent the leading cause of death in MDS.[1] Life-threatening bleeding caused by thrombocytopenia is another complication directly attributable to marrow failure.[1] The most frequent presentation, however, is anemia.[3] Red blood cell transfusion dependence and the resulting iron overload may lead to additional organ complications, particularly in the heart, live,r and endocrine organs.[4,5]

For most patients with MDS, chemotherapy alone is not a viable treatment option. Only about 40% of patients will achieve remissions, which are generally of short duration.[6–8] For high-risk patients with MDS, 3-year survival rates after chemotherapy are in the range of only 5%.[9]

Currently the only therapy with proven curative potential for MDS is hematopoietic stem cell transplantation (HSCT),[10–13] with long-term survival rates between 25% and 70%.[14–17] However, HSCT carries a risk of toxicity and potentially fatal complications, particularly in older patients. Given the frequently slow progression in low-risk MDS, the risk of treatment-related mortality (TRM) must be carefully weighed against the potential benefits of transplantation. Patient characteristics, timing of transplantation,

This work was supported in part by NIH grant HL036444, Bethesda, MD.
a Clinical Research Division, Fred Hutchinson Cancer Research Center, 1100 Fairview Avenue N, D1-100, Seattle, WA 98109-1024, USA
b Department of Medicine, University of Washington School of Medicine, 1959 NE Pacific Street, Seattle, WA 98195, USA
* Corresponding author. Clinical Research Division, Fred Hutchinson Cancer Research Center, 1100 Fairview Avenue N, D1-100, Seattle, WA 98109-1024.
E-mail address: jdeeg@fhcrc.org

Hematol Oncol Clin N Am 24 (2010) 407–422
doi:10.1016/j.hoc.2010.02.003
0889-8588/10/$ – see front matter © 2010 Elsevier Inc. All rights reserved.

hemonc.theclinics.com

and choice of conditioning regimen have to be considered. Thus, the questions are: transplantation for whom, when, and how? Should induction chemotherapy be given before HSCT? What should be the source of stem cells? Should the graft be T-cell depleted? How can one optimize the rate of engraftment and the graft-versus-tumor effect (GvT) while minimizing the incidence of graft-versus-host disease (GvHD) and TRM? The present article focuses on these questions.

GENERAL CONSIDERATIONS

MDS originates in hematopoietic stem or precursor cells, and the goal of HSCT is to replace those cells and their progeny with cells from a healthy donor. Successful allogeneic HSCT requires that (1) healthy donor cells are able to establish themselves (engraft) in patients, and (2) the abnormal (malignant) cells responsible for the patients' disease are eliminated or inactivated.

To allow donor cell engraftment it is generally necessary that patients are conditioned (ie, the immunologic barrier, which protects the body against intrusion by foreign organisms or cells, must be overcome).[18] T-cell mediated host-versus-graft reactions seem to be the main cause of rejection, in addition to natural killer (NK)-cell effects.[19,20]

Conditioning can include various immunosuppressive drugs, chemotherapeutic agents or irradiation, and new regimens are continuously being developed and tested. Regimens are often categorized as conventional/high-dose (myeloablative conditioning), reduced intensity (RIC), or low-dose/non-myeloablative conditioning.[21] However, a review of the literature shows that there is a spectrum of regimens that basically form a continuum,[22] and any categorization must remain artificial. Nevertheless, it is clear that the extent of toxicity correlates with conditioning intensity, and in general the probability of relapse is higher the lower the regimen intensity.[23] This correlation is particularly true with transplantation for advanced disease. An important potential advantage of RIC is the ability of autologous marrow function to recover if the donor graft is rejected.

An undesired consequence of currently used conditioning regimens is that the defense against infectious organisms is also disrupted, and the fact that most conditioning regimens damage the anatomic tissue barriers (skin, mucosa) further enhances the risk of infections. This consequence was one rationale for the development of RIC regimens, which cause less tissue toxicity than conventional high-dose regimens, which in turn translates into lower acute non-relapse mortality (NRM). The development of these RIC regimens has also allowed to offer HSCT to older individuals who, until recently, were not considered transplant candidates,[23,24] and TRM in various HSCT regimens has steadily declined in recent years.[25,26]

A second purpose of the conditioning regimen is to ablate the abnormal cells responsible for patients' disease. Although the conditioning regimens are generally effective in killing a large proportion of tumor cells, we rely on the immuno-therapeutic effect of donor cells for complete disease eradication. The lower the conditioning intensity, the more the patients' cure will depend upon this GvT effect.[22] In clinical studies, there is a strong correlation of GvT effect and GvHD, in particular chronic GvHD.[18,27] Although recent research suggests that it may be possible to separate a GvT effect from the reactions that cause GvHD,[28,29] clinically we have yet to show that such a separation is possible. Even if patients achieve remissions following HSCT, relapse remains a problem, especially in advanced MDS.[30,31] The immunologic effects of HSCT, and consequently the risk of relapse and GvHD, depend upon the conditioning regimen, the nature of the graft (ie, degree of human leukocyte antigen

[HLA]-match), stem-cell source (bone marrow, peripheral blood or umbilical cord blood), and GvHD prophylaxis, among others.

Only about 25% of patients will have HLA identical sibling donors (or matched related donors other than a sibling). However, large volunteer donor banks have been set up, and currently, an HLA-matched unrelated donor can be identified for about 50% to 60% of Caucasians; the proportion is lower for African Americans, and may be as low as 10% in some ethnic minorities.[32,33] If a patient and sibling have inherited the same paternal and maternal chromosomes 6, they should be genotypically identical for HLA-A, -B, -C, -DR, and –DQ (ie, show a "10 out of 10" match). The only exception would be if a crossover has occurred. When we search for unrelated donors and typing by high resolution is available, we have the same objective of finding a "10 out of 10 match." Lesser degrees of matching may be acceptable for some indications. With increasing degrees of mismatching, there is a higher probability of non-engraftment (particularly with HLA-C disparities) and a higher probability of GVHD. For patients without an HLA-matched related or unrelated donor, cord blood cells, or cells from a haploidentical-related donor may offer alternatives.[34–36] Cord blood has the advantage of immaturity, allowing to transplant HLA-mismatched cells without a significant increase in GvHD incidence. A drawback is the limited number of cells available, often associated with a marked delay in engraftment.[37] The use of two units of cord blood or in vitro expansion of the cord blood before infusion has partially overcome this limitation.[38–40]

Initial results with haploidentical HSCT are encouraging. Graft failure presents only a minor problem, and GvHD rates have been surprisingly low, with relapse-free survival (RFS) and NRM comparing favorably with results from other HLA nonidentical transplants.[35] It is clear, of course, that in addition to HLA antigens, so-called non-HLA and minor antigens (which are presented by HLA antigens) are involved in allogeneic interactions and GVHD[18] (otherwise, no GVHD should be observed in HLA-genotypically identical sibling transplants). It is currently not routine to type donor and patient for those minor antigens.

In addition, research in recent years has shown that antigens typically expressed on NK cells, in particular killer-cell immunoglobulin-like receptor (KIR) antigens, are involved in donor/host interactions and may play an essential role in tumor cell elimination.[19]

RISK ASSESSMENT AND SCORING

Several MDS scoring systems have been developed and are used to identify patients who are likely to benefit from HSCT.

Multiparameter Prognostic Scoring Systems

The International Prognostic Scoring System (IPSS),[2] used widely to assess patient prognosis, has also proven a reliable indicator of the probability of transplant success. The higher the IPSS score, the lower RFS.[11,41] A major point of criticism is that the instrument's predictions are based on data from time of diagnosis,[42] although one recent study showed that if recalculated at the time of transplantation, the IPSS retained its predictive power.[41] The more recently developed World Health Organization (WHO) Prognostic Scoring System (WPSS)[5] includes WHO classification, karyotype, and transfusion dependence. In contrast to the IPSS it allows for real-time assessment of prognosis. A recent study validated its applicability to HSCT.[43]

Another recent addition is the Simplified MDS Risk Score[44] that includes poor performance status, older age, thrombocytopenia, anemia, increased marrow blasts, leukocytosis, chromosome 7 or complex (≥ 3) abnormalities, and earlier transfusions as adverse risk factors. It has been validated for secondary MDS and a cohort of de novo patients with MDS.[45] Whether this system is truly simpler than others remains to be seen, but its value might lie in the fact that it incorporates performance status, which in turn might reflect comorbidities. A possible relevance in the context of HSCT remains to be determined.

Cytogenetics

Patients' karyotype is the most powerful predictor of RFS after HSCT for MDS.[2,43,46] This has led Armand and colleagues[47] to reexamine the cytogenetic risk stratification of MDS in regards to the impact on transplant outcome. Their data, recently validated in a multicenter analysis, indicate that patients with MDS can be separated into two groups, good/intermediate versus poor-risk cytogenetics, with significantly differing outcome post-HSCT.[42,48]

Flow Cytometry

Several studies have analyzed immunophenotypic aberrancies of MDS marrow cells and determined their prognostic relevance.[49,50] Wells and colleagues[51] developed a flow scoring system and showed a correlation of the severity of flow-cytometric aberrancies and the probability of relapse after HSCT. This was true even for patients with less than 5% marrow blasts at the time of HSCT.[49] Presumably, differences in gene expression underlie the observed immunophenotypic abnormalities, and gene expression profiling has been shown to predict the risk for progression of MDS to AML.[52]

Transfusion Dependence and Iron Overload

Several recent studies[53–59] suggest that transfusion dependence (reflected in the WPSS) and iron overload have a negative impact on outcome after HSCT. The significance of elevated ferritin levels, however, is controversial, as ferritin may be elevated for various reasons, in particular inflammation. As such, a high ferritin level may reflect a different underlying disease process, rather than iron overload, although iron can contribute to inflammation. Liver iron content seems to be a more specific marker of iron overload,[60,61] with noninvasive assessment procedures being developed.[56,58] Treatment of iron overload may improve outcome following HSCT,[55,58] although this is a matter of controversy.

Transfusion dependence is also linked to marrow fibrosis, the presence of which has long been recognized as being associated with accelerated disease progression in patients with MDS. Recent studies[58] confirm those findings, and one study at least has shown a negative impact of fibrosis on post-HSCT outcome, particularly in patients with more advanced MDS.[62]

Age and Comorbidity

Until the mid 1990s few patients over 55 years were offered allogeneic HSCT[63] because of higher NRM in older patients. As only about 25% of patients with MDS are younger than 60 years,[2,64] efforts have focused on reducing the elevated risk of NRM associated with older age by modifying conditioning regimens (as discussed earlier), supportive care, and complication management.[63] Recent successfully transplanted cohorts included patients with median ages of 55 to 60 years, with some patients older than 70 years.[63]

Much of the negative impact of age on prognosis appears to be caused by the frequency of comorbid conditions with older age.[41] Sorror and colleagues[65] developed a HCT-specific comorbidity index (HCT-CI) for risk assessment before transplantation, introducing objective laboratory and functional testing data, thereby modifying the Charlson Comorbidity Index.[66] The instrument has been validated for patients with lymphoma and myeloma,[67] and for a mixed patient sample.[68] A multivariate analysis showed that the HCT-CI had greater predictive power for toxicities, NRM and overall survival after RIC HSCT than the Karnofksy Performance Score (KPS), but these findings were not confirmed in a Canadian study.[69] However, the instruments measure two distinct patient characteristics, as evidenced by their weak correlation with each other. A combination of comorbidity and performance status assessment allows a more refined risk stratification for HSCT.[65]

TIMING OF TRANSPLANTATION

Determining the optimal timing of HSCT for MDS has proven difficult since it involves weighing the benefit of early transplantation (reduced risk of disease progression and relapse) with high TRM (in some studies as high as 20%–25%), especially in patients in whom disease progression (even without HSCT) may be slow.[2,11]

Generally, shorter disease duration before HSCT is linked to improved overall survival, decreased TRM and increased RFS. Lower blast count (based on French-American-British (FAB) classification) and younger age are also linked to more favorable outcome.[70] Cutler and colleagues used a Markov model, involving a non-transplantation cohort and two patient cohorts receiving HLA-identical sibling transplants after high-dose conditioning, to determine the optimal timing of HSCT for MDS. They showed that patients with high or intermediate-2 risk by IPSS did benefit from early transplantation, whereas transplantation should be delayed for low-risk patients until evidence of disease progression. Intermediate-1 patients should probably be evaluated on a case by case basis.[71] Although this analysis was restricted to patients transplanted from HLA-identical siblings, most transplant centers also apply this approach to patients transplanted from unrelated donors.[72]

Al-Ali and colleagues found that outcome after allogeneic (and autologous) HSCT was best if transplantation was performed between 6 to 12 months after diagnosis, with higher overall survival and lower TRM than observed in patients transplanted later. They attributed the negative effect of later transplantation to frequent blood transfusion, longer duration of pancytopenias, and increased risk for progression during the waiting period for HSCT.[73]

If transplantation has to be delayed, for example because of a lengthy search for an unrelated donor (median time 2–3 months[74]; median time from diagnosis to HSCT 12.9 months in the US[75]; median search duration 22 days for 549 patients in Germany[76]), bridging treatment with hypomethylating agents may delay progression to AML before HSCT.[72] Such a strategy is especially relevant for patients who have MDS with IPSS intermediate-2 or high-risk disease, where the average time to AML progression may be short.[2]

PRETRANSPLANT INDUCTION CHEMOTHERAPY AND THE USE OF HYPOMETHYLATING DRUGS

Studies linking elevated pretransplant blast counts to increased risk for relapse[17] have led to investigations into the benefit of pretransplant induction chemotherapy[30,77] for RFS after HSCT. Induction chemotherapy plays an important role in autologous HSCT, because this transplant modality requires that patients be in remission[46]; for allogeneic HSCT, the indication is less clear. Several retrospective studies suggest that patients who achieve remission after induction chemotherapy have a lower risk of relapse after HSCT than patients who do not respond to induction chemotherapy.[72,78,79] It is still controversial whether this approach affects RFS.[78,80,81]

It is conceivable that the effect of pretransplant chemotherapy consists in selecting treatment-sensitive patients.[43] To address these questions, the European Group for Blood and Marrow Transplantation (EBMT) is currently conducting a prospective randomized phase III trial investigating the impact of pre-HSCT induction therapy on relapse rates after HSCT (EBMT Study code: Allo-MDS2x2).

Hypomethylating agents are emerging as an alternative to classic induction chemotherapy.[72] In a recent retrospective study of therapy before allogeneic HSCT, overall survival, RFS, and cumulative incidence of relapse after 1 year were 47%, 41%, and 20%, respectively, for patients with MDS (and chronic myelogenous leukemia [CML]) receiving 5-azacytidine, compared with 60%, 51%, and 32% for non-5-azacytidine treated patients. Pretransplant administration of 5-azacytidine resulted in a trend to reduced risk of relapse.[82] In 17 patients with MDS, the hypomethylating drug 2-deoxy-5-azacytidine (decitabine) did not negatively affect toxicity after HSCT, and disease downstaging may improve HSCT outcome.[83] However, responses to both, 5-azacytidine and decitabine are often delayed; in cases requiring urgent action (eg, due to high risk for progression), induction chemotherapy may be preferable.[30]

CONDITIONING REGIMENS

Intensive research in recent years has been geared toward minimizing the toxicity while optimizing the efficacy of conditioning regimens. However, there is no one-size-fits-all conditioning regimen.[46] Instead, conditioning should be tailored to diagnosis, disease stage, patient age, prior therapy, comorbidities, and the other components of HSCT, such as donor and stem cell source.[11,31]

Although conventional conditioning is associated with a lower risk for relapse,[30] its toxicity makes it unsuitable for many patients with comorbidities, and it is generally only offered to patients younger than 65 or 60 years with suitable related or unrelated donors, respectively.[11] For MDS patients over 60 years,[64] and those with comorbidities, RIC is a viable alternative. Although it is associated with a higher risk for relapse, this is possibly offset by lower TRM,[84,85] thereby offering equivalent overall survival and RFS,[30,46,84–86] although no prospective randomized study of comparable patients has been conducted so far. Even patients older than 70 years have been transplanted successfully using RIC.[87,88] These results from retrospective studies should be interpreted with caution, because of likely bias in patient selection.[85,89,90] Only prospective studies will allow a definite comparison.

DONOR SELECTION

The policy at most centers currently is to search for HLA-identical siblings. If no sibling is available, then an attempt is made to identify HLA-matched unrelated donors. Cord blood is being used as a third option. However, various centers have focused their research on the use of cord blood and might use this source of stem cells even instead of searching for a living unrelated donor. Further, efforts are underway to use haploidentical transplants more frequently since preliminary observations suggest a low rejection frequency and a surprisingly low incidence of GVHD. However, this approach must be considered investigational, and further data are required before firm recommendations can be made.

STEM CELL SOURCE AND MANIPULATION

Stem cells obtained by bone marrow (BM) aspiration, umbilical cord blood cells (UCB), and granulocyte colony stimulating factor (G-CSF) mobilized peripheral blood progenitor cells (PBPC) lead to different outcomes, because of different GvHD and GvT effects, the number and nature of cells transplanted, and the relative maturity or activation of cells.[18]

A retrospective EBMT study,[91] in agreement with data from FHCRC,[12] showed that the use of G-CSF mobilized PBPC for HSCT from related donors in patients with MDS was associated with lower treatment failure rates (relapse and refractory disease) than the use of marrow in all MDS subgroups except refractory anemia. Data from a recent Markov decision model of choice between BM and PBPC grafts in HLA-matched related donor HSCT[92] involving 1111 adult subjects conditioned with high-dose regimens and given unmanipulated grafts, showed significantly higher survival and better quality of life with PBPC, mainly because of lower risk of relapse, despite a higher incidence of GvHD. How PBSC compares with BM in unrelated HSCT is controversial,[93,94] but a randomized prospective study in unrelated transplant recipients was just recently completed and results are pending (Blood and Marrow Transplant Clinical Trials Network protocol 0201).

A third option is, as discussed, the use of UCB transplantation.[34,37,39,95,96] The introduction of two-unit transplants[39] has helped to overcome restrictions associated with the low cell dose of UCB units,[95] and in vitro expansion of UCB is emerging as a further option.[38] Few studies are available on the use of UCB in MDS.[97]

WHAT CAN PATIENTS WITH MYELODYSPLASTIC SYNDROMES EXPECT FROM TRANSPLANTATION?

As discussed, many factors influence the outcome of HSCT. Two recent reviews offer a comprehensive compilation of current results. Kindwall-Keller and Isola[97] reviewed results of 24 studies that used high-dose conventional transplant conditioning and 30 studies that used RIC between 2000 and 2008. Oliansky and colleagues[46] attempted an "evidence based review" which included articles published between 1990 and 2008. Following below is a discussion of selected reports.

Warlick and colleagues[30] studied 84 subjects transplanted with marrow from related or unrelated donors or cord blood, following conditioning with conventional or RIC regimens. At 1 year, overall survival was 48%, cumulative relapse incidence 23%, and RFS 38%. The corresponding figures at 5 years were 31%, 25% and 29%, respectively. TRM at one year was 39%, and the incidence of acute GvHD was 43% for grades II-IV. The incidence of chronic GvHD at 1 year was 15%. RFS did not differ significantly by graft source or conditioning regimen. The probability of relapse was 18% for subjects with less than or equal to 5% myeloblasts at HSCT and 35% for subjects with greater than or equal to 5% blasts. In subjects with less than 5% blasts, conventional conditioning was associated with a lower risk of relapse compared with RIC (9% vs 31%), but the difference was not significant in subjects with more than 5% blasts. Conditioning intensity did not affect overall survival or RFS.

A study by de Witte and colleagues[25] included an EBMT registry cohort of 374 subjects with refractory anemia (RA) or RA with ringed sideroblasts (RARS) receiving HLA-matched grafts after various conditioning regimens. At 4 years, overall survival was 52%, RFS 48%, relapse 15%, and NRM 37%. After adjusting for confounding factors, multivariate analysis showed increased risk for relapse after RIC compared with conventional conditioning, with a hazard ratio (HR) of 2.8. However, overall survival and RFS did not differ, because of lower NRM after RIC, with a HR of 0.8. HSCT from unrelated donors was associated with a lower relapse risk (HR 0.6), but higher NRM (HR 1.4) and overall survival did not differ significantly from that with related donors. Outcome did not differ between BM and PBSC grafts, whereas

T-cell depletion was associated with higher NRM. Older age and transplantation more than 12 months after diagnosis adversely affected outcome.

An FHCRC study[98] analyzed outcomes in 257 subjects with secondary MDS, including 103 whose disease had progressed to AML. Grades II-IV acute GvHD occurred in 67% of subjects, and 57% developed chronic GvHD. The 5-year incidence of relapse was 33% for therapy-related acute myeloid leukemia (tAML), 36% for refractory anemia with excess blasts (RAEB) and 12% for RA/RARS. The 5-year RFS was 29% overall, 19% for tAML, 25% for RAEB, and 41% for RA/RARS. Outcomes were compared with results in 339 subjects transplanted for de novo MDS/tAML. Multivariate analysis failed to show significant differences between the two cohorts after adjusting for cytogenetic risk. Relapse probability and RFS significantly correlated with disease stage ($P<.001$) and karyotype ($P<.001$). Subjects receiving unrelated donor transplants (n = 122) had a lower risk of relapse ($P = .003$) and higher RFS ($P = .02$) compared with those receiving grafts from related donors. Conditioning with (targeted) busulfan and cyclophosphamide ([t]BUCY) (n = 93) was associated with the highest RFS (43%) and lowest NRM (28%).

In a retrospective multicenter study, Martino and colleagues[85] analyzed HSCT outcomes in 836 subjects with MDS transplanted from HLA-identical sibling donors after RIC (n = 215) or conventional conditioning (n = 621). For the conventional and RIC cohorts, 3-year NRM was 32% versus 22%, overall survival 45% versus 41%, and RFS 41% versus 33%. The cumulative incidence of acute GvHD was 58% versus 43% at 100 days posttransplantation. Within 1 year, chronic GvHD developed in 52% versus 45% of subjects. Lack of complete remission before HSCT ($P = .001$), poor-risk karyotype ($P = .03$), diagnosis of tAML ($P = .03$), and age older than 50 years ($P = .05$) negatively affected RFS.

Lim and colleagues[99] prospectively evaluated the outcomes of 75 subjects undergoing alemtuzumab-based RIC followed by unrelated donor HSCT. Actuarial 3-year TRM, RFS and overall survival, respectively, were 24%, 55%, and 59% for subjects with refractory cytopenia with multilineage dysplasia (RCMD) (n = 28) and 44%, 18% and 18%, respectively, for patients with RAEB 1 and 2 (n = 15). In multivariate analysis, HLA-mismatch adversely affected TRM, RFS, and overall survival. Disease status at transplantation and comorbidity significantly influenced overall survival.

MANAGING RELAPSE AFTER HEMATOPOIETIC STEM CELL TRANSPLANTATION

Although TRM after HSCT has progressively declined over the past decade, because of intensive efforts aimed at optimizing conditioning regimens, relapse has remained a major problem in all reports, but more so with RIC. Whether post-HSCT monitoring for disease progression or recurrence will be useful in instituting therapy for minimal residual disease (MRD), found helpful in other diseases, remains to be shown. BM cyto- and histomorphology, cytogenetic monitoring, polymerase chain reaction-assessment of molecular markers, assessment of donor-host chimerism, and immunophenotyping[100] have all been applied.

In a recent study, MRD was found to significantly influence outcome after HSCT.[101] MRD was assessed by counting cells with a leukemia associated phenotype as determined by flow-cytometry 100 days after transplant. Not surprisingly, subjects with low MRD ($<10^{-3}$) had better overall survival (73% vs 25%) and RFS (74% vs 17%) compared with those with high MRD ($\geq 10^{-3}$). Subjects with low tumor burden and GvHD might benefit from intensified immunosuppression, reaping the benefit of reduced GvHD while running only a small risk of relapse caused by reduced GvL effects.[101]

Various teams have administered preemptive donor lymphocyte infusions in patients with relapse.[102–108] It is not clear, however, how effective such a strategy will be eventually. Chemotherapy has generally been disappointing, and second HSCT in adults have been associated with a low success rate.[109]

AUTOLOGOUS HEMATOPOIETIC STEM CELL TRANSPLANTATION

If no suitable matched donor is available, autologous transplantation of stem cells harvested during remission may be an option. Autologous HSCT has the advantage of transplantation without the risk for GvHD. Unfortunately, this also means the absence of a GvT effect, and consequently, increased risk for relapse.[73,110,111] With the development of UCB transplants and the use of haploidentical donors autologous transplants are being used rather infrequently in patients with MDS.

SUMMARY

Hematopoietic stem cell transplantation is currently the only treatment modality with proven curative potential for MDS. With the development of reduced-intensity conditioning regimens, it has been possible to offer HSCT to patients in the seventh and even eighth decade of life, an important consideration in view of age distribution of MDS. Further, the development of large unrelated donor registries, the availability of cord blood as a source of stem cells, and, most recently, the renewed interest in using haploidentical donors for transplantation allows to offer HSCT to a growing number of patients. Although 20% to 25% of patients may suffer from chronic medical problems after HSCT, more than 70% report their quality of life as being "good to excellent" 1 to 2 years after transplantation.[92] It is clear, however, that despite all progress that has been made, with some patients now followed for more than 25 years after successful transplantation, disease recurrence and GVHD remain major hurdles. Great hopes are placed on immunotherapy after transplantation, but progress has been slow. With the availability of approved drugs for the treatment of MDS, ongoing studies are exploring the incorporation of those agents into the overall transplant approach. It will be of interest to follow the impact of pretransplant therapy and posttransplant adjuvant treatment with hypomethylating agents or lenalidomide on long-term success.

REFERENCES

1. Steensma DP, Bennett JM. The myelodysplastic syndromes: diagnosis and treatment [review]. Mayo Clin Proc 2006;81:104–30.
2. Greenberg P, Cox C, LeBeau MM, et al. International scoring system for evaluating prognosis in myelodysplastic syndromes. Blood 1997;89:2079–88 [erratum appears in Blood 1998;91(3):1100].
3. Greenberg PL, Baer MR, Bennett JM, et al. Myelodysplastic syndromes: clinical practice guidelines in oncology. J Natl Compr Canc Netw 2006;4:58–77 [erratum appears in J Natl Compr Canc Netw 2006;4(3): table of contents Note: dosage error in text].
4. Gattermann N. The treatment of secondary hemochromatosis. Dtsch Arztebl Int 2009;106:499–504.
5. Malcovati L, Germing U, Kuendgen A, et al. Time-dependent prognostic scoring system for predicting survival and leukemic evolution in myelodysplastic syndromes. J Clin Oncol 2007;25:3503–10.
6. de Witte T, Suciu S, Peetermans M, et al. Intensive chemotherapy for poor prognosis myelodysplasia (MDS) and secondary acute myeloid leukemia (sAML) following MDS of more than 6 months duration. A pilot study by the Leukemia

Cooperative Group of the European Organisation for Research and Treatment in Cancer (EORTC-LCG). Leukemia 1995;9:1805–11.

7. Estey E, Thall P, Beran M, et al. Effect of diagnosis (refractory anemia with excess blasts, refractory anemia with excess blasts in transformation, or acute myeloid leukemia [AML]) on outcome of AML-type chemotherapy. Blood 1997; 90:2969–77.

8. Ruutu T, Hanninen A, Jarventie G, et al. Intensive chemotherapy of poor prognosis myelodysplastic syndromes (MDS) and acute myeloid leukemia following MDS with idarubicin and cytarabine. Leuk Res 1997;21:133–8.

9. Beran M. Intensive chemotherapy for patients with high-risk myelodysplastic syndrome [review]. Int J Hematol 2000;72:139–50.

10. Nachtkamp K, Kundgen A, Strupp C, et al. Impact on survival of different treatments for myelodysplastic syndromes (MDS). Leuk Res 2009;33:1024–8.

11. Scott B, Deeg HJ. Hemopoietic cell transplantation as curative therapy of myelodysplastic syndromes and myeloproliferative disorders. Best Pract Res Clin Haematol 2006;19:519–22.

12. Deeg HJ, Storer B, Slattery JT, et al. Conditioning with targeted busulfan and cyclophosphamide for hemopoietic stem cell transplantation from related and unrelated donors in patients with myelodysplastic syndrome. Blood 2002;100:1201–7.

13. de Lima M, Anagnostopoulos A, Munsell M, et al. Nonablative versus reduced-intensity conditioning regimens in the treatment of acute myeloid leukemia and high-risk myelodysplastic syndrome: dose is relevant for long-term disease control after allogeneic hematopoietic stem cell transplantation. Blood 2004; 104:865–72.

14. Deeg HJ. Hematopoietic cell transplantation for myelodysplastic syndrome and myeloproliferative disorders. In: Appelbaum FR, Forman SJ, Negrin RS, et al, editors. Thomas' hematopoietic cell transplantation. Oxford, UK: Wiley-Blackwell; 2009. p. 827–44.

15. de Lima M, Giralt S. Allogeneic transplantation for the elderly patient with acute myelogenous leukemia or myelodysplastic syndrome [review]. Semin Hematol 2006;43:107–17.

16. de Witte T, Hermans J, Vossen J, et al. Haematopoietic stem cell transplantation for patients with myelo-dysplastic syndromes and secondary acute myeloid leukaemias: a report on behalf of the Chronic Leukaemia Working Party of the European Group for Blood and Marrow Transplantation (EBMT). Br J Haematol 2000;110:620–30.

17. Sierra J, Pérez WS, Rozman C, et al. Bone marrow transplantation from HLA-identical siblings as treatment for myelodysplasia. Blood 2002;100:1997–2004.

18. Welniak LA, Blazar BR, Murphy WJ. Immunobiology of allogeneic hematopoietic stem cell transplantation [review]. Annu Rev Immunol 2007;25:139–70.

19. Yu J, Venstrom JM, Liu XR, et al. Breaking tolerance to self, circulating natural killer cells expressing inhibitory KIR for non-self HLA exhibit effector function after T cell-depleted allogeneic hematopoietic cell transplantation. Blood 2009;113:3875–84.

20. Ruggeri L, Capanni M, Urbani E, et al. Effectiveness of donor natural killer cell alloreactivity in mismatched hematopoietic transplants. Science 2002;295: 2097–100.

21. Bacigalupo A, Ballen K, Rizzo D, et al. Defining the intensity of conditioning regimens: working definitions. Biol Blood Marrow Transplant 2009;15:1628–33.

22. Deeg HJ, Maris MB, Scott BL, et al. Optimization of allogeneic transplant conditioning: not the time for dogma. Leukemia 2006;20:1701–5.

23. Baron F, Sandmaier BM. Current status of hematopoietic stem cell transplantation after nonmyeloablative conditioning. Curr Opin Hematol 2005;12: 435–43.
24. Valcarcel D, Martino R. Reduced intensity conditioning for allogeneic hematopoietic stem cell transplantation in myelodysplastic syndromes and acute myelogenous leukemia [review]. Curr Opin Oncol 2007;19:660–6.
25. de Witte T, Brand R, van Biezen A, et al. Allogeneic stem cell transplantation for patients with refractory anaemia with matched related and unrelated donors: delay of the transplant is associated with inferior survival. Br J Haematol 2009;146:627–36.
26. Castro-Malaspina H, Harris RE, Gajewski J, et al. Unrelated donor marrow transplantation for myelodysplastic syndromes: outcome analysis in 510 transplants facilitated by the National Marrow Donor Program. Blood 2002; 99:1943–51.
27. Laport GG, Sandmaier BM, Storer BE, et al. Reduced-intensity conditioning followed by allogeneic hematopoietic cell transplantation for adult patients with myelodysplastic syndrome and myeloproliferative disorders. Biol Blood Marrow Transplant 2008;14:246–55.
28. Kawase T, Matsuo K, Kashiwase K, et al. HLA mismatch combinations associated with decreased risk of relapse: implications for the molecular mechanism. Blood 2009;113:2851–8.
29. Michalek J, Collins RH, Durrani HP, et al. Definitive separation of graft-versus-leukemia- and graft-versus-host-specific CD4+ T cells by virtue of their receptor beta loci sequences. Proc Natl Acad Sci U S A 2003;100:1180–4.
30. Warlick ED, Cioc A, DeFor T, et al. Allogeneic stem cell transplantation for adults with myelodysplastic syndromes: importance of pretransplant disease burden. Biol Blood Marrow Transplant 2009;15:30–8.
31. Ramakrishnan A, Deeg HJ. Allogeneic hematopoietic cell transplantation for patients with myelodysplastic syndrome and myeloproliferative disorders. In: Soiffer RJ, editor. Hematopoietic stem cell transplantation. Totowa (NJ): Humana Press; 2008. p. 167–82.
32. Rocha V, Locatelli F. Searching for alternative hematopoietic stem cell donors for pediatric patients [review]. Bone Marrow Transplant 2008;41:207–14.
33. Petersdorf EW. Hematopoietic cell transplantation from unrelated donors. In: Appelbaum FR, Forman SJ, Negrin RS, et al, editors. Thomas' hematopoietic cell transplantation. Oxford (UK): Wiley-Blackwell; 2009. p. 675–91.
34. Brunstein CG, Weisdorf DJ. Future of cord blood for oncology uses. Bone Marrow Transplant; prepublished online 5 October; 2009. DOI:10.1038/bmt.2009.286.
35. Aversa F. Haploidentical haematopoietic stem cell transplantation for acute leukaemia in adults: experience in Europe and the United States [review]. Bone Marrow Transplant 2008;41:473–81.
36. Luznik L, O'Donnell PV, Symons HJ, et al. HLA-haploidentical bone marrow transplantation for hematologic malignancies using nonmyeloablative conditioning and high-dose, post-transplantation cyclophosphamide. Biol Blood Marrow Transplant 2008;14:641–50.
37. Koh LP, Chao NJ. Umbilical cord blood transplantation in adults using myeloablative and nonmyeloablative preparative regimens [review]. Biol Blood Marrow Transplant 2004;10:1–22.
38. Kelly SS, Sola CB, de Lima M, Ex vivo expansion of cord blood. Bone Marrow Transplant 9999; pre-published online 5 October 2009. DOI:10.1038/bmt.2009.284.

39. Barker JN, Weisdorf DJ, Defor TE, et al. Transplantation of 2 partially HLA-matched umbilical cord blood units to enhance engraftment in adults with hematologic malignancy. Blood 2005;105:1343–7.

40. Delaney C, Gutman JA, Appelbaum FR. Cord blood transplantation for haematological malignancies: conditioning regimens, double cord transplant and infectious complications [review]. Br J Haematol 2009;147:207–16.

41. Lee J-H, Lee J-H, Lim S-N, et al. Allogeneic hematopoietic cell transplantation for myelodysplastic syndrome: prognostic significance of pre-transplant IPSS score and comorbidity. Bone Marrow Transplant 9999; pre-published online 10 August 2009. DOI:10.1038/bmt.2009.190.

42. Armand P, Kim HT, Cutler CS, et al. A prognostic score for patients with acute leukemia or myelodysplastic syndromes undergoing allogeneic stem cell transplantation. Biol Blood Marrow Transplant 2008;14:28–35.

43. Alessandrino EP, Della Porta MG, Bacigalupo A, et al. WHO classification and WPSS predict posttransplantation outcome in patients with myelodysplastic syndrome: a study from the Gruppo Italiano Trapianto di Midollo Osseo (GITMO). Blood 2008;112:895–902.

44. Kantarjian H, O'Brien S, Ravandi F, et al. Proposal for a new risk model in myelodysplastic syndrome that accounts for events not considered in the original International Prognostic Scoring System. Cancer 2008;113:1351–61.

45. Breccia M, Cannella L, Stefanizzi C, et al. WPSS versus simplified myelodysplastic syndrome risk score: which is the best tool for prediction of survival in myelodysplastic patients? Leuk Res 2009;33:e93–4.

46. Oliansky DM, Antin JH, Bennett JM, et al. The role of cytotoxic therapy with hematopoietic stem cell transplantation in the therapy of myelodysplastic syndromes: an evidence-based review. Biol Blood Marrow Transplant 2009;15:137–72.

47. Armand P, Kim HT, DeAngelo DJ, et al. Impact of cytogenetics on outcome of de novo and therapy-related AML and MDS after allogeneic transplantation. Biol Blood Marrow Transplant 2007;13:655–64.

48. Armand P, Deeg HJ, Kim HT, et al. Multicenter validation study of a transplantation-specific cytogenetics grouping scheme for patients with myelodysplastic syndromes. Bone Marrow Transplant; pre-published online 28 September 2009. DOI:10.1038/bmt.2009.253.

49. Scott BL, Wells DA, Loken MR, et al. Validation of a flow cytometric scoring system as a prognostic indicator for posttransplantation outcome in patients with myelodysplastic syndrome. Blood 2008;112:2681–6.

50. Stetler-Stevenson M, Arthur DC, Jabbour N, et al. Diagnostic utility of flow cytometric immunophenotyping in myelodysplastic syndrome. Blood 2001;98:979–87.

51. Wells DA, Benesch M, Loken MR, et al. Myeloid and monocytic dyspoiesis as determined by flow cytometric scoring in myelodysplastic syndrome correlates with the IPSS and with outcome after hemopoietic stem cell transplantation. Blood 2003;102:394–403.

52. Mills KI, Kohlmann A, Williams PM, et al. Microarray-based classifiers and prognosis models identify subgroups with distinct clinical outcomes and high risk of AML transformation of myelodysplastic syndrome. Blood 2009;114:1063–72.

53. Kataoka K, Nannya Y, Hangaishi A, et al. Influence of pretransplantation serum ferritin on non-relapse mortality after myeloablative and nonmyeloablative

allogeneic hematopoietic stem cell transplantation. Biol Blood Marrow Transplant 2009;15:195–204.

54. Maradei SC, Maiolino A, de Azevedo AM, et al. Serum ferritin as risk factor for sinusoidal obstruction syndrome of the liver in patients undergoing hematopoietic stem cell transplantation. Blood 2009;114:1270–5.

55. Lee JW, Kang HJ, Kim EK, et al. Effect of iron overload and iron-chelating therapy on allogeneic hematopoietic SCT in children. Bone Marrow Transplant; pre-published online 27 April 2009. DOI:10.1038/bmt.2009.88.

56. Busca A, Falda M, Manzini P, et al. Iron overload in patients receiving allogeneic hematopoietic stem cell transplantation: quantification of iron burden by super-conducting quantum interference device (SQUID) and therapeutic effectiveness of phlebotomies. Biol Blood Marrow Transplant; pre-published online 18 September 2009. DOI:10.1016/j.bbmt.2009.09.011.

57. Mahindra A, Bolwell B, Sobecks R, et al. Elevated pretransplant ferritin is associated with a lower incidence of chronic graft-versus-host disease and inferior survival after myeloablative allogeneic haematopoietic stem cell transplantation. Br J Haematol 2009;146:310–6.

58. Cazzola M, Della Porta MG, Malcovati L. Clinical relevance of anemia and transfusion iron overload in myelodysplastic syndromes [review]. Hematology Am Soc Hematol Educ Program 2008;166–75.

59. Armand P, Kim HT, Cutler CS, et al. Prognostic impact of elevated pretransplantation serum ferritin in patients undergoing myeloablative stem cell transplantation. Blood 2007;109:4586–8.

60. Sucak GT, Yegin ZA, Ozkurt ZN, et al. The role of liver biopsy in the workup of liver dysfunction late after SCT: is the role of iron overload underestimated? Bone Marrow Transplant 2008;42:461–7.

61. Strasser SI, Kowdley KV, Sale GE, et al. Iron overload in bone marrow transplant recipients. Bone Marrow Transplant 1998;22:167–73.

62. Scott BL, Storer BE, Greene JE, et al. Marrow fibrosis as a risk factor for post-transplant outcome in patients with advanced MDS or AML with multilineage dysplasia. Biol Blood Marrow Transplant 2007;13:345–54.

63. Marcondes M, Deeg HJ. Hematopoietic cell transplantation for patients with myelodysplastic syndromes (MDS): when, how and for whom? Best Pract Res Clin Haematol 2008;21:67–77.

64. Ma X, Does M, Raza A, et al. Myelodysplastic syndromes: incidence and survival in the United States. Cancer 2007;109:1538–42.

65. Sorror M, Storer B, Sandmaier BM, et al. Hematopoietic cell transplantation-co-morbidity index and Karnofsky performance status are independent predictors of morbidity and mortality after allogeneic nonmyeloablative hematopoietic cell transplantation. Cancer 2008;112:1992–2001.

66. Charlson ME, Pompei P, Ales KL, et al. A new method of classifying prognostic comorbidity in longitudinal studies: development and validation. J Chronic Dis 1987;40:373–83.

67. Farina L, Bruno B, Patriarca F, et al. The hematopoietic cell transplantation co-morbidity index (HCT-CI) predicts clinical outcomes in lymphoma and myeloma patients after reduced-intensity or non-myeloablative allogeneic stem cell transplantation. Leukemia 2009;23:1131–8.

68. Kataoka K, Nannya Y, Ueda K, et al. Differential prognostic impact of pretransplant comorbidity on transplant outcomes by disease status and time from transplant: a single Japanese transplant centre study Bone Marrow Transplant; pre-published online 17 August 2009. DOI:10.1038/bmt.2009.194.

69. Guilfoyle R, Demers A, Bredeson C, et al. Performance status, but not the hematopoietic cell transplantation comorbidity index (HCT-CI), predicts mortality at a Canadian transplant center. Bone Marrow Transplant 2009;43:133–9.

70. Runde V, de Witte T, Arnold R, et al. Bone marrow transplantation from HLA-identical siblings as first-line treatment in patients with myelodysplastic syndromes: early transplantation is associated with improved outcome. Chronic Leukemia Working Party of the European Group for Blood and Marrow Transplantation. Bone Marrow Transplant 1998;21:255–61.

71. Cutler CS, Lee SJ, Greenberg P, et al. A decision analysis of allogeneic bone marrow transplantation for the myelodysplastic syndromes: delayed transplantation for low-risk myelodysplasia is associated with improved outcome. Blood 2004;104:579–85.

72. Kindwall-Keller T, Isola LM. The evolution of hematopoietic SCT in myelodysplastic syndrome [review]. Bone Marrow Transplant 2009;43:597–609.

73. Al Ali HK, Brand R, van Biezen A, et al. A retrospective comparison of autologous and unrelated donor hematopoietic cell transplantation in myelodysplastic syndrome and secondary acute myeloid leukemia: a report on behalf of the Chronic Leukemia Working Party of the European Group for Blood and Marrow Transplantation (EBMT). Leukemia 2007;21:1945–51.

74. Howe CWS, Radde-Stepaniak T. Hematopoietic cell donor registries. In: Thomas ED, Blume KG, Forman SJ, editors. Hematopoietic cell transplantation. Boston: Blackwell Science; 1999. p. 503–12.

75. Karanes C, Nelson GO, Chitphakdithai P, et al. Twenty years of unrelated donor hematopoietic cell transplantation for adult recipients facilitated by the National Marrow Donor Program [review]. Biol Blood Marrow Transplant 2008;14:8–15.

76. Hirv K, Bloch K, Fischer M, et al. Prediction of duration and success rate of unrelated hematopoietic stem cell donor searches based on the patient's HLA-DRB1 allele and DRB1-DQB1 haplotype frequencies. Bone Marrow Transplant 2009; 44:433–40.

77. Maris MB, Sandmaier BM, Storer BE, et al. Allogeneic hematopoietic cell transplantation after fludarabine and 2 Gy total body irradiation for relapsed and refractory mantle cell lymphoma. Blood 2004;104:3535–42.

78. Scott BL, Storer B, Loken M, et al. Pretransplantation induction chemotherapy and posttransplantation relapse in patients with advanced myelodysplastic syndrome. Biol Blood Marrow Transplant 2005;11:65–73.

79. Yakoub-Agha I, de La Salmonière P, Ribaud P, et al. Allogeneic bone marrow transplantation for therapy-related myelodsyplastic syndrome and acute myeloid leukemia: a long-term study of 70 patients-report of the French Society of bone marrow transplantation. J Clin Oncol 2000;18:963–71.

80. Nakai K, Kanda Y, Fukuhara S, et al. Value of chemotherapy before allogeneic hematopoietic stem cell transplantation from an HLA-identical sibling donor for myelodysplastic syndrome. Leukemia 2005;19:396–401.

81. de Lima M, Couriel D, Thall PF, et al. Once-daily intravenous busulfan and fludarabine: clinical and pharmacokinetic results of a myeloablative, reduced-toxicity conditioning regimen for allogeneic stem cell transplantation in AML and MDS. Blood 2004;104:857–64.

82. Pidala J, Kim J, Field T, et al. Infliximab for managing steroid-refractory acute graft-versus-host disease. Biol Blood Marrow Transplant 2009;15:1116–21.

83. De Padua SL, de Lima M, Kantarjian H, et al. Feasibility of allo-SCT after hypomethylating therapy with decitabine for myelodysplastic syndrome. Bone Marrow Transplant 2009;43:839–43.

84. Alyea EP, Kim HT, Ho V, et al. Impact of conditioning regimen intensity on outcome of allogeneic hematopoietic cell transplantation for advanced acute myelogenous leukemia and myelodysplastic syndrome. Biol Blood Marrow Transplant 2006;12:1047–55.

85. Martino R, Iacobelli S, Brand R, et al. Retrospective comparison of reduced-intensity conditioning and conventional high-dose conditioning for allogeneic hematopoietic stem cell transplantation using HLA-identical sibling donors in myelodysplastic syndromes. Blood 2006;108:836–46.

86. Scott BL, Sandmaier BM, Storer B, et al. Myeloablative vs nonmyeloablative allogeneic transplantation for patients with myelodysplastic syndrome or acute myelogenous leukemia with multilineage dysplasia: a retrospective analysis. Leukemia 2006;20:128–35.

87. Maris M, Storb R. The transplantation of hematopoietic stem cells after non-myeloablative conditioning: a cellular therapeutic approach to hematologic and genetic diseases. Immunol Res 2003;28:13–24.

88. Platzbecker U, Ehninger G, Schmitz N, et al. Reduced-intensity conditioning followed by allogeneic hematopoietic cell transplantation in myeloid diseases [review]. Ann Hematol 2003;82:463–8.

89. Sorror ML, Maris MB, Storb R, et al. Hematopoietic cell transplantation (HCT)-specific comorbidity index: a new tool for risk assessment before allogeneic HCT. Blood 2005;106:2912–9.

90. Sorror M, Maris M, Baron F, et al. A modified hematopoietic cell transplantation (HCT)-specific co-morbidity index [abstract #1146]. Blood 2004;104(Part 1): 324a–5a.

91. Guardiola P, Runde V, Bacigalupo A, et al. Retrospective comparison of bone marrow and granulocyte colony-stimulating factor-mobilized peripheral blood progenitor cells for allogeneic stem cell transplantation using HLA identical sibling donors in myelodysplastic syndromes. Blood 2002;99:4370–8.

92. Pidala J, Anasetti C, Kharfan-Dabaja MA, et al. Decision analysis of peripheral blood versus bone marrow hematopoietic stem cells for allogeneic hematopoietic cell transplantation. Biol Blood Marrow Transplant 2009;15:1415–21.

93. Pulsipher MA, Chitphakdithai P, Miller JP, et al. Adverse events among 2408 unrelated donors of peripheral blood stem cells: results of a prospective trial from the National Marrow Donor Program. Blood 2009;113:3604–11.

94. Eapen M, Logan BR, Confer DL, et al. Peripheral blood grafts from unrelated donors are associated with increased acute and chronic graft-versus-host disease without improved survival. Biol Blood Marrow Transplant 2007;13: 1461–8.

95. Rocha V, Gluckman E. Improving outcomes of cord blood transplantation: HLA matching, cell dose and other graft- and transplantation-related factors. Br J Haematol 2009;147:262–74.

96. Ooi J. The efficacy of unrelated cord blood transplantation for adult myelodysplastic syndrome. Leuk Lymphoma 2006;47:599–602.

97. Harrison SJ, Cook G, Nibbs RJ, et al. Immunotherapy of multiple myeloma: the start of a long and tortuous journey [review]. Expert Rev Anticancer Ther 2006;6: 1769–85.

98. Chang CK, Storer BE, Scott BL, et al. Hematopoietic cell transplantation in patients with myelodysplastic syndrome or acute myeloid leukemia arising from myelodysplastic syndrome: similar outcomes in patients with de novo disease and disease following prior therapy or antecedent hematologic disorders. Blood 2007;110:1379–87.

99. Lim ZY, Ho AY, Ingram W, et al. Outcomes of alemtuzumab-based reduced intensity conditioning stem cell transplantation using unrelated donors for myelodysplastic syndromes. Br J Haematol 2006;135:201–9.

100. Bacher U, Zander AR, Haferlach T, et al. Minimal residual disease diagnostics in myeloid malignancies in the post transplant period [review]. Bone Marrow Transplant 2008;42:145–57.

101. Diez-Campelo M, Perez-Simon JA, Perez J, et al. Minimal residual disease monitoring after allogeneic transplantation may help to individualize post-transplant therapeutic strategies in acute myeloid malignancies. Am J Hematol 2009;84:149–52.

102. Warlick ED, O'Donnell PV, Borowitz M, et al. Myeloablative allogeneic bone marrow transplant using T cell depleted allografts followed by post-transplant GM-CSF in high-risk myelodysplastic syndromes. Leuk Res 2008;32:1439–47.

103. Campregher PV, Gooley T, Scott BL, et al. Results of donor lymphocyte infusions for relapsed myelodysplastic syndrome after hematopoietic cell transplantation. Bone Marrow Transplant 2007;40:965–71.

104. Rizzieri DA, Koh LP, Long GD, et al. Partially matched, nonmyeloablative allogeneic transplantation: clinical outcomes and immune reconstitution. J Clin Oncol 2007;25:690–7.

105. Spitzer TR. Haploidentical stem cell transplantation: the always present but overlooked donor. Hematology Am Soc Hematol Educ Program 2005;390–5.

106. Depil S, Deconinck E, Milpied N, et al. Donor lymphocyte infusion to treat relapse after allogeneic bone marrow transplantation for myelodysplastic syndrome. Bone Marrow Transplant 2004;33:531–4.

107. Kang Y, Chao NJ, Aversa F. Unmanipulated or CD34 selected haplotype mismatched transplants [review]. Curr Opin Hematol 2008;15:561–7.

108. Lim ZY, Pearce L, Ho AY, et al. Delayed attainment of full donor chimaerism following alemtuzumab-based reduced-intensity conditioning haematopoietic stem cell transplantation for acute myeloid leukaemia and myelodysplastic syndromes is associated with improved outcomes Br J Haematol; 2007 138:517–526. DOI:10.1111/j.1365–2141.2007.06676.x.

109. Shaw BE, Mufti GJ, Mackinnon S, et al. Outcome of second allogeneic transplants using reduced-intensity conditioning following relapse of haematological malignancy after an initial allogeneic transplant. Bone Marrow Transplant 2008; 42:783–9.

110. de Witte T, Oosterveld M, Muus P. Autologous and allogeneic stem cell transplantation for myelodysplastic syndrome [review]. Blood Rev 2007;21:49–59.

111. Oosterveld M, Suciu S, Verhoef G, et al. The presence of an HLA-identical sibling donor has no impact on outcome of patients with high-risk MDS or secondary AML (sAML) treated with intensive chemotherapy followed by transplantation: results of a prospective study of the EORTC, EBMT, SAKK and GIMEMA Leukemia Groups (EORTC study 06921). Leukemia 2003;17:859–68.

Novel Therapies for Myelodysplastic Syndromes

David P. Steensma, MD

KEYWORDS

- Myelodysplastic syndromes • Histone deacetylase inhibitors
- Clofarabine • Ezatiostat • Farnesyltransferase inhibitors
- Laromustine

The myelodysplastic syndromes (MDS), a diverse collection of neoplastic disorders characterized by marrow failure and a risk of clonal progression, were long considered an unexciting backwater of hematology practice, because of a lack of effective therapies other than supportive care or allogeneic stem cell transplantation.[1] However, United States Food and Drug Administration (FDA) approval of three drugs for MDS-related indications (azacitidine [Vidaza] in 2004; lenalidomide [Revlimid] in 2005; and decitabine [Dacogen] in 2006), followed by a 2007 report that azacitidine treatment improves median survival of higher-risk patients with MDS by 9 months, began to change the biomedical community's perceptions of these difficult disorders.[2–5]

No longer are MDS viewed solely with a sense of therapeutic nihilism. Today, more than 300 clinical trials, using more than 50 experimental compounds, are actively recruiting patients with MDS to improve patients' quality of life and alter the natural history of disease (**Box 1**). Other studies of novel compounds and combinations of drugs have recently completed enrollment and results will soon be reported, while additional biologically interesting molecules are in late preclinical stages of development.[6,7]

Despite a new sense of optimism and an exciting flurry of investigative activity, the therapeutic gains achieved have been modest. Even the encouraging 9-month median increase in survival with azacitidine treatment still represents less than 5% of the 15.4-year life expectancy for a 65-year-old American man without MDS.[8] Furthermore, the clinical, cytogenetic, and molecular heterogeneity of MDS, and the high proportion of patients with these syndromes who are elderly and frail, remain challenging obstacles to rapid clinical trial accrual and successful drug development. Much about MDS pathobiology remains mysterious, which impedes development of targeted therapies;

Dr Steensma has participated in advisory boards for Genzyme, Eisai, and Celgene.
Department of Hematologic Malignancies, Dana-Farber Cancer Institute, 44 Binney Street, Suite D1B30, Boston, MA 02115, USA
E-mail address: david_steensma@dfci.harvard.edu

Hematol Oncol Clin N Am 24 (2010) 423–441
doi:10.1016/j.hoc.2010.02.010   hemonc.theclinics.com
0889-8588/10/$ – see front matter © 2010 Elsevier Inc. All rights reserved.

Box 1
Clinical trials currently recruiting patients with myelodysplastic syndromes

Trials using FDA-approved agents for MDS-related indications, either alone or in combination

Azacitidine

    Monotherapy (including an oral formulation): four trials

    With histone deacetylases (HDAC) inhibitors (vorinostat, valproate, panobinostat, belinostat, MS-275): six trials

    With lenalidomide: two trials

    With thalidomide: one trial

    With chemotherapy: one trial

    With bortezomib: one trial

Decitabine

    Monotherapy (including an oral formulation): four trials

    With HDAC inhibitors: two trials

    With gemtuzumab: one trial

    With clofarabine: one trial

    With lenalidomide: one trial

    With arsenic and vitamin C: one trial

    With tretinoin: one trial

    With cytotoxic chemotherapy: one trial

Lenalidomide

    Monotherapy: eight trials

    With or without epoetin alfa: one trial

    With romiplostim: one trial

    With stem cell factor: one trial

    With vaccine: three trials

Iron chelation with deferasirox or deferoxamine: seven trials

Trials using drugs that are FDA-approved for conditions other than MDS

Alemtuzumab + cyclosporine A: one trial

Arsenic trioxide + vitamin C: one trial

ATG + cyclosporine A: two trials

Bendamustine: one trial

Bevacizumab: one trial

Bexarotene: one trial

Bortezomib, alone or in combinations other than with azacitidine: three trials

Calcitriol + dexamethasone: one trial

Clofarabine

    Monotherapy: six trials

    With decitabine or cytarabine: two trials

Cytotoxic chemotherapy: two trials

    With HDAC inhibitor: two trials

    With tipifarnib or gemtuzumab: one trial

Dasatinib: one trial

Eltrombopag: two trials

Erythropoiesis-stimulating agents (monotherapy): four trials

Everolimus (RAD001)

    Monotherapy: one trial

    With PKC412 (protein kinase C inhibitor): one trial

Romiplostim

    Monotherapy: two trials

    With lenalidomide: one trial

Sorafenib

    Monotherapy: two trials

    With chemotherapy: two trials

    With clofarabine: one trial

    With vorinostat: one trial

Vorinostat monotherapy: one trial

Trials using HDAC inhibitor monotherapy (other than vorinostat)

    Belinostat: one trial

    JNJ-26481585: one trial

    NVP-LBH 589: three trials

    SNDX-275 (MS-275): two trials

Trials using agents not yet FDA approved for any condition

ABT-888 [PARP inhibitor] + chemotherapy: one trial

Afibercept [anti-VEGF agent]: one trial

ARRY-614 [multikinase inhibitor]: one trial

AT9283 [Aurora kinase inhibitor]: one trial

Cediranib (AZD2171) [VEGF inhibitor]: one trial

CP-4055 [cytarabine prodrug]: one trial

DB-67 (AR-67) [camptothecin]: two trials

Ezatiostat (TLK199) [glutathione S1 analog]: one trial

Gimatecan (ST1481) [topoisomerase inhibitor]: one trial

GTI-2040 [ribonucleotide reductase antisense oligonucleotide]: one trial

HuM195 [humanized anti-CD33 antibody]: two trials

IMC-A12 [IGF-1R monoclonal antibody] + temsirolimus: one trial

INCB018424 [JAK2 inhibitor]: one trial

Laromustine (cloretazine) [novel alkylator] + cytarabine: one trial

MLN4924 [Nedd8 activating enzyme inhibitor]: one trial

MLN8237 [Aurora kinase inhibitor]: one trial

MultiStemA [manufactured stem cell product]: one trial

NOV-002 [chemoprotectant]: one trial

ON 01910.Na [cyclin D1 inhibitor]: five trials

PF-04449913 [Hedgehog inhibitor]: one trial

Sapacitabine (CYC682) [nucleoside analog]: one trial

SB1518 [JAK2 inhibitor]: one trial

SNS-595 [topoisomerase II inihibitor and DNA damage causing agent]: one trial

STA-9090 [Hsp90 inhibitor]: one trial

TAK-901 [Aurora kinase inhibitor]: one trial

Tipifarnib [farnesyltransferase inhibitor]: one trial

UCN-01 [staurosporine analog] + perifosine [modulator of membrane permeability]: one trial

Vaccine approaches (nontransplant): 11 trials

Data from www.clinicaltrials.gov. Accessed August 27, 2009.

Of 432 trials returned by a search for "Recruiting," "Investigational," and "MDS," 91 trials were excluded because they were recruiting only patients with diseases other than with MDS, or were testing supportive therapies not designed to alter blood counts or the underlying condition (eg, massage therapy, bisphosphonates, or antiemetics). Additionally, 96 trials studying various aspects of stem cell transplantation (eg, conditioning regimens, stem cell product manipulation, and maintenance approaches) are not listed here.

even the precise mechanisms of action of the three FDA-approved medications are currently unclear.

This article discusses five different types of agents currently undergoing clinical trials in MDS: (1) histone deacetylase inhibitors; (2) the purine nucleoside clofarabine; (3) the glutathione S-transferase analog ezatiostat (TLK199); (4) the novel alkylating agent laromustine (cloretazine); and (5) the farnesyltransferase inhibitor tipifarnib. This sample is by no means comprehensive, but these classes of agents are representative of contemporary developmental therapeutic approaches to MDS. Most of these medications have also been studied in patients with acute myeloid leukemia (AML), and AML data are discussed later. Trial results in patients with myeloproliferative neoplasms are beyond the scope of the present discussion, however, because the clinical problems encountered in patients with myeloproliferative neoplasms, such as primary myelofibrosis (eg, splenomegaly, constitutional symptoms, and thrombohemorrhagic events), are less common in MDS.

HISTONE DEACETYLASE INHIBITORS
Histone Modification and Biologic Effects

Octamers of histone proteins are the chief protein component of chromatin. Histones play an important structural role in the eukaryotic nucleus, binding DNA with a similar topology to a spool wound with thread. Yet, histones are not merely inert DNA packaging material: they are dynamic proteins, undergoing numerous posttranslational modifications, including methylation, acetylation, ubiquitination, phosphorylation, and SUMOylation (modifications collectively called the "histone code"), which can result in changes in the accessibility of associated DNA to transcription, and alter interactions of the nucleosome with chromatin-associated proteins.[9–11]

One of the most important histone posttranslational modifications is acetylation of lysine residues of histone subunit H3.[12] Acetylation at lysine residues 9 or 14 (ie, K9 and K14) can result in transcriptional activation of the DNA associated with the acetylated histone; such acetylation is catalyzed by histone lysine acetyltransferases (KATs). In contrast, acetyl groups are removed by histone deacetylases (HDACs), of which there are four classes with at least 11 enzyme members, with both class-specific and enzyme-specific biologic effects.[11,13-15]

Although there is no direct evidence yet of specific regions of pathologic histone deacetylation in MDS, clinical success in MDS with the methylation modifiers azacitidine and decitabine led investigators to consider the therapeutic possibilities of alteration of HDAC activity also, because histone acetylation and DNA hypomethylation are coupled and alter gene expression in a complementary manner.[6,12,16] In a perhaps naive view (but potentially a correct one, at least in part), inhibition of HDACs could shift the balance in favor of KAT enzyme activity, resulting in increased histone acetylation and consequent increased transcriptional activity of tumor suppressor genes, thereby eliminating neoplastic cells that are dependent on transcriptional silencing of tumor suppressors.[7,10,17]

The reality is almost certainly more complex. Despite their name, HDACs have a number of nonhistone protein targets for deacetylation, including nuclear and cytoplasmic proteins that regulate processes altered in neoplasia, such as apoptosis, differentiation, and cell proliferation.[6,18] As for azacitidine and decitabine, which inhibit DNA methyltransferases and act by epigenetic mechanisms (See the article by Jean-Pierre Issa elsewhere in this issue for further exploration of this topic.), but also damage DNA in a fashion similar to traditional cytotoxic drugs, any therapeutic effects of HDAC inhibitors should not be attributed to reawakening silenced tumor suppressors without convincing evidence. In addition, transcriptional profiling experiments indicate that expression of only a small proportion of genes (<5%) is altered by HDAC inhibition, raising further questions about whether the most likely clinical effect of this class of drugs is a result of changing gene expression, or something else.[15]

HDAC Inhibitors as a Drug Class

Pharmaceutical companies have developed a number of HDAC inhibitors with varying potency and chemical structural class (**Table 1**), and dozens of clinical trials with these agents are currently enrolling patients with hematologic malignancies or solid tumors.[14] Some compounds inhibit specific HDAC enzymes, such as entinostat (SNDX-275/MS-275) or MGCD0103 (MethylGene), which selectively inhibit only class I HDACs (ie, HDACs 1, 2, 3, and 8). Other agents, such as panobinostat (NVP-LBH589), inhibit HDACs more broadly.[15] It is not clear whether class specificity is a desirable property of an HDAC inhibitor, but it is possible that inhibition of certain classes of enzyme and not others could alter the repertoire of cytoplasmic proteins modified, and effect the adverse event profile.[6] In clinical trials, most HDAC inhibitors have been associated with gastrointestinal side effects, severe fatigue, and thrombocytopenia as the most common treatment-related adverse events. QTc monitoring is also recommended, although clinically significant QTc prolongation has proved uncommon.

Vorinostat (suberoylanilide hydroxamic acid, Zolinza) was the first, HDAC inhibitor to receive formal regulatory approval; the FDA licensed vorinostat in 2006 for treatment of patients with cutaneous T-cell lymphoma.[18] Romidepsin was approved for the same indication in November 2009. Investigators have also "repurposed" as HDAC inhibitors several drugs that were originally developed and approved for other indications, after those drugs were serendipitously found during screening programs to have HDAC inhibitory activity. Examples include valproic acid, an anticonvulsant, and sodium phenylbutyrate, an agent used to treat patients with congenital urea cycle disorders.

Table 1
HDAC inhibitors in clinical trials in neoplasia

HDAC Inhibitor	Sponsor	Chemical Class	Data in MDS or AML?
Valproic acid[a]	Multiple suppliers	Branched short-chain fatty acid	Yes, Phase II
Sodium phenylbutyrate and phenylacetate[a]	Ucyclyd	Aromatic short-chain fatty acid	Yes, Phase II
AN-9/ pivaloyloxymethyl butyrate[b]	Titan	Aliphatic short-chain fatty acid	No
FK228/FR901228/ depsipeptide/ romidepsin	Gloucester (now part of Celgene)	Tetrapeptide	Yes, Phase II
ITF2357/givinostat	Italfarmaco	Hydroxamic acid	No
JNJ-26481585	Centocor OrthoBiotech	Hydroxamic acid	No
NVP-LBH589/ panobinostat	Novartis	Hydroxamic acid	Yes, Phase I/II
NVP-LAQ824/ dacinostat	Novartis	Hydroxamic acid	No
PCI-24781	Pharmacyclics	Hydroxamic acid	No
PXD101/belinostat	Curagen and Topotarget A/S	Hydroxamic acid	Yes, Phase II
SAHA/vorinostat[a]	Merck	Hydroxamic acid	Yes, Phase II
CI-994/ N-acetyldinaline	Pfizer	Benzamide	No
MGCD0103[c]	MethylGene	Benzamide	Yes, Phase I/II
SNDX-275/MS-275/ entinostat	Syndax	Benzamide	Yes, Phase I; Phase III ongoing

[a] As of this writing, SAHA/vorinostat and romidepsin are the only HDAC inhibitors to have achieved Food and Drug Administration approval for treatment of a neoplasm: cutaneous T-cell lymphoma. Sodium phenylbutyrate and sodium phenylacetate (Buphenyl and Ammonul) are marketed as orphan drugs, but for hyperammonemia related to urea cycle disorders rather than neoplasia. Valproic acid is used as an anticonvulsant and mood-stabilizing agent.
[b] Development discontinued because of adverse events.
[c] Partial clinical hold since August 2008 because of pericardial effusion adverse event.

The drug development strategy pursued by different HDAC inhibitor sponsors has varied, depending on preclinical signals and marketing considerations. Some developmental programs are focusing on solid tumors or, given the success of vorinostat in cutaneous T-cell lymphoma, on lymphoproliferative disorders. Other sponsors, having noted the success of azacitidine and decitabine for MDS, are performing trials in the MDS and AML settings (most trials to date have enrolled both higher-risk MDS and AML patients). Agents for which there are at least preliminary data in MDS and AML include entinostat; belinostat (PXD101); romidepsin (FK228/FR901229/depsipepide); panobinostat; MGCD0103; valproic acid; and sodium phenylbutyrate.

Entinostat (SNDX-275/MS-275)
A Phase I study of oral entinostat in 38 patients with acute leukemia found that the maximum tolerated dose (MTD) was 8 mg/m^2 administered once weekly for 4 weeks every 6 weeks.[19] Adverse events included somnolence, unsteady gait (the

dose-limiting toxicity [DLT]), and severe fatigue; gastrointestinal side effects, hypoalbuminemia, and hypocalcemia were also observed. No objective clinical responses were seen, however, indicating that entinostat has limited activity as monotherapy in leukemia.

In May 2009, the Eastern Cooperative Oncology Group (ECOG) suspended accrual to intergroup Phase III protocol ECOG E1905 after the study met its initial target enrollment of at least 152 patients. In the E1905 protocol, patients with higher-risk MDS, chronic myelomonocytic leukemia (CMML) with a white blood count less than 12 × 10^9/L, or AML with trilineage dysplasia and white blood count less than 30 × 10^9/L were randomized to receive either azacitidine at a nonstandard dose of 50 mg/m^2 subcutaneously daily for 10 days every 28 days, or subcutaneous azacitidine using that same nonstandard schedule plus oral entinostat, 4 mg/m^2, on days 3 and 10 of each treatment cycle. Because single-agent activity of HDAC inhibitors in MDS may be limited, this study will answer the important question of whether HDAC inhibitors might instead augment response to hypomethylating agents. In a Phase I study of 27 patients with MDS, AML, or CMML that used the same azacitidine-entinostat combination used in E1905, 12 patients responded, including two complete remissions.[20] Results of the E1905 study are expected by 2010.

Belinostat (PXD101)

After a Phase I study in patients with solid tumors identified the MTD of belinostat as 1000 mg/m^2 administered intravenously once daily over 30 minutes for 5 consecutive days every 21 days, another Phase I belinostat study enrolled 16 patients with advanced hematologic malignancies (none had MDS or leukemia).[21] This study identified fatigue and neurotoxicity as the most common treatment-related adverse events; no formal tumor responses were seen, but two patients with multiple myeloma developed transient tumor lysis and associated grade 4 renal insufficiency.

The National Cancer Institute–sponsored Phase 2 Consortium recently suspended accrual to a Phase II study of belinostat that was enrolling patients with MDS-associated cytopenias whose disease had failed to respond to azacitidine. There were no complete or partial responses meeting International Working Group MDS response criteria. As with entinostat, belinostat seems to have limited efficacy as a single agent in MDS; however, it is still possible that these agents might have a role in combination therapy.

Romidepsin (FK228/depsipeptide)

In a Phase II study of 12 patients, 9 with AML and 3 with MDS, romidepsin was administered intravenously at a dose of 18 mg/m^2 on day 1 and day 5 every 21 days, the MTD that had been identified in solid tumor studies with romidepsin.[22] The investigators observed no consistent changes in histone acetylation in primary cells after romidepsin use. One patient with AML experienced a complete response. Recurrent adverse events included febrile neutropenia, thrombocytopenia, nausea, and asymptomatic hypophosphatemia.

The authors of the report of this Phase II study, in a commendably honest admission (particularly in view of the lamentable contemporary tendency to describe any nonlethal regimen as "well-tolerated," and all regimens as "worthy of further study" regardless of response rate) concluded, "depsipeptide monotherapy has limited clinical activity in unselected AML/MDS patients." On November 5, 2009, romidepsin was approved by the US FDA for the treatment of cutaneous T cell lymphoma.

Panobinostat (NVP-LBH589)

A Phase I/II study of oral panobinostat in advanced hematologic malignancies identified 60 mg administered once weekly as the MTD in patients with AML, with the DLT being fatigue (drug-associated grade 4 thrombocytopenia and neutropenia were also common).[23] Among 26 evaluable patients at the time of a preliminary report of that study (65 patients with AML were enrolled), there were two complete responses. A case report described a patient with AML who experienced tumor lysis syndrome during panobinostat monotherapy.[24] Panobinostat data in patients with MDS have not yet been reported. As for some other HDAC inhibitors, thrombocytopenia may make it difficult to combine panobinostat with azacitidine or decitabine in MDS.

Valproic acid

Valproic acid specifically inhibits HDAC2. In most studies of valproic acid used as a HDAC inhibitor, the dose has been adjusted to achieve serum concentrations of 50 to 100 μg/mL, equivalent to 0.347 to 0.694 mM, levels at which HDAC inhibition is present (concentrations of >0.25 mM increase histone H4 acetylation), but not maximal (HDAC inhibition is "massive" at concentrations of 2 mM).[25] The main limitation of valproic acid as an antineoplastic agent is that in doses required to attain sustained levels associated with robust HDAC inhibition, neurotoxicity can be problematic.[26] For instance, in a Phase II study of MDS-CMML using valproic acid plus 13-*cis*-retinoic acid and 1,25-dihydroxyvitamin D, 8 (42%) of 19 enrolled patients had to discontinue therapy because of adverse events, whereas only 3 patients (16%) experienced a measurable response.[27]

In a Phase II study of 75 patients with MDS, AML, or CMML treated with valproic acid (initially as monotherapy in 66 patients, followed by all-*trans*-retinoic acid as a potential differentiating agent in nonresponders), 1 patient achieved a complete response, 1 achieved a partial response, and 12 patients achieved a major erythroid response (19% overall response rate).[28] Overall, the adverse events with doses used in this study were mild, with four patients developing tremor and three patients experiencing reversible thrombocytopenia. The specific contribution of all-*trans*-retinoic acid to the observed responses is unclear. A 26-patient Phase II trial of the same drug combination in patients with poor-risk leukemia resulted in no complete responses.[29]

Valproic acid has also been used in combination with decitabine and azacitidine. In a Phase I/II study of 54 patients with MDS (N = 10) or leukemia, 8 patients (15%) responded to a decitabine and valproic acid combination for a median of 7 months.[30] These responses were associated with an increase in histone H3 and H4 acetylation. The contribution of the decitabine alone to the responses, however, is unclear. A randomized study of 67 evaluable patients with MDS, AML, or CMML attempted to isolate the effect of the valproic acid by comparing decitabine at a dose of 20 mg/m² daily for 5 consecutive days every 28 days with the same decitabine regimen plus valproic acid.[26] There was no significant difference in the response rate in the decitabine monotherapy arm compared with the combined therapy arm, and neurotoxicity was common in the arm that included valproic acid. In a Phase II trial of the combination of azacitidine and valproic acid, which enrolled 62 patients with MDS or CMML, the response rate observed was not higher than the rate expected with azacitidine alone.[31]

Sodium phenylbutyrate

Sodium phenylacetate has HDAC inhibitory properties, but is rarely used clinically because of its musky, foul odor (it can be isolated from the defensive glands of the aptly named stinkpot turtle). Sodium phenylbutyrate is a less offensive prodrug of sodium phenylacetate.

A pilot study enrolled 23 patients with AML or MDS, and administered sodium phenylbutyrate by continuous intravenous infusion for 7 days out of 14, or 21 consecutive days out of 28.[32] Two patients achieved hematologic improvement, and the DLT was somnolence. In a small Phase II study that enrolled eight patients with AML and two with MDS, standard 7-day subcutaneous injections of azacitidine, followed by 5 days of sodium phenylbutyrate given intravenously at a dose of 200 mg/kg/d, led to partial response or stable disease in five patients.[33] Most (>80%) patients experienced somnolence and injection site reactions. Histone H4 reacetylation did not correlate with clinical response.

Because of the inconvenient administration schedules required to achieve biologically effective serum concentrations, sodium phenylbutyrate is not being developed further as an HDAC inhibitor in MDS.

MGCD0103

A Phase I study of oral MGCD0103 enrolled 29 patients with either MDS (N = 7) or AML (N = 22) and determined that the MTD for this agent is 60 mg/m^2 administered three times weekly.[34] Three patients (10%) in this Phase I study experienced reduction in marrow blasts to less than 5%, whereas DLTs included fatigue and gastrointestinal effects (nausea, vomiting, or diarrhea). Drug-induced histone acetylation was detected, and was dose dependent.

Subsequently, a Phase I/II study enrolled 37 evaluable patients with MDS (N = 6) or AML (N = 31) and combined a standard azacitidine schedule with MGCD0103.[35] When used in combination, the MTD of MGCD0103 was found to be 90 mg/m^2 administered three times weekly, slightly higher than the MTD determined in the monotherapy Phase I trial. Eleven patients (30%) experienced a response, including nine complete responses, with or without hematopoietic recovery. This complete response rate is somewhat higher than might be expected with azacitidine alone, but numbers of treated patients are small.

A follow-up randomized study of azacitidine with or without MGCD0103 was planned, but unfortunately an adverse event of hemodynamically significant pericardial effusion led the FDA to put a partial clinical hold on the development of this agent in August 2008, preventing accrual of new patients to open clinical studies. Shortly thereafter, the drug's sponsor, Celgene, who had acquired the agent when purchasing Pharmion in March 2008, terminated a collaborative agreement with MethylGene, so that MethylGene reacquired the rights to MGCD0103.[20,36] As of this writing, the FDA hold is still in effect, and the developmental future of this compound is uncertain.

Vorinostat

The reason that vorinostat and other HDAC inhibitors are clinically active in T-cell lymphoma is unclear. It is possible that the clinical effects of vorinostat may not result from HDAC activity, but may be a consequence of acetylation of cytoplasmic proteins instead.

In a Phase I study of oral vorinostat enrolling 31 patients with AML and 3 with MDS, the MTD was determined to be 200 mg twice daily or 250 mg three times daily.[37] DLTs included fatigue and gastrointestinal side effects; grade 3 or 4 thrombocytopenia was seen in 12% of patients. Four complete responses were seen, including two with incomplete hematopoietic recovery, all in patients with AML.

There is also preliminary experience with vorinostat used in combination with decitabine, albeit exclusively in AML. In a Phase I study of sequential dosing of 5-day intravenous decitabine schedules and 14-day oral vorinostat in 30 evaluable patients with relapsed or refractory leukemia, one patient experienced a brief complete remission (5 weeks), and four patients enjoyed a reduction in bone marrow blast proportion.[38]

Summary: HDAC Inhibitors

The HDAC inhibitors seem to have limited single-agent activity in MDS. Combination regimens are currently considered more promising. Given the potential of some HDAC inhibitors to cause thrombocytopenia, their use in combination with other cytopenia-inducing agents, such as azacitidine or decitabine, must be approached cautiously, and may ultimately limit the use of this class of drugs.

The sequence of administration of HDAC inhibitors relative to other agents may also be important. For example, in vitro data indicate that administering azacitidine before the HDAC inhibitor entinostat maximizes biologic synergy, whereas administration of entinostat followed by azacitidine is less effective.[20] These schedule questions will also have to be addressed in clinical trials.

CLOFARABINE

Clofarabine (Clolar and Evoltra) is a halogenated purine nucleoside analog with structural similarities to both cladribine and fludarabine (**Fig. 1**), drugs that are FDA-approved for hairy cell leukemia and as a second-line treatment for chronic lympho-cytic leukemia, respectively. Both fludarabine and cladribine have some activity in myeloid neoplasms. Fludarabine has been used for patients with poor-risk AML or higher-risk MDS as part of the FLAG-idarubicin induction regimen, whereas cladribine can reduce splenomegaly in myeloproliferative neoplasms, and reports of two recent provocative large Phase III studies from a Polish cooperative group indicated that add-ing cladribine to the standard 7 + 3 induction therapy for AML improved both remis-sion rates and overall survival, compared with 7 + 3 alone.[39–41]

The proposed mechanism of action of clofarabine in neoplasia includes not just incorporation into DNA with induction of apoptosis, but also inhibition of ribonucleo-tide reductase and DNA synthesis.[42] Clofarabine was approved by the FDA in 2004 for relapsed-refractory acute lymphoblastic leukemia in children. The approved pedi-atric dose, a 2-hour intravenous infusion of 52 mg/m^2 daily for 5 consecutive days, has been too toxic in adults, where tolerable administered doses have typically ranged from 30 to 40 mg/m^2 daily for 5 consecutive days.

As with many myelosuppressive cytotoxic drugs, there is more information available about clofarabine's effects in AML than in MDS. The most recent and promising results in the AML setting are from the CLASSIC II study, which enrolled 112 patients with higher-risk AML, including 36% with an antecedent pre-AML hematologic disorder. The overall response rate in the CLASSIC II study was 46%, with 38% complete responses and 8% complete responses with incomplete platelet recovery.[43] During the first 30 days of treatment, 9.8% of patients died. Adverse effects included grade 4 neutropenia in 46% of patients, thrombocytopenia in 67%, and febrile neutro-penia in 39%; nonhematologic events included nausea (62%, mostly grade 1 or 2); diarrhea; hepatotoxicity; and nephrotoxicity. Grade 3 or higher elevations of bilirubin occurred in 12 patients (11%); hepatic transaminases in 23%; and creatinine in 6%.

Based on these results, clofarabine's sponsor, Genzyme, has applied to the FDA for regulatory approval to expand the clofarabine label to include treatment of elderly patients with AML. On September 1, 2009, the agency's Oncology Drugs Advisory Committee (ODAC) voted nine to three in favor of requiring randomized controlled trial data before approval of an expanded clofarabine label, with the three dissenting members being the three hematologists on the ODAC panel.[44] The optimal control therapy for a clofarabine randomized trial in AML is unclear, because there is currently no widely accepted standard of care for patients who are elderly or have serious comorbidities, and who are not candidates for the usual 7 + 3 induction regimen.

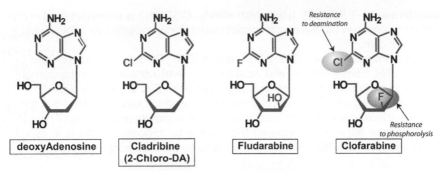

| deoxyAdenosine | Cladribine (2-Chloro-DA) | Fludarabine | Clofarabine |

Fig. 1. Comparison of clofarabine structure with other purine nucleoside analogs. The chlorine molecule at position 2 of the imidazole ring prevents deamination, whereas the fluorine molecule attached to the ribose sugar prevents degradation by purine nucleoside phosphorylase and stabilizes the compound. (*Data from* Secrist JA 3rd, Shortnacy AT, Montgomery JA. Synthesis and biological evaluations of certain 2-halo-2'-substituted derivatives of 9-beta-D-arabinofuranosyladenine. J Med Chem 1988;31:405–10; and Montgomery JA, Shortnacy-Fowler AT, Clayton SD, et al. Synthesis and biologic activity of 2'-fluoro-2-halo derivatives of 9-beta-D-arabinofuranosyladenine. J Med Chem 1992;35:397–40.)

The MD Anderson Cancer Center enrolled 61 patients with higher-risk MDS or CMML on a randomized Phase II study of intravenous versus oral clofarabine; 64% of enrolled patients had been failed by previous hypomethylating agent therapy.[45] Among the 24 evaluable patients in the oral clofarabine arm, most of whom received 30 mg/m²/d orally for 5 days every 4 to 6 weeks, 9 patients (37%) achieved a complete response, with or without platelet recovery, using AML response criteria rather than MDS criteria. For the 36 evaluable patients who received intravenous clofarabine, the complete response rate was similar at 44%. Six patients died on study because of infections; all were on the intravenous arm. Seven patients developed acute renal failure.

A clinical trial led by the author of this article, and a similar clinical trial conducted at the University of Utah, used extended dosing oral clofarabine, administered at a low doses ($\leq$5 mg/day) for 10 or 14 consecutive days. Unfortunately, the 14-day study closed because of prolonged thrombocytopenia in the first two cohorts enrolled, and thrombocytopenia requiring dose reduction was also seen in the 10-day study, so a shorter-course oral regimen, such as that used by the MD Anderson investigators, seems more attractive for future studies.

Cladribine and especially fludarabine are commonly used in reduced-intensity stem cell transplantation condition regimens. In a pilot study in patients with MDS and AML, however, a transplant conditioning regimen of intravenous clofarabine (40 mg/m²/d for 5 consecutive days) with cytarabine and antithymocyte globulin was not sufficiently myelosuppressive to ensure donor cell engraftment.[46] The study was closed after three of the first seven patients enrolled died within 32 days of stem cell infusion. A conditioning regimen combining clofarabine with melphalan and alemtuzumab caused unexpected renal toxicity, but a transplant conditioning regimen combining clofarabine with busulfan seems more promising.[47–49]

EZATIOSTAT (TLK199)

Ezatiostat (TLK199, TER199, Telintra) is a glutathione analog that exerts biologic effects by indirect activation of Jun-N-terminal kinase (JNK). Ezatiostat's principal metabolites are TLK 235, TLK236, and TLK117; TLK117 binds to glutathione

S-transferase P1-1 (GST P1-1) with high affinity. GST P1-1 is overexpressed in many neoplasms, and may have important growth regulatory properties by its binding to and inhibition of JNK.[50,51]

TLK117 interaction with GST P1-1 causes GST P1-1 to dissociate from JNK, releasing JNK from inhibition and activating it, with consequent enhancement of growth and maturation of hematopoietic progenitors (**Fig. 2**); notably, GST P1-1 null mice have leukocytosis.[52] At least one cell line experiment has suggested that chronic exposure of leukemia cells to ezatiostat can result in growth potentiation of neoplastic cells, but other experiments indicate that ezatiostat triggers apoptosis in leukemic cells, or induces sensitivity of transformed cells to differentiating agents.[51–53]

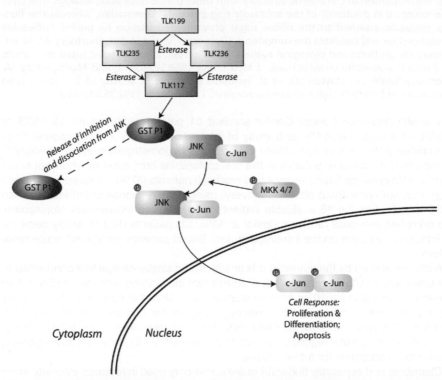

Fig. 2. Mechanism of action of ezatiostat (TLK199). Ezatiostat (TLK199) is a prodrug that undergoes de-esterification to TLK235 and TLK236, and subsequently additional de-esterification to TLK117, the active metabolite. TLK117 selectively binds to and inhibits glutathione S transferase π (GST P1), facilitating dissociation of GST P1 from Jun kinase (JNK), which is in turn bound to c-Jun. JNK is phosphorylated and activated, potentially by MAPK kinases 4 and 7 (MKK 4/7). JNK then phosphorylates c-Jun, which dimerizes and translocates to the nucleus. Phosphorylated c-Jun also dimerizes with c-Fos (not shown) to form the AP-1 early response transcription factor. Activated c-Jun, either as homodimer or heterodimer with c-Fos, has diverse cellular effects, including alteration of rates of cell growth and differentiation, and (with prolonged activation) increased apoptosis. (*Data from* Raza A, Galili N, Callander N, et al. Phase 1-2a multicenter dose-escalation study of ezatiostat hydrochloride liposomes for injection (Telintra(R), TLK199), a novel glutathione analog prodrug in patients with myelodysplastic syndrome. J Hematol Oncol 2009;2:20; and McIlawin CC, Townsend DM, Tew KD. Glutathione S-transferase polymorphisms: cancer incidence and therapy. Oncogene 2006;25:1639–48.)

A Phase I/II study explored intravenous liposomal ezatiostat in 54 patients with MDS, using a variety of doses and schedules.[52] Trilineage responses were observed in 4 (25%) of 16 patients who had trilineage cytopenias, whereas erythroid hematologic improvement was observed in 9 (24%) of 38 evaluable anemic patients, neutrophil improvement in 11 (42%) of 26 neutropenic patients, and platelet improvement in 12 (50%) of 24 thrombocytopenic patients. Most adverse events were mild, and were potentially attributable to the liposomal preparation (eg, back pain, chills, nausea, bone pain, and diarrhea) rather than ezatiostat.

The sponsor of ezatiostat, Telik, has also developed an oral preparation of this agent. In a Phase I study of oral ezatiostat in 45 patients with lower-risk MDS, daily doses of up to 6000 mg of ezatiostat tablets days 1 to 7 of a 21-day cycle were tolerated without development of a DLT.[50] Seventeen hematologic responses were observed, most at the higher end of the dose range. Adverse events were low-grade and almost all gastrointestinal: nausea (65% of patients); diarrhea (43%); vomiting (31%); constipation (13%); and abdominal pain (9%). A Phase II trial of ezatiostat in MDS is ongoing, and a Phase III trial is planned. Combination approaches could also be considered, especially because ezatiostat can revert the multidrug resistance phenotype in vitro.[54]

LAROMUSTINE (CLORETAZINE)

Laromustine (cloretazine, VNP40101M, Onrigin) is a sulfonylhydrazine prodrug for 90CE, a chloroethylating agent that alkylates DNA guanine bases at the O6 position.[55] What is unique about laromustine compared with other alkylators is that intracellular metabolism of 90CE releases methyl isocyanate, which inhibits O6-alkyl-guanine transferase, preventing repair of the specific type of DNA damage caused by 90CE.

As for clofarabine, there are more data on laromustine in the AML setting than in patients with MDS. A multicenter Phase II study of laromustine enrolled patients 60 years of age or older with previously untreated de novo AML (N = 44), secondary AML (N = 45), or high-risk MDS (N = 15), and administered laromustine as a single 600 mg/m² intravenous infusion.[56] A second induction was allowed for patients without evidence of clinical progression or complete remission, and a consolidation cycle of laromustine, 400 mg/m² intravenously, was administered to responders. Adverse events were similar to those expected for AML induction chemotherapy, with a 30-day mortality of 18%. Overall, 28% of patients achieved complete response, and 4% had a complete response with incomplete platelet recovery. A study of laromustine in 44 evaluable patients with relapsed AML less than 12 months after an initial remission, however, showed almost no activity, with a 4% complete remission rate and 9% 30-day mortality in this very high-risk patient group.[57]

Laromustine has also been combined with cytarabine in the acute leukemia setting, but there are no trials of this combination in MDS specifically. In a Phase I study that enrolled 37 evaluable patients with treatment-refractory leukemia, the MTD was determined to be 600 mg/m² of laromustine, combined with 1.5 g/m²/d of a continuous infusion of cytarabine for 3 days.[58] In the combination study, the complete response rate was 27%.

Laromustine was reviewed by the ODAC of the FDA on September 1, 2009, for potential approval for treatment of elderly patients with AML. The panel voted 13 to 0 to recommend randomized clinical trial data before consideration of FDA approval of laromustine, and the panel also expressed concern about busulfan-like pulmonary toxicity observed in a subset of patients.[36] Because the drug's sponsor, Vion, declared bankruptcy in December 2009 the future of this compound is uncertain.

TIPIFARNIB

Tipifarnib (R115777, Zarnestra) is one of two farnesyltransferase inhibitors currently in development; the other is lonafarnib (SCH66336, Sarasar), which is primarily being studied in patients with solid tumors. Farnesyltransferase is an enzyme that is important for membrane attachment of the Ras oncogene; constitutive Ras activation and Ras overactivity contributes to cell proliferation and survival in a wide variety of neoplasms, including some patients with AML or MDS (especially those with secondary, treatment-related disease).[59,60] A number of cell lines, including those that lack Ras mutations, are sensitive to farnesyltransferase inhibitors. Presumably, inhibition of farnesylation of other proteins besides Ras accounts for these compounds' activity in cells with wild-type Ras. Among other non–Ras-related biologic activities, tipifarnib and lonafarnib inhibit the P-glycoprotein multidrug resistance gene product.[60]

In 2005, tipifarnib's sponsor, Johnson and Johnson, applied for regulatory approval for tipifarnib to treat patients with AML over age 65, but this application was denied by the FDA. Development of this compound in myeloid neoplasms, however, including MDS, continues. In a Phase II study of oral tipifarnib, administered to 27 evaluable patients with MDS at a dose of 600 mg twice daily for 4 weeks out of every 6-week cycle, three patients (11%) responded, two complete responses and one partial response.[61] The most common adverse events included myelosuppression, rash, fatigue, and gastrointestinal upset; dose reduction to 300 mg twice daily was required in 41% of patients. A follow-up multicenter Phase II study reported in 2007 enrolled 82 patients with higher-risk MDS, who received tipifarnib 300 mg orally twice daily for 21 days of each 28-day cycle.[62] Using International Working Group criteria, there were 12 (15%) complete responses, and 14 (17%) of patients experienced hematologic improvements. The drug was also active in higher-risk MDS when given in an alternate-week schedule.[63]

A small study of lonafarnib in 12 evaluable patients with MDS showed no responses.[64]

SUMMARY

The results demonstrate that a broad range of intracellular pathways are potential therapeutic targets in MDS. Although HDAC inhibitors seem to have limited activity in MDS and AML when used as single agents, their activity in combination regimens continues to be explored. Because thrombocytopenia has been seen in Phase I/II trials with most HDAC inhibitors, this adverse event may be especially problematic when combining HDAC inhibitors with hypomethylating drugs. Platelet support with the new thrombopoietin agonists (eltrombopag and romiplostim) is one possible way of addressing this limitation. A variety of doses and schedules need to be tested to find the optimal combination. If the results of the ECOG E1905 study are negative, enthusiasm for studying HDAC inhibitors in MDS may diminish.

Clofarabine and laromustine are active cytotoxic drugs in AML and probably also in higher-risk MDS. Both agents experienced a developmental setback, however, at FDA ODAC meetings in September 2009. In currently used doses and schedules, these two agents are likely to be used primarily in higher-risk MDS patients and in those patients with AML who are not good candidates for 7 + 3 induction regimen. For example, in MDS, cytoreduction of patients with excess blasts, especially before stem cell transplantation, is a potential role for these agents. ODAC made it clear that randomized clinical trial data are necessary for either drug to achieve regulatory approval in the United States, but the optimal comparison therapy for a randomized trial in AML or

MDS is not clear. Approval in AML alone may be important, because it may open the door for off-label use in higher-risk MDS, especially if a compendium listing is achieved.

Ezatiostat seems to be well-tolerated as chronic therapy and may be useful for improving cytopenias in a subset of lower-risk MDS patients. Because of the ezatiostat drug mechanism augmenting JNK/c-Jun signaling, careful assessment of rates of AML emergence seems prudent, although safety concerns have not emerged in Phase I and Phase II testing.

Finally, tipifarnib is an active agent in higher-risk MDS and AML, but faces a challenging regulatory approval process given the denial of approval for elderly AML in 2005. The relative infrequency of Ras mutations in MDS is not a serious obstacle, because responses to farnesyltransferase inhibitors have been seen in patients with wild-type Ras. Given the degree of myelosuppression associated with tipifarnib, it seems that high-risk patients refractory to other agents is the optimal MDS group to treat with this drug.

ACKNOWLEDGMENTS

I thank Daniel DeAngelo, MD, PhD, for helpful review of the manuscript.

REFERENCES

1. Steensma DP, Bennett JM. The myelodysplastic syndromes: diagnosis and treatment. Mayo Clin Proc 2006;81:104.
2. Fenaux P, Mufti GJ, Hellstrom-Lindberg E, et al. Efficacy of azacitidine compared with that of conventional care regimens in the treatment of higher-risk myelodysplastic syndromes: a randomised, open-label, phase III study. Lancet Oncol 2009;10:223.
3. Kantarjian H, Issa JP, Rosenfeld CS, et al. Decitabine improves patient outcomes in myelodysplastic syndromes: results of a phase III randomized study. Cancer 2006;106:1794.
4. List A, Dewald G, Bennett J, et al. Lenalidomide in the myelodysplastic syndrome with chromosome 5q deletion. N Engl J Med 2006;355:1456.
5. Silverman LR, Demakos EP, Peterson BL, et al. Randomized controlled trial of azacitidine in patients with the myelodysplastic syndrome: a study of the cancer and leukemia group B. J Clin Oncol 2002;20:2429.
6. Gore SD, Hermes-DeSantis ER. Future directions in myelodysplastic syndrome: newer agents and the role of combination approaches. Cancer Control 2008; 15(Suppl):40.
7. Griffiths EA, Gore SD. DNA methyltransferase and histone deacetylase inhibitors in the treatment of myelodysplastic syndromes. Semin Hematol 2008;45:23.
8. Anonymous. Life expectancy in the United States. Centers for Disease Control. Available at: http://www.cdc.gov/nchs/data/hus/hus08.pdf. Accessed August 30, 2009.
9. Godde JS, Ura K. Cracking the enigmatic linker histone code. J Biochem 2008; 143:287.
10. Lawless MW, Norris S, O'Byrne KJ, et al. Targeting histone deacetylases for the treatment of disease. J Cell Mol Med 2009;13:826.
11. Santini V, Gozzini A, Ferrari G. Histone deacetylase inhibitors: molecular and biological activity as a premise to clinical application. Curr Drug Metab 2007;8:383.
12. Yang XJ, Seto E. Lysine acetylation: codified crosstalk with other posttranslational modifications. Mol Cell 2008;31:449.

13. Kortenhorst MS, Carducci MA, Shabbeer S. Acetylation and histone deacetylase inhibitors in cancer. Cell Oncol 2006;28:191.
14. Moradei O, Vaisburg A, Martell RE. Histone deacetylase inhibitors in cancer therapy: new compounds and clinical update of benzamide-type agents. Curr Top Med Chem 2008;8:841.
15. Stimson L, Wood V, Khan O, et al. HDAC inhibitor-based therapies and haematological malignancy. Ann Oncol 2009;20:1293.
16. Figueroa ME, Skrabanek L, Li Y, et al. MDS and secondary AML display unique patterns and abundance of aberrant DNA methylation. Blood 2009;114(16): 3448–58.
17. Kuendgen A, Lubbert M. Current status of epigenetic treatment in myelodysplastic syndromes. Ann Hematol 2008;87:601.
18. Cang S, Ma Y, Liu D. New clinical developments in histone deacetylase inhibitors for epigenetic therapy of cancer. J Hematol Oncol 2009;2:22.
19. Gojo I, Jiemjit A, Trepel JB, et al. Phase 1 and pharmacologic study of MS-275, a histone deacetylase inhibitor, in adults with refractory and relapsed acute leukemias. Blood 2007;109:2781.
20. Gore SD, Jiemjit A, Silverman LB, et al. Combined methyltransferase/histone deacetylase inhibition with 5-azacitidine and MS-275 in patients with MDS, CMMoL and AML: clinical response, histone acetylation and DNA damage. ASH Annual Meeting Abstracts 2006;108:517.
21. Gimsing P, Hansen M, Knudsen LM, et al. A phase I clinical trial of the histone deacetylase inhibitor belinostat in patients with advanced hematological neoplasia. Eur J Haematol 2008;81:170.
22. Klimek VM, Fircanis S, Maslak P, et al. Tolerability, pharmacodynamics, and pharmacokinetics studies of depsipeptide (romidepsin) in patients with acute myelogenous leukemia or advanced myelodysplastic syndromes. Clin Cancer Res 2008;14:826.
23. Ottmann OG, Spencer A, Prince HM, et al. Phase IA/II study of oral panobinostat (lbh589), a novel pan- deacetylase inhibitor (DACi) demonstrating efficacy in patients with advanced hematologic malignancies. ASH Annual Meeting Abstracts 2008;112:958.
24. Kalff A, Shortt J, Farr J, et al. Laboratory tumor lysis syndrome complicating LBH589 therapy in a patient with acute myeloid leukemia. ASH Annual Meeting Abstracts 2006;108:4554.
25. Gottlicher M, Minucci S, Zhu P, et al. Valproic acid defines a novel class of HDAC inhibitors inducing differentiation of transformed cells. EMBO J 2001;20:6969.
26. Issa JP, Castoro R, Ravandi-Kashani F, et al. Randomized phase ii study of combined epigenetic therapy: decitabine vs. decitabine and valproic acid in MDS and AML. ASH Annual Meeting Abstracts 2008;112:228.
27. Siitonen T, Timonen T, Juvonen E, et al. Valproic acid combined with 13-cis retinoic acid and 1,25-dihydroxyvitamin D3 in the treatment of patients with myelodysplastic syndromes. Haematologica 2007;92:1119.
28. Kuendgen A, Knipp S, Fox F, et al. Results of a phase 2 study of valproic acid alone or in combination with all-trans retinoic acid in 75 patients with myelodysplastic syndrome and relapsed or refractory acute myeloid leukemia. Ann Hematol 2005;84(Suppl 13):61.
29. Bug G, Ritter M, Wassmann B, et al. Clinical trial of valproic acid and all-trans retinoic acid in patients with poor-risk acute myeloid leukemia. Cancer 2005;104:2717.
30. Garcia-Manero G, Kantarjian HM, Sanchez-Gonzalez B, et al. Phase 1/2 study of the combination of 5-aza-2'-deoxycytidine with valproic acid in patients with leukemia. Blood 2006;108:3271.

31. Voso MT, Santini V, Finelli C, et al. Valproic acid at therapeutic plasma levels may increase 5-azacytidine efficacy in higher risk myelodysplastic syndromes. Clin Cancer Res 2009;15:5002.
32. Gore SD, Weng LJ, Figg WD, et al. Impact of prolonged infusions of the putative differentiating agent sodium phenylbutyrate on myelodysplastic syndromes and acute myeloid leukemia. Clin Cancer Res 2002;8:963.
33. Maslak P, Chanel S, Camacho LH, et al. Pilot study of combination transcriptional modulation therapy with sodium phenylbutyrate and 5-azacytidine in patients with acute myeloid leukemia or myelodysplastic syndrome. Leukemia 2006;20:212.
34. Garcia-Manero G, Assouline S, Cortes J, et al. Phase 1 study of the oral isotype specific histone deacetylase inhibitor MGCD0103 in leukemia. Blood 2008;112:981.
35. Garcia-Manero G, Yang AS, Klimek V, et al. Phase I/II study of MGCD0103, an oral isotype-selective histone deacetylase (HDAC) inhibitor, in combination with 5-azacitidine in higher-risk myelodysplastic syndrome (MDS) and acute myelogenous leukemia (AML). ASH Annual Meeting Abstracts 2007;110:444.
36. Anonymous. Methylgene press release October 27, 2008. Available at: http://www.fiercebiotech.com/press-releases/methylgene-reacquires-rights-mgcd0103-celgene-implements-plan-focus-development-propr. Accessed February 17, 2010.
37. Garcia-Manero G, Yang H, Bueso-Ramos C, et al. Phase 1 study of the histone deacetylase inhibitor vorinostat (suberoylanilide hydroxamic acid [SAHA]) in patients with advanced leukemias and myelodysplastic syndromes. Blood 2008;111:1060.
38. Ravandi F, Faderl S, Thomas D, et al. Phase I study of suberoylanilide hydroxamic acid (SAHA) and decitabine in patients with relapsed, refractory or poor prognosis leukemia. ASH Annual Meeting Abstracts 2007;110:897.
39. Faoro LN, Tefferi A, Mesa RA. Long-term analysis of the palliative benefit of 2-chlorodeoxyadenosine for myelofibrosis with myeloid metaplasia. Eur J Haematol 2005;74:117.
40. Holowiecki J, Grosicki S, Kyrcz-Krzemien S, et al. Addition of cladribine to the standard daunorubicine - cytarabine (DA 3+7) remission induction protocol (DAC) contrary to adjunct of fludarabine (DAF) improves the overall survival in untreated adults with acute myeloid leukemia aged up to 60 Y: a multicenter, randomized, phase III PALG AML 1/2004 DAF/DAC/DA study in 673 patients. ASH Annual Meeting Abstracts 2008;112:133.
41. Parker JE, Pagliuca A, Mijovic A, et al. Fludarabine, cytarabine, G-CSF and idarubicin (FLAG-IDA) for the treatment of poor-risk myelodysplastic syndromes and acute myeloid leukaemia. Br J Haematol 1997;99:939.
42. Kantarjian HM, Jeha S, Gandhi V, et al. Clofarabine: past, present, and future. Leuk Lymphoma 1922;48:2007.
43. Erba HP, Kantarjian H, Claxton DF, et al. Phase II study of single agent clofarabine in previously untreated older adult patients with acute myelogenous leukemia (AML) unlikely to benefit from standard induction chemotherapy. ASH Annual Meeting Abstracts 2008;112:558.
44. Anonymous. FDA Advisory Committee recommends randomized trial to support proposed indication for clolar in adult AML. Genzyme Press; September 1, 2009. Available at: http://www.genzyme.com/corp/media/GENZ%20PR-090109.asp. Accessed September 22, 2009.
45. Faderl S, Garcia-Manero G, Ravandi F, et al. Oral (po) and intravenous (iv) clofarabine for patients (pts) with myelodysplastic syndrome (MDS). ASH Annual Meeting Abstracts 2008;112:222.

46. Martin MG, Uy GL, Procknow E, et al. Allo-SCT conditioning for myelodysplastic syndrome and acute myeloid leukemia with clofarabine, cytarabine and ATG. Bone Marrow Transplant 2009;44:13.

47. Andersson BS, de Lima M, Popat U, et al. Allogeneic stem cell transplantation (allo-sct) for relapsed, refractory myeloid leukemia and MDS using clofarabine (clo) +/- fludarabine (flu) with iv busulfan (bu) as conditioning therapy. Presented at the 2009 BMT Tandem Meeting. Tampa, Florida, February, 2009. [Abstract #238].

48. Magenau J, Pawarode A, Buck T, et al. Conditioning with clofarabine and busulfan x 4 (clobu4) for non-remission hematologic malignancies including AML is well tolerated, facilitates secure engraftment, and exhibits significant anti-tumor activity. Presented at the 2009 BMT Tandem Meeting. Tampa, Florida, February, 2009. [Abstract #287].

49. van Besien K, Kline J, Godley L, et al. Phase I-II study of clofarabine-melphalan-alemtuzumab conditioning for allogeneic hematopoietic cell transplantation (HCT) in patients with advanced hematologic malignancies: unexpected renal toxicity. Presented at the 2009 BMT Tandem Meeting. Tampa, Florida, February, 2009. [Abstract #290].

50. Raza A, Galili N, Smith S, et al. Phase 1 multicenter dose-escalation study of ezatiostat hydrochloride (TLK199 tablets), a novel glutathione analog prodrug, in patients with myelodysplastic syndrome. Blood 2009;113:6533.

51. Ruscoe JE, Rosario LA, Wang T, et al. Pharmacologic or genetic manipulation of glutathione S-transferase P1-1 (GSTpi) influences cell proliferation pathways. J Pharmacol Exp Ther 2001;298:339.

52. Raza A, Galili N, Callander N, et al. Phase 1-2a multicenter dose-escalation study of ezatiostat hydrochloride liposomes for injection (Telintra(R), TLK199), a novel glutathione analog prodrug in patients with myelodysplastic syndrome. J Hematol Oncol 2009;2:20.

53. Gate L, Lunk A, Tew KD. Resistance to phorbol 12-myristate 13-acetate-induced cell growth arrest in an HL60 cell line chronically exposed to a glutathione S-transferase pi inhibitor. Biochem Pharmacol 2003;65:1611.

54. O'Brien ML, Vulevic B, Freer S, et al. Glutathione peptidomimetic drug modulator of multidrug resistance-associated protein. J Pharmacol Exp Ther 1999;291:1348.

55. Pigneux A. Laromustine, a sulfonyl hydrolyzing alkylating prodrug for cancer therapy. IDrugs 2009;12:39.

56. Giles F, Rizzieri D, Karp J, et al. Cloretazine (VNP40101M), a novel sulfonylhydrazine alkylating agent, in patients age 60 years or older with previously untreated acute myeloid leukemia. J Clin Oncol 2007;25:25.

57. Giles F, Verstovsek S, Faderl S, et al. A phase II study of cloretazine (VNP40101M), a novel sulfonylhydrazine alkylating agent, in patients with very high risk relapsed acute myeloid leukemia. Leuk Res 2006;30:1591.

58. Giles F, Verstovsek S, Thomas D, et al. Phase I study of cloretazine (VNP40101M), a novel sulfonylhydrazine alkylating agent, combined with cytarabine in patients with refractory leukemia. Clin Cancer Res 2005;11:7817.

59. Feldman EJ. Farnesyltransferase inhibitors in myelodysplastic syndrome. Curr Hematol Rep 2005;4:186.

60. Medeiros BC, Landau HJ, Morrow M, et al. The farnesyl transferase inhibitor, tipifarnib, is a potent inhibitor of the MDR1 gene product, P-glycoprotein, and demonstrates significant cytotoxic synergism against human leukemia cell lines. Leukemia 2007;21:739.

61. Kurzrock R, Albitar M, Cortes JE, et al. Phase II study of R115777, a farnesyl transferase inhibitor, in myelodysplastic syndrome. J Clin Oncol 2004;22:1287.
62. Fenaux P, Raza A, Mufti GJ, et al. A multicenter phase 2 study of the farnesyltransferase inhibitor tipifarnib in intermediate- to high-risk myelodysplastic syndrome. Blood 2007;109:4158.
63. Kurzrock R, Kantarjian HM, Blascovich MA, et al. Phase I study of alternate-week administration of tipifarnib in patients with myelodysplastic syndrome. Clin Cancer Res 2008;14:509.
64. Ravoet C, Mineur P, Robin V, et al. Farnesyl transferase inhibitor (lonafarnib) in patients with myelodysplastic syndrome or secondary acute myeloid leukaemia: a phase II study. Ann Hematol 2008;87:881.

Myelodysplastic Syndromes Classification and Risk Stratification

Rami S. Komrokji, MD[a],*, Ling Zhang, MD[a], John M. Bennett, MD[b]

KEYWORDS

• FAB • World Health Organization • IPSS
• Myelodysplastic syndromes

Myelodysplastic syndromes (MDS) are bone marrow failure disorders with resultant cytopenias and a tendency to progress to acute myeloid leukemia (AML). The diagnosis of the disease requires demonstration of cytologic dysplasia in one or more of the different bone marrow cell lines.[1,2]

MDS is more than one disease or subsets of disorders with different driving biologic features that share a common pathologic phenotype "dysplasia." The classification of MDS directly reflects the understanding of the disease and it has been an evolving process over many years.

At the beginning of the past century the observation was made that a group of patients had a form of anemia refractory to available treatments at that time. The term "anemia pseudoaplastica" was one of the earliest descriptions for MDS.[3] In the late 1940s, it was thought that the disease progresses to leukemia and the term "preleukemia" was applied.[4] The definition was expanded to include multilineage cytopenia in the 1950s.[5] It not until the 1970s when Saarni and Linman[6] recognized the disease as a primary bone marrow disorder characterized by decreased hematopoietic precursor maturation and bone marrow hypercellularity. The French-American-British group (FAB) coined the term "myelodysplastic syndromes" in a series of proposals on the acute leukemias in 1976 and later expanded the FAB classification in the 1980s.[7,8] The next advancement in classification and risk stratification was in 1997 with the introduction of the International Prognostic Scoring System (IPSS).[9] Under the auspice of the World Health Organization (WHO) a distinguished panel of more than 100 hematologists and hematopathologists revised the MDS classification

[a] H. Lee Moffitt Cancer Center and Research Institute, 12902 Magnolia Drive, Tampa, FL 33612, USA
[b] James P. Wilmot Cancer Center, Strong Memorial Hospital, 601 Elmwood Avenue, Rochester, NY 14642, USA
* Corresponding author.
E-mail address: rami.komrokji@moffitt.org

Hematol Oncol Clin N Am 24 (2010) 443–457
doi:10.1016/j.hoc.2010.02.004   hemonc.theclinics.com
0889-8588/10/$ – see front matter © 2010 Elsevier Inc. All rights reserved.

and published the WHO MDS classification in 1999.[10–12] In the last decade the evolution of the classification progressed more rapidly with better technologies to understand the disease biology. New prognostic models were introduced, such as the WHO Prognostic Scoring System (WPSS),[13] and the WHO classification was refined.

In this modern era, risk stratification based more on biology is crucial. A better classification will allow the tailoring of treatments toward more homogenous groups of patients. Newer therapies may help in the exploration of underlying disease biology and enhance classification.

DIAGNOSTIC CRITERIA FOR MDS

The general recommendations for diagnosis of MDS include demonstration of cytologic dysplasia in one or more cell lines in patients with persistent or progressive cytopenia or demonstration of increased myeloblasts (5%–19%) (**Fig. 1**).[14] MDS remains a diagnosis of exclusion. In certain cases MDS diagnosis can be made without clear evidence of morphologic dysplasia, such as chronic myelomonocytic leukemia (CMML) if monocytes are persistently elevated or if a recurrent cytogenetic abnormality is detected in patients with sustained unexplained cytopenia ("presumptive MDS" by WHO 2008 criteria).

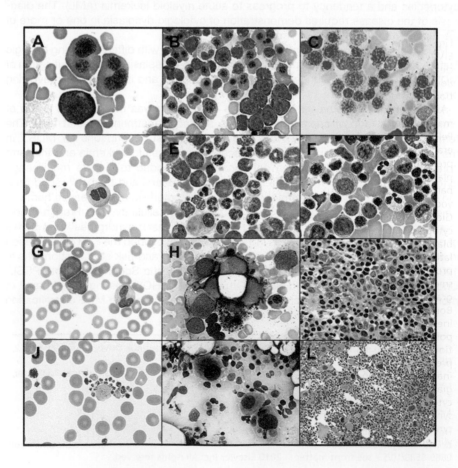

It is still recommended to perform a 500-cell differential, eliminating lymphocytes and plasma cells for the count. The dysplasia in each cell line is noted and the percentage of blasts is calculated. If the absolute percentage of erythroid precursors is 50% or greater, the percentage of blasts is based on the nonerythroid precursors. Iron stains are essential to address the percentage of ring sideroblasts. The bone marrow core biopsy could complement the bone marrow aspirate in several aspects,[1] such as cellularity; dysmegakaryopoiesis; and identifying clusters of abnormal localization of immature precursors, which are immature cells myeloblasts or promyelocytes (displaced from the paratrabecular area to the intertrabecular areas). In addition, the reticulin stain provides additional information about the degree of reticulin fibrosis, which can add prognostic information.[15] Conventional cytogenetics obtained from bone marrow aspirate could be complemented by interphase fluorescence in situ hybridization tests that could be obtained from bone marrow or peripheral blood (PB) samples.

MDS PATHOLOGIC CLASSIFICATIONS
FAB Classification

The FAB classification was the first attempt at systemic classification of the disease based on observations and understanding of the disease at that time. It was known

Fig. 1. Morphologic findings of myelodysplasia in peripheral blood and bone marrow. (*A*) Erythroid precursors displaying cytoplasmic to nuclear maturation asynchrony and multinucleation in bone marrow aspirate smear (Wright-Giemsa stain, original magnification ×). (*B*) Bone marrow aspirate with erythroid hyperplasia, left-shifted and megaloblastoid maturation, occasional nuclear budding, and binucleation (Wright-Giemsa, original magnification ×). (*C*) Numerous ringed-sideroblasts are highlighted by Prussian-blue iron stain in bone marrow aspirate (original magnification ×). (*D*) Circulating granulocytes showing pseudo–Pelger-Huët change with hyposegmentation and hypogranulation in cytoplasm in peripheral blood smear (May-Gruenwald–Giemsa, original magnification ×). (*E*) Dysmyelopoiesis presenting with hyposegmentation or hypersegmentation, abnormal distribution of cytoplasmic granules or patch loss of granules in myeloid cells, ringed formed nuclei, and giant band or metamyelocyte in bone marrow aspirate. A micomekaryocytes or "dwarf megakaryocyte" with single nucleus is also noted representative of dysmegakaryopoisis (Wright-Giemsa, original magnification ×). (*F*) Myeloid dysplasia with marked hypogranulation, cytoplasmic to nuclear maturation asynchrony with increased immature precursors-myeloblasts noted in bone marrow aspirate (Wright-Giemsa, original magnification ×). (*G*) Circulating blasts with round-to-oval nucleus, lacy chromatin, one to more than one very prominent nucleoli, and a small amount of cytoplasm are identified in peripheral blood smear. There is a single Auer rod noted in the cytoplasm of one blast. Background of hypogranulated granulocytes is present (May-Gruenwald–Giemsa, original magnification ×). (*H*) Bone marrow aspirate containing small-to-large blasts with fine chromatin, visible to prominent nucleoli and scant to some amount of basophilic cytoplasm admixed with dysplastic polychromatic normoblasts showing nuclear budding (Wright-Giemsa, original magnification ×). (*I*) Bone marrow core biopsy showing nonparatrabecular located immature myeloid precursors in cluster-abnormal localization of immature precursors (hematoxylin-eosin, original magnification ×). (*J*) Dysplastic platelets displaying variable size and shape, including giant hypogranulated platelets (original magnification ×). (*K*) Medium-sized megakaryocytes with single lobated nucleus characterized in 5q- syndrome, subtype of myelodysplastic syndrome (original magnification ×). (*L*) Representative bone marrow core biopsy of 5q-syndrome with moderately increased in single or hypolobated megakaryocytes (hematoxylin-eosin, original magnification ×).

that some patients present with a disease that bore some resemblance to AML, but did not have as many myeloblasts in the bone marrow. The disease resulted in alteration in maturation of the three major cell lines, manifesting as pancytopenia. It was also observed that the rate of disease progression was highly variable: some patients never evolved to acute leukemia, whereas others unfortunately did quickly.[7] The original FAB classification included two of the subtypes of what are now called MDS refractory anemia with excess blasts (RAEB) and CMML.[7]

In 1982, a revision of the FAB classification was published. This was based on the accumulating experience with larger number of cases reviewed and observations of different subsets, which have dysplasia as a common feature but had a distinct clinical outcome. This revision included five subgroups: (1) refractory anemia (RA), (2) refractory anemia with ring sideroblasts (RARS), (3) RAEB, (4) RAEB in transformation (RAEB-t), and (5) CMML (**Table 1**).[8]

The RA included any patient with anemia or variant cytopenias with less than 5% myeloblasts and less than 15% ring sideroblasts. The RARS group included patients who demonstrated 15% or more ring sideroblasts (iron from the Greek) where iron stains in necklace fashion around the nucleus. RARS case reports were originally described in 1956.[16] It was later noted that some patients had pure sideroblastic anemia, whereas others had dysplasia in other cell lines and in general had higher risk to transform to AML.[17] RAEB included patients with 5% to 20% myeloblasts in the bone marrow or 1% to 4% blasts on PB, whereas RAEB-t described patients with 20% to 30% myeloblasts in the bone marrow and greater than or equal to 5% blasts on PB or with presence of Auer rods. Finally, CMML was defined by persistent absolute monocytosis on PB (more than $1 \times 10^9/L$). The FAB group suggested distinguishing two CMML subtypes: myelodysplastic CMML (white blood cell [WBC] count $<13 \times 10^9/L$) and myeloproliferative CMML (WBC count $\geq 13 \times 10^9/L$).

Table 1
MDS classification

FAB	WHO	WHO 2008	Dysplasia	BM Blasts %	PB Blasts %
RA	RA	RCUD			
	MDS-U	RA	Erythroid	<5	<1
	RCMD	RN, RT	Nonerythroid	<5	<1
	Del5q MDS	RCMD	Erythroid + other	<5	<1
		Isolated del 5q	Erythroid + mega	<5	<1
		MDS-U	Unilineage + pancytopneia or RCMD/RCUD with 1% PB blasts	<5	1
RARS	RARS	RARS	Erythroid only	<5	< 1
	RCMD-RS	RCMD-RS	Erythroid + other (all >15% ring sideroblasts)	<5	< 1
RAEB	RAEB-1	RAEB-1	≥1 lineage	5–9	2–4
	RAEB-2	RAEB-2	≥1 lineage	10–19	5–19 Auer rods
RAEB-t	AML	AML	Myeloid ± other	≥20	
CMML	MDS/MPD	MDS/MPN	Variable >1 × 10⁹/L monocytosis	<20	
	CMML	CMML			
	JMML	JMML			
	aCML	BCR/Abl neg CML			
	MDS/MPD-U	MDS/MPD-U			

The FAB classification could clearly differentiate outcome between the low-risk group (RA, RARS) and high-risk group (RAEB, RAEB-t) with median overall survival ranging from 5 to 6 years for low risk compared with less than 1 year for the least favorable forms (**Fig. 2**A, B). The classification, however, had several limitations. It did not address the importance of unilineage versus multilineage dysplasia, it did not provide any role for cytogenetic classification, RAEB included a large heterogeneous category and RAEB-t represented a gray area between MDS and AML, and CMML behavior and outcome were not well characterized.

WHO Classification

The WHO classification was an attempt to address some of the shortcomings of the FAB classification creating more homogenous subtypes.[11] The following are the highlights of WHO classification (see **Table 1**).[18]

Recognition of unilineage versus multilineage dysplasia

RA and RARS were divided based on line of dysplasia. Pure RA or RARS was redefined when dysplasia is truly limited to erythroid cell line. The separate categories

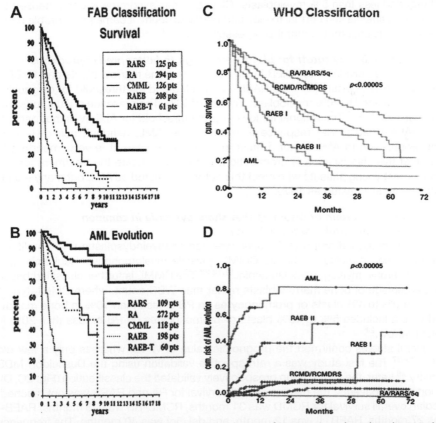

Fig. 2. Survival (*A*) and freedom (*B*) from AML evolution of MDS patients based on the FAB classification (Kaplan-Meier curves). (*C, D*) Survival and freedom from AML evolution of MDS patients related to their WHO classification subgroup (Kaplan-Meier curves). (*Modified from* Germing U, Strupp C, Kuendgen A, et al. Prospective validation of the WHO proposals for the classification of myelodysplastic syndromes. Haematologica 2006;91:1596–604. *Obtained from* Haematologica/ the Hematology Journal website http://www.haematologica.org.

refractory cytopenia with multilineage dysplasia and refractory cytopenia with multilineage dysplasia and ring sideroblasts (RCMD-RS) were added when more than 10% dysplastic changes are seen in either myeloid or megakaryocytic cell line in addition to the erythroid dysplasia.

This was based on logical observations where presence of multilineage dysplasia carries a worse prognosis even in presence of sideroblasts.[19,20] A higher frequency and different cytogenetic complexity were reported in patients with RAEB and RCMD compared with RA and RARS. The presence of cytogenetic abnormalities was noted in 39.3% in RA and RARS compared with 50.4% in RCMD patients.[21] Some studies showed the presence of clonal cell subpopulations in the PB and bone marrow of RCMD but not in RA and RARS or del(5q) patients.[22] The WHO recognized cases with unilineage or bilineage myeloid or megakaryocytic dysplasia without erythroid dysplasia but they were categorized as MDS unclassified.[11,12,23]

Introduction of cytogenetic information as first attempt of better biologic classification

The WHO classification recognized 5q syndrome as a distinct subgroup with isolated del (5q) and less than 5% myeloblasts. Clinically, this syndrome is characterized by macrocytic anemia and normal to elevated platelets count. It carries a favorable prognosis and it is uncommon that it progresses to AML.[11,12,23]

Refining the arbitrary cutoff for blasts percentage to better predict prognosis

The RAEB was divided into RAEB I with 5% to 9% bone marrow blasts and RAEB II with 10% to 19% blasts.[11,23] The RAEB-t is omitted and the threshold for diagnosing AML was lowered to 20% myeloblasts instead of 30%. The presence of Auer rods was disregarded.[11,12,23] The rational for lowering the threshold for AML was that patients with RAEB-t had similar response to treatment as AML, although acknowledging that progression to AML is not a must in each single case. It is very important to note that this classification is prognostic but does not dictate the treatment for this group; most young patients who meet this cutoff are treated as AML but many elderly patients are still treated as MDS.

Recognition of a group of disorders that share dysplasia in common but also may have proliferative behavior

This newly proposed group of diseases was named myelodysplastic-myeloproliferative disorders. It included chronic CMML, juvenile myelomonocytic leukemia, and atypical chronic myelogenous leukemia.[11,12,23] The CMML is further classified based the percentage of bone marrow blasts rather than WBC count, where CMML type 1 included 0% to 4% blasts or promonocytes on PB or less than 10% in bone marrow and type 2 included 5% to 19% blasts or promonocytes on PB or less than 20% in bone marrow.[24]

Several studies confirmed the prognostic value of WHO, whereas only a few did not.[15,25–27] The first study was a retrospective validation using the Dusseldorf MDS registry.[28] Later, the same group prospectively validated the classification (**Fig. 2**C, D). Among 1095 patients, the median overall survival for RA and RARS was not reached, median overall survival for RCMD was 31 months, RCMD-RS was 28 months, RAEB-I was 27 months, RAEB- II was 12 month, and del (5q) was 40 months. The frequency of AML progression 2 years after diagnosis was RA, 0%; RARS, 8%; RCMD, 9%; RCMD-RS, 12%; RAEB- I, 13%; RAEB- II, 40%; and 5q, 8%.[29]

The WHO introduction of multilineage dysplasia may also have therapeutic implications. Differences in response rates to erythropoietin-stimulating agents and growth factors among different WHO subtypes were reported. The response rate was 67%

in RA versus 50% in RCMD. More difference was observed between RARS (75%) and RCMD-RS (9%) (P value 0.003).[30]

Revised WHO Classification (2008)

For the first time, the WHO 2008 classification proposes diagnosis of "presumptive MDS" in cases with persistent clinical cytopenias without dysplasia if certain cytogenetic abnormalities are present. The WHO categorizes this entity under MDS-U. Although not part of the WHO classification, the term "idiopathic cytopenia of unknown significance" is applied if patients had persistent cytopenias without alternative explanation, no dysplasia, and without the specific cytogenetic abnormalities.[31,32] **Box 1** summarizes the revisions under WHO 2008 classification (see **Table 1**).[31,32]

OTHER MDS GROUPS

Two MDS variants occur with sufficient frequency to warrant discussion: hypocellular MDS and MDS with myelofibrosis.[38,39] Neither of these entities is incorporated in the classification. A relatively hypocellular bone marrow adjusted for age may be identified in approximately 10% of MDS cases. The challenge on diagnosis is to distinguish those cases from aplastic anemia.[40] Hypocellular MDS has yet to be shown to alter

---

Box 1
The revisions under WHO 2008 classification

1. The revision recognizes less common cases of MDS with unilineage nonerythroid dysplasia. Instead of RA, the term "refractory cytopenia with unilineage dysplasia" (RCUD) is introduced. This category includes RA, refractory neutropenia (RN), and refractory thrombocytopenia (RT). RCUD includes cases where dysplasia is demonstrated in $\geq 10\%$ of one cell line. The patients have unicytopenia or bicytopenia but not pancytopenia.

2. Patients with pancytopenia and unilineage dysplasia, patients with no overt dysplasia but cytogenetic evidence of MDS, and cases of RCUD or RCMD with PB blasts of 1% and bone marrow blasts less than 5% and peripheral blasts are subsets of cases still categorized as MDS-U.

3. The term "5q syndrome" is less emphasized in the new WHO classification given that lenalidomide therapeutic benefit is the same for patients with 5q syndrome or isolated del 5(q).

4. The revised classification further refines the blasts percent cutoff in higher-risk disease. RAEB-1 now includes cases with 2%–4% PB blasts and RAEB-II includes 5%–19% PB blasts. Auer rods presence regardless of blast percentage qualifies RAEB-II or CMML-2 classification.[33]

5. Most cases of MDS with myelofibrosis (MDS-F) are RAEB cases. Accurate estimate of blasts percentage is difficult and fibrosis is associated with worse outcome.

6. The MDS-MPN category is also refined. The name is changed to myelodysplastic syndromes–myeloproliferative neoplasm (MDS-MPN). Provisional entity of RARS-T (refractory anemia with ring sideroblasts with thrombocytosis) is proposed. Up to 60% of patients harbor the JAK2 V617F mutation. The platelet threshold is 450,000/mm³ and more.[34] This group of patients tends to have indolent course similar to RARS. Atypical CML is renamed as atypical CML, BCR/ABL-1 negative to emphasize importance of obtaining those tests.[35] A subset of patients with CMML and eosinophilia who are associated with genetic abnormalities including PDGFR are better classified as myeloid neoplasms with eosinophilia. Those patients can respond to imaitinb mesylate therapy.[36]

7. Provisional entity of refractory cytopenia of childhood is proposed.[37]

disease course or prognosis, but some studies suggest benefit from immunosuppressive therapeutics.[38] In contrast, MDS associated with marrow fibrosis (MDS-F) has a more aggressive clinical course with poor outcome and higher rate of AML transformation.[39] This subgroup is observed in 10% to 17% of cases. This is an important subtype to recognize given that even in the absence of increased blasts it portends an unfavorable prognosis. The WHO recognized that most MDS-F are high risk and probably RAEB but it is difficult to get an adequate estimate of blast percentage.

MDS RISK STRATIFICATION

The FAB and WHO, although informative about prognosis, were not widely used to tailor treatment strategies. In the past, patients with higher blast percentage (ie, RAEB) were treated more like AML. The WHO system reproducibility outside academic centers had also been a challenge. Risk stratification models are widely used to gear therapy. In general, patients are divided into "lower risk MDS" where goals of treatment are improving quality of life and minimizing transfusions and "higher risk group" where the goal of treatment is to try to alter the natural history of the disease and AML progression. It becomes clear to the reader that several different models have been proposed each with its own advantages and shortcomings. An international effort is ongoing to update and address many of those issues.

IPSS

The IPSS was developed by the international MDS risk analysis workshop.[9] Data were pooled from seven previous studies that used independent risk-based prognostic systems. Seven prior studies were included where 816 patients were evaluated. In the univariate analysis age, gender, cytogenetics, FAB classification, cytopenia, hemoglobin levels, platelets, and bone marrow blasts were statistically significant prognostic variables for survival. Absolute neutrophilic count was a significant prognostic variable for AML progression in addition to the mentioned variables. In multivariate analysis age, gender, cytogenetics, cytopenia, and bone marrow blasts were the only significant independent prognostic variables. The prognostic model and the scoring system were built based on blast count, degree of cytopenia, and blast percentage. Risk scores were weighted relative to their statistical power. Based on the sum of the risk scores patients were divided into four risk groups (Table 2).

The IPSS is currently the most widely used classification and risk stratification system. It can guide treating physicians to select therapy. The IPSS has several shortcomings. The scoring system was developed in a cohort of untreated patients and often the estimated median survival does not represent outcome of patients treated with current approved treatments. The model was designed to be applied at time of diagnosis and was not intended to be a flexible model that could be applied at different points, although in fairness it had been useful at different disease stages including pretransplant. Finally, the model does not count for multilineage dysplasia or degree of cytopenia.

WHO Prognostic Scoring System

The WPSS is a dynamic scoring system and can be used at any time during disease course.[13] The model incorporated WHO subtype rather than blast percentage, transfusion requirements rather number of cytopenia, and used IPSS cytogenetic risk stratification (Table 3). The major limitation in its wide application had been lack of WHO subtype description in many of the bone marrow pathology reports. The WPSS only indirectly accounts for other cytopenias or their degree.

Table 2
International prognostic scoring system

	Score Value				
Prognostic Indicator	0	0.5	1	1.5	2
Bone Marrow Blasts (%)	<5	5–10	—	11–20	21–30
Karyotype[a]	Good	Intermediate	Poor	—	—
Cytopenias[b]	0–1	2–3	—	—	—

	IPSS			
	Low	Intermediate 1	Intermediate 2	High
Score	0	0.5–1	1.5–2	>2.5
Percent MDS	33	38	22	7
Median Survival (Months)[c]	5.7	3.5	1.1	0.4
Progression to AML (25%)[c]	9.4	3.3	1.1	0.2

[a] Karyotype: Good→ Normal (46XX or XY); -Y; del(5q); del(20) [*alone*] Intermediate→*All* that is not Poor or Good (*Other*) Poor→ Complex (>3); Chromosome 7 anomalies.
[b] Cytopenia: ANC <1800; Hemoglobin <10; Platelets <100.
[c] Without therapy.
Data from Greenberg P, Cox C, Lebeau MM, et al. International scoring system for evaluating prognosis in myelodysplastic syndromes. Blood 1997;89:2079–88 and Warren EH, Greenberg P, Riddell SR. Cytotoxic T-lymphocyte-defined human minor histocompatibility antigens with a restricted tissue distribution. Blood 1998;2197–207.

NEW MODELS FOR RISK STRATIFICATION

To address some of the discussed shortcomings of the IPSS and WPSS, newer risk models have been proposed. One study analyzed data of 1915 patients.[41] A new

Table 3
WHO prognostic scoring system

Variable	0	1	2	3
WHO Category	RA RARS 5q	RCMD RCMD-RS	RAEB-1	RAEB-2
Karyotype	Good	Intermediate	Poor	
Transfusion Requirement	No	Regular		

Karyotype as defined per IPSS
RBC transfusion dependency was defined as having at least 1 RBC transfusion every 8 wk over a period of 4 mo.

Risk Group	Score	Median OS (mo)	AML Progression (2 y Cumulative Probability)
Very Low	0	141	0.03
Low	1	66	0.06
Intermediate	2	48	0.21
High	3–4	26	0.38
Very High	5–6	9	0.80

Data from Malcovati L, Germing U, Kuendgen A, et al. Time-dependent prognostic scoring system for predicting survival and leukemic evolution in myelodysplastic syndromes. J Clin Oncol 2007;25(23):3503–10.

model was proposed accounting for variables not included in prior models, such as age, performance status, and severity of thrombocytopenia. The model could distinguish outcome of four distinct groups (**Table 4**). This model allowed inclusion of therapy-related MDS, previously treated MDS patients, and CMML patients. Moreover, if one applies this model to a group of patients classified as low or intermediate 1 risk group by IPSS one could identify a subset of patients who really carry worse outcome (**Fig. 3**). It is important to study if this group of patients should be treated similar to patients with higher-risk IPSS. Another model was published by Garcia-Manero and colleagues[42] focusing on further risk-stratifying patients classified as low or intermediate 1 risk by IPSS. Another study classified patients into four categories (based on cytopenia-dysplasia criteria)[27]: (1) unilineage cytopenia with unilineage dysplasia, (2) multilineage cytopenia with unilineage dysplasia, (3) unilineage cytopenia with multilineage dysplasia, and (4) multilineage cytopenia with multilineage dysplasia. The median overall survival was 109, 90, 68, and 25 months, respectively. This classification was able further to refine prediction of outcome within each (IPSS) group (low risk, intermediate 1, and intermediate 2). IPSS, however, was not able to identify significant difference among each of those groups.

CMML Risk Stratification

Patients with CMML have variable prognosis.[43] The median overall survival for those patients is 2 to 3 years. Patients with myeloproliferative CMML have better outcome

Table 4		
New proposed MDS risk model		
Prognostic Factor		**Point**
Performance Status ≥ 2		2
Age ≥ 65		2
Age 60–64		1
Platelets ($\times 10^9$/L)		
<30		3
30–49		2
50–199		1
Hgb <12 g/dL		2
Bone Marrow Blasts %		
11–29		2
5–10		1
WBC >20 $\times 10^9$/L		2
Chromosome 7 Abnormality or Complex Cytogenetics		3
Prior Transfusion		1
Risk Group	**Score**	**Median Overall Survival (mo)**
Low	0–4	54
Intermediate 1	5–6	25
Intermediate 2	7–8	14
High	9->10	6

Modified from Kantarjian H, O'brien S, Ravandi F, et al. Proposal for a new risk model in myelodysplastic syndrome that accounts for events not considered in the original International Prognostic Scoring System. Cancer 2008;113:1351–61; with permission.

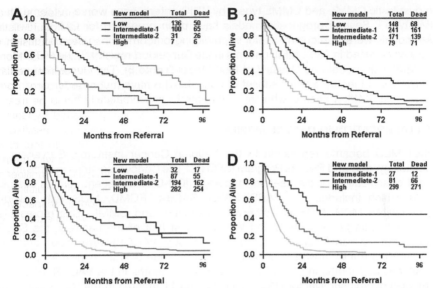

Fig. 3. Survival according to the new prognostic myelodysplastic syndrome risk model in each of the four International Prognostic Scoring System risk subsets: low risk (*A*), intermediate-1 risk (*B*), intermediate-2 risk (*C*), and high risk (*D*). (*From* Kantarjian H, O'brien S, Ravandi F, et al. Proposal for a new risk model in myelodysplastic syndrome that accounts for events not considered in the original International Prognostic Scoring System. Cancer 2008;113:1351–61; with permission.)

Table 5
CMML risk models

Risk Factor (One Point Each)	Dusseldorf CMML Risk Model	MD Anderson CMML Risk Model
Hgb	<9 g/dL	<12 g/dL
Blasts %	>5	>10
LDH	Abnormal	—
Platelets	<100,000	—
Immature myeloid precursors in PB	—	>0%
Absolute lymphocytes	—	<2500

Risk Group	Score Sum Dusseldorf	MD Anderson	Median Overall Survival (mo) Dusseldorf	MD Anderson
Low	0	0,1	93	36
Intermediate 1	1–2	2	26	16
Intermediate 2	—	3	—	13
High	3–4	4	11	9

Data from Germing U, Kundgen A, Gattermann N. Risk assessment in chronic myelomonocytic leukemia (CMML). Leuk Lymph 2004;45:1311–18.

than dysplastic CMML and CMML type II by WHO criteria have worse outcome than CMML type I. Several prognostic models have been proposed for CMML. Two of those models were particularly useful in predicting outcome when several of those models were tested in 288 CMML patients in the Dusseldorf registry[43]: the MD Anderson CMML risk model and Dusseldorf Risk Model (**Table 5**). The Dusseldorf model particularly can identify a small subset of patients who have much better prognosis than average CMML patients, who are only treated symptomatically.[43]

MDS CLASSIFICATION IN DATA REGISTRIES

In 2001 MDS became reportable to the National Cancer Institute's Surveillance, Epidemiology, and End Results Program (SEER).[44] The Cancer registries use the international classification of diseases for oncology (ICD-O). The recent version used is ICD-O3, which includes RA, RARS, RAEB, RAEB-t, RCMD, MDS with del(5q), therapy-related MDS, MDS not otherwise specified, and CMML. This represents work in transition between FAB and WHO. Almost half of the cases in the SEER data and the Veteran Affairs Central Cancer Registry (VACCR) were coded unfortunately as MDS not otherwise specified.[44–46] The median overall survival for patients with RA was 28 months in the SEER data and 41.4 months in the VACCR. Similarly, the median overall survival for RAEB patients was 11 months in the SEER data and 8 months in the VACCR database.[44,46] IPSS is not included in any of those registries.

SUMMARY

The classification of MDS continues to evolve as more is learned about the disease. The FAB was the first systemically to classify the disease and it served its purpose well for several years. The WHO and its refinement are clear additions and a step forward. Several risk stratification models are available to predict outcome. Currently, IPSS is most widely used for treatment decisions. Newly introduced models are flexible and account for other variables. There is a clear need for a standard and uniform risk stratification model to be used in clinical practice and clinical trials. It is hoped that in the near future classification and risk stratification will further advance incorporating molecular profiling and biologic signatures.

REFERENCES

1. Bennett JM, Komrokji R, Kouides P. The myelodysplastic syndromes. In: Abeloff MD, Armitage JO, Niederhuber JE, editors. Clinical oncology. New York: Churchill Livingstone; 2004. p. 2849–81.
2. Kouides PA, Bennett JM. Understanding the myelodysplastic syndromes. Oncologist 1997;2(6):389–401.
3. Luzzatto A. Sull anemia grave megaloblastica senza reporto ematologico corrispondente (anemia pseudoaplastica). Riv Veneta di sc Med Venezia 1907;47: 193–212.
4. Hamilton-Paterson JL. Pre-leukemia anemia. Acta Hematologica 1949;2:309.
5. Block M, Jacobson LO, Bethard WF. Preleukemic acute human leukemia. JAMA 1953;152:1018.
6. Saarni MI, Linman JW. Preleukemia: the hematological syndrome preceding acute leukemia. Am J Med 1973;55:38–48.
7. Bennett JM, Catovsky D, Daniel MT, et al. Proposals for the classification of the acute leukaemias. French-American-British (FAB) Co-operative Group. Br J Haematol 1976;33(4):451–8.

8. Bennett JM, Catovsky D, Daniel MT, et al. Proposals for the classification of the myelodysplastic syndromes. Br J Haematol 1982;51(2):189–99.
9. Greenberg P, Cox C, Lebeau MM, et al. International scoring system for evaluating prognosis in myelodysplastic syndromes. Blood 1997;89(6):2079–88.
10. Harris NL, Jaffe ES, Diebold J, et al. World Health Organization classification of neoplastic diseases of the hematopoietic and lymphoid tissues: report of the Clinical Advisory Committee meeting-Airlie House, Virginia, November 1997. J Clin Oncol 1999;17(12):3835–49, 1999(12):3835–49.
11. Bennett JM. World Health Organization classification of the acute leukemias and myelodysplastic syndrome. Int J Hematol 2000;72(2):131–3.
12. Vardiman JW, Harris NL, Brunning RD. The World Health Organization (WHO) classification of the myeloid neoplasms. Blood 2002;100(7):2292–302.
13. Malcovati L, Germing U, Kuendgen A, et al. Time-dependent prognostic scoring system for predicting survival and leukemic evolution in myelodysplastic syndromes. J Clin Oncol 2007;25(23):3503–10.
14. Valent P, Horny HP, Bennett JM, et al. Definitions and standards in the diagnosis and treatment of the myelodysplastic syndromes: consensus statements and report from a working conference. Leuk Res 2007;31(6):727–36.
15. Malcovati L, Della Porta MG, Cazzola M. Predicting survival and leukemic evolution in patients with myelodysplastic syndrome. Haematologica 2006;91(12): 1588–90.
16. Bjorkman SE. Chronic refractory anemia with sideroblastic bone marrow: a study of four cases. Blood 1956;11(3):250–9.
17. Gattermann N, Aul C, Schneider W. Two types of acquired idiopathic sideroblastic anaemia (AISA). Br J Haematol 1990;74(1):45–52.
18. Komrokji R, Bennett J. What is "WHO"? Myelodysplastic syndromes classification. Clin Leuk 2008;2(1):20–7.
19. Rosati S, Mick R, Xu F, et al. Refractory cytopenia with multilineage dysplasia: further characterization of an unclassifiable myelodysplastic syndrome. Leukemia 1996;10(1):20–6.
20. Balduini CL, Guarnone R, Pecci A, et al. Multilineage dysplasia without increased blasts identifies a poor prognosis subset of myelodysplastic syndromes. Leukemia 1998;12(10):1655–6.
21. Bernasconi P, Klersy C, Boni M, et al. World Health Organization classification in combination with cytogenetic markers improves the prognostic stratification of patients with de novo primary myelodysplastic syndromes. Br J Haematol 2007;137(3):193–205.
22. Cermak J, Belickova M, Krejcova H, et al. The presence of clonal cell subpopulations in peripheral blood and bone marrow of patients with refractory cytopenia with multilineage dysplasia but not in patients with refractory anemia may reflect a multistep pathogenesis of myelodysplasia. Leuk Res 2005;29(4):371–9.
23. Komrokji R, Bennett JM. The myelodysplastic syndromes: classification and prognosis. Curr Hematol Rep 2003;2(3):179–85.
24. Bennett JM, Brunning RD, Vardiman JW. Myelodysplastic syndromes: from French-American-British to World Health Organization: a commentary. Blood 2002;99(8):3074–5.
25. Lorand-Metze I, Pinheiro MP, Ribeiro E, et al. Factors influencing survival in myelodysplastic syndromes in a Brazilian population: comparison of FAB and WHO classifications. Leuk Res 2004;28(6):587–94.
26. Nosslinger T, Reisner R, Koller E, et al. Myelodysplastic syndromes, from French-American-British to World Health Organization: comparison of

classifications on 431 unselected patients from a single institution. Blood 2001; 98(10):2935–41.

27. Verburgh E, Achten R, Louw VJ, et al. A new disease categorization of low-grade myelodysplastic syndromes based on the expression of cytopenia and dysplasia in one versus more than one lineage improves on the WHO classification. Leukemia 2007;21(4):668–77.

28. Germing U, Gattermann N, Strupp C, et al. Validation of the WHO proposals for a new classification of primary myelodysplastic syndromes: a retrospective analysis of 1600 patients. Leuk Res 2000;24(12):983–92.

29. Germing U, Strupp C, Kuendgen A, et al. Prospective validation of the WHO proposals for the classification of myelodysplastic syndromes. Haematologica 2006;91(12):1596–604.

30. Howe RB, Porwit-Macdonald A, Wanat R, et al. The WHO classification of MDS does make a difference. Blood 2004;103(9):3265–70.

31. Brunning RD, Orazi A, Germing U. Myelodysplastic syndromes/neoplasms overview. In: Swerdlow SH, Campo E, Harris NL, et al, editors. WHO Classification of tumours of haematopoietic and lymphoid tissues. 4th edition. Lyon (France): IARC; 2008. p. 88–93.

32. Komrokji R, Bennett JM. What is "WHO"?: myelodysplastic syndrome classification and prognosis. Alexandria (VA): ASCO Educational Book; 2009. p. 413–19.

33. Orazi A, Brunning RD, Hasserjian RP. Refractory anemia with excess blasts. In: Swerdlow SH, Campo E, Harris NL, et al, editors. WHO classification of tumours of haematopoietic and lymphoid tissues. 4th edition. Lyon (France): IARC; 2008. p. 100–1.

34. Vardiman JW, Bennett JM, Bain BJ. Myelodysplastic/myeloproliferative neoplasm, unclassifiable. In: Swerdlow SH, Campo E, Harris NL, et al, editors. WHO classification of tumours of haematopoietic and lymphoid tissues. 4th edition. Lyon (France): IARC; 2008. p. 85–6.

35. Vadiman JW, Bennett JM, Bain RJ. Atypical Chronic myleoid leukemia, BCR-ABL1 negative. In: Swerdlow SH, Campo E, Harris NL, et al, editors. WHO classification of tumours of haematopoietic and lymphoid tissues. 4th edition. Lyon (France): IARC; 2008. p. 80–1.

36. Orazi A, Bennett JM, Germing U. Chronic myelomonocytic leukemia. In: Swerdlow SH, Campo E, Harris NL, et al, editors. WHO classification of tumours of haematopoietic and lymphoid tissues. 4th edition. Lyon (France): IARC; 2008. p. 76–9.

37. Baumann I, Niemeyer CM, Bennett JM. Childhood myelodysplastic syndrome. In: Swerdlow SH, Campo E, Harris NL, et al, editors. WHO classification of tumours of haematopoietic and lymphoid tissues. 4th edition. Lyon (France): IARC; 2008. p. 104–7.

38. Lim ZY, Killick S, Germing U, et al. Low IPSS score and bone marrow hypocellularity in MDS patients predict hematological responses to antithymocyte globulin. Leukemia 2007;21(7):1436–41.

39. Della Porta MG, Malcovati L, Boveri E, et al. Clinical relevance of bone marrow fibrosis and CD34-positive cell clusters in primary myelodysplastic syndromes. J Clin Oncol 2009;27(5):754–62.

40. Young NS, Calado RT, Scheinberg P. Current concepts in the pathophysiology and treatment of aplastic anemia. Blood 2006;108(8):2509–19.

41. Kantarjian H, O'brien S, Ravandi F, et al. Proposal for a new risk model in myelodysplastic syndrome that accounts for events not considered in the original International Prognostic Scoring System. Cancer 2008;113(6):1351–61.

42. Garcia-Manero G, Shan J, Faderl S, et al. A prognostic score for patients with lower risk myelodysplastic syndrome. Leukemia 2007;22(3):538–43.
43. Germing U, Kundgen A, Gattermann N. Risk assessment in chronic myelomonocytic leukemia (CMML). Leuk Lymphoma 2004;45(7):1311–8.
44. Ma X, Does M, Raza A, et al. Myelodysplastic syndromes: incidence and survival in the United States. Cancer 2007;109(8):1536–42.
45. Rollison DE, Howlader N, Smith MT, et al. Epidemiology of myelodysplastic syndromes and chronic myeloproliferative disorders in the United States, 2001-2004, using data from the NAACCR and SEER programs. Blood 2008;112(1):45–52.
46. Komrokji RS, Matacia-Murphy GM, Ali NH, et al. Outcome of patients with myelodysplastic syndromes in the veterans administration population. Leuk Res 2010;34(1):59–62.

Prognostic Classification and Risk Assessment in Myelodysplastic Syndromes

Mario Cazzola, MD*, Luca Malcovati, MD

KEYWORDS

- Myelodysplastic syndrome • Acute myeloid leukemia
- Anemia • Transfusion • Prognosis

Myelodysplastic syndromes (MDS) are clonal hematopoietic stem cell disorders characterized by ineffective hematopoiesis, peripheral cytopenias, and substantial risk for progression to acute myeloid leukemia (AML).[1–3] They typically occur in elderly people with a median age at diagnosis ranging between 65 and 75 years in most series, and the annual incidence exceeds 20 per 100,000 persons more than 70 years of age.[2]

Myelodysplastic syndromes were defined and classified in 1982 by the French American British group.[4] In 2001 the World Health Organization (WHO) classification of myeloid neoplasms was developed[5]; this classification has been updated in 2008.[6] The current diagnostic approach includes peripheral blood and bone marrow morphology (to evaluate abnormalities of peripheral blood cells and hematopoietic precursors); bone marrow biopsy (to assess marrow cellularity, fibrosis and topography); and cytogenetics (to identify nonrandom chromosomal abnormalities). The combination of overt marrow dysplasia and clonal cytogenetic abnormality allows a conclusive diagnosis of MDS, but this is found in only a portion of patients.[1] Although bone marrow biopsy may be considered too invasive for elderly patients, it provides

This review article is based on a presentation given by Mario Cazzola at an education session on myelodysplastic syndromes of the 14th Congress of the European Hematology Association (EHA), Berlin, Germany, June 5 to7, 2009. This presentation was reported in the meeting proceedings (Cazzola M, Malcovati L. Risk-adapted treatment of myelodysplastic syndromes. Hematology Education 2009;3:181). The authors wish to thank EHA for its permission to reproduce parts of the above report.

Department of Hematology Oncology, Medical School, University of Pavia, Fondazione IRCCS Policlinico San Matteo, Pavia 27100, Italy

* Corresponding author.

E-mail address: mario.cazzola@unipv.it

Hematol Oncol Clin N Am 24 (2010) 459–468

doi:10.1016/j.hoc.2010.02.005

extremely useful diagnostic and prognostic information regarding cellularity,[7] fibrosis,[8] and CD34-positive cell topography.[8]

PROGNOSTIC FACTORS IN MYELODYSPLASTIC SYNDROMES

The clinical heterogeneity of myelodysplastic syndromes is best illustrated by the observation that these disorders range from indolent conditions with a near-normal life expectancy to forms approaching AML.[1] A risk-adapted treatment strategy is mandatory for conditions showing a highly variable clinical course, and definition of the individual risk has been based so far on the use of prognostic scoring systems.

In 1997, Greenberg and coworkers[9] developed the International Prognostic Scoring System (IPSS), based on bone marrow blasts, cytogenetic abnormalities, and number of cytopenias (**Table 1**). The IPSS was derived from a multivariate analysis of hematological characteristics of 816 subjects at clinical onset, also including subjects with 20% to 30% marrow blasts, now considered as having AML. Despite these limitations, IPSS proved to be useful for predicting survival and acute leukemic risk in individuals with MDS and has been incorporated to the design and analysis of therapeutic trials in these disorders.[10]

In 2001, the WHO formulated a new classification of MDS based on uni- or multilineage dysplasia, bone marrow blast count, and distinctive cytogenetic features.[5] This proposal was shown to provide a relevant prognostic information, and was largely confirmed in the updated classification 2008.[6,11] In particular, among patients with MDS without excess blasts, an isolated involvement of the erythroid lineage was found to be associated with a better prognosis compared with multilineage dysplasia.

In a study on the prognostic significance of the WHO classification,[12] the authors found that the IPSS retained significance within the WHO subgroups. However, when accounting for blast percentage using WHO categories, the only other IPSS

Table 1
International prognostic scoring system for myelodysplastic syndromes

Variable	Variable Scores				
	0.0	0.5	1.0	1.5	2.0
Bone marrow blasts (%)	<5	5–10	—	11–20	21–30
Karyotype[a]	Good	Intermediate	Poor	—	—
Cytopenias[b]	0/1	2/3	—	—	—

Definition of the individual patient's risk group

Risk Group	Score	Median Survival (Years)	Median Times to 25% AML Evolution
Low	0	5.7	9.4
Intermediate 1	0.5–1.0	3.5	3.3
Intermediate 2	1.5–2.0	1.2	1.1
High	≥2.5	0.4	0.2

[a] Good: normal, -Y, del(5q), del(20q); poor: complex (≥3 abnormalities) or chromosome 7 anomalies; intermediate: other abnormalities.
[b] Cytopenias were defined as a hemoglobin level of less than 10 g/dL, an absolute neutrophil count of less than 1.5×10^9/L, and a platelet count of less than 100×10^9/L.
Data from Greenberg P, Cox C, LeBeau MM, et al. International scoring system for evaluating prognosis in myelodysplastic syndromes. Blood 1997;89:2079.

variable adding prognostic information was found to be cytogenetics. The authors also found that transfusion dependency had a significant effect on survival in multivariable analysis.[12] **Fig. 1** illustrates the important impact of transfusion dependency on survival of MDS patients.[13] The authors concluded that transfusion dependency could be considered as an independent indicator of the severity of the disease, and consequently an independent prognostic factor. Analyzing pre-transfusion hemoglobin levels in independent cohorts of subjects, transfusion-dependency was shown to recognize a homogeneous population including about 95% of subjects with less than 9 g/dL. These data are in agreement with the results of a recent study by Greenberg and coworkers,[14] indicating that the severity of anemia at diagnosis is of additive prognostic value to IPSS in survival.

Several mechanisms may concur to determine the negative impact of severe anemia on the clinical outcome of patients with MDS. The severity of anemia likely reflects more severe marrow failure and more aggressive disease. In addition, chronic anemia is known to be associated with increased mortality and morbidity per se in older adults, especially when associated with chronic heart failure.[15] Furthermore, cardiac dysfunction can result from transfusional iron overload developing in adulthood.[16–18]

THE WORLD HEALTH ORGANIZATION CLASSIFICATION-BASED PROGNOSTIC SCORING SYSTEM

In collaboration with the Duesseldorf colleagues, the authors developed a prognostic model that accounted for the WHO categories, cytogenetics, and transfusion dependency.[19] This WHO classification-based Prognostic Scoring System (WPSS) was able

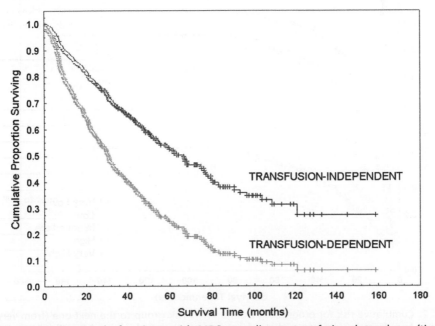

Fig. 1. Overall survival of patients with MDS according to transfusion-dependency (time-dependent model). (*Data from* Malcovati L. Impact of transfusion dependency and secondary iron overload on the survival of patients with myelodysplastic syndromes. Leuk Res 2007;31(Suppl 3):S2.)

to classify patients into five risk groups showing different survivals and probabilities of leukemic evolution. WPSS was shown to predict survival and leukemia progression at any time during follow-up, and may therefore be used for implementing risk-adapted treatment strategies. **Fig. 2** illustrates the risk for progressing from a WPSS risk group to the next one or to acute myeloid leukemia over time.

More recently, the authors found that bone marrow fibrosis identifies a distinct subgroup of MDS with multilineage dysplasia, high transfusion requirement, and poor prognosis, and represents an independent prognostic factor that may be useful in clinical decision making.[8] Within patients stratified according to IPSS and WPSS categories, bone marrow fibrosis involved a shift to a one-step more advanced risk group.[8] As indicated in **Table 2**, grade 2 to 3 marrow fibrosis can therefore be used to better define the individual patient's risk group within the WPSS.

Accounting for multilineage dysplasia, transfusion dependency and bone marrow fibrosis within the WPSS categorization allows defining the prognosis of the individual patient with MDS more accurately as compared with the IPSS categorization. This accuracy is mainly noticeable for patients belonging to the IPSS low or intermediate-1 risk groups (**Table 3**) (ie, those patients who pose most difficulties in therapeutic decision making).

DYNAMIC PROGNOSTIC ASSESSMENT IN MYELODYSPLASTIC SYNDROMES

A critical point in assessing the prognostic value of disease-related variables is that most of them are subject to changes during the natural history of the disease. By

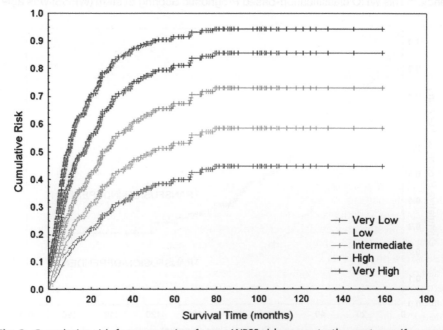

Fig. 2. Cumulative risk for progressing from a WPSS risk group to the next one (from very low to low, from low to intermediate, from intermediate to high, and from high to very high) or from the very high risk group to acute myeloid leukemia. (*Data from* Cazzola M, Malcovati L. Risk-adapted treatment of myelodysplastic syndromes. Hematology Education 2009;3:181.)

Table 2
WPSS and bone marrow fibrosis as criteria for predicting likelihood of survival and risk for leukemic evolution in the individual patient with myelodysplastic syndrome

Calculation of the WPSS Score and Evaluation of Bone Marrow Fibrosis

	Variable Scores			
Variable	0	1	2	3
WHO category	RA, RARS, MDS with isolated deletion (5q)	RCMD	RAEB-1	RAEB-2
Karyotype[a]	Good	Intermediate	Poor	—
Transfusion requirement[b]	Absent	Present	—	—
Bone marrow fibrosis[c]	The presence of grade 2–3 bone marrow fibrosis involves a shift to a one-step more advanced risk group after accounting for WHO category, karyotype, and transfusion requirement.			

Definition of the individual patient's risk group

Risk Group	Score	Median Survival (Years)	Risk of Leukemic Evolution
Very low	0	>10	<10% at 15 y
Low	1 (or score 0 plus marrow fibrosis)	>5	10%–20% at 5 y
Intermediate	2 (or score 1 plus marrow fibrosis)	~4	30%–40% at 5 y
High	3–4 (or score 2 plus marrow fibrosis)	~2	30% at 3 y
Very high	5–6 (or score 3–4 plus marrow fibrosis)	~1	>50% at 1 y

Abbreviations: RA, refractory anemia; RAEB-1, refractory anemia with excess blasts-1; RAEB-2, refractory anemia with excess blasts-2; RARAS, refractory anemia with ringed sideroblasts; RCMD, refractory cytopenia with multilineage dysplasia.
[a] Good: normal, -Y, del(5q), del(20q); Poor: complex, chromosome 7 anomalies; Intermediate: other chromosomal abnormalities.
[b] Transfusion dependency: at least one transfusion every 8 weeks over a period of 4 months.
[c] Bone marrow fibrosis should be evaluated according to the European consensus criteria.
Data from Cazzola M, Malcovati L. Risk-adapted treatment of myelodysplastic syndromes. Hematology Education 2009;3:181.

applying a Cox regression model with time-dependent covariates, the WPSS was also shown to stratify survival and leukemia progression at any time during the clinical course of the disease. According to this model, patients are classified into a risk group at the time of diagnosis, and when they show progression to a different WHO subgroup, develop new cytogenetic abnormalities, or become transfusion-dependent, they will change WPSS category according to the resulting score. As a result, the new WPSS score provides an updated estimate of survival and risk for leukemic evolution.

The time dependency of WPSS appears to be particularly relevant in low-risk MDS, where delayed treatment strategies may be adopted in the clinical practice. A clinical decision analysis from the International Bone Marrow Transplant Registry demonstrated that life expectancy of patients with low-risk MDS who have HLA-identical siblings was higher when transplantation was delayed as long as the patients remained in the low-risk groups, but performed before the development of AML.[20] The dynamic WPSS appears potentially useful for this type of clinical decision making, and was recently proven to significantly stratify the outcome of patients with MDS receiving allogeneic stem cell transplantation.[21]

Table 3
Comparison of two different risk assessment systems (IPSS and WPSS) in 258 subjects with MDS

IPSS Risk Group	No. of Subjects	Median Overall Survival[a]	WPSS Risk Group	No. of Subjects (%)	Median Overall Survival[b]
Low	71	68	Very low	26 (37)	141
			Low	23 (32)	66
			Intermediate	16 (23)	48
			High	6 (8)	26
Intermediate 1	122	42	Very low	6 (5)	141
			Low	23 (19)	66
			Intermediate	42 (34)	48
			High	33 (27)	26
			Very high	18 (15)	9
Intermediate 2	47	14	Intermediate	1 (2)	48
			High	25 (53)	26
			Very high	21 (45)	9
High	18	5	High	1 (6)	26
			Very high	17 (94)	9

Within each IPSS risk group, patients have been stratified according to WPSS criteria, taking into account WHO category, karyotype, transfusion dependency, and bone marrow fibrosis as indicated in **Table 2**.

[a] *Data from* Greenberg P, Cox C, LeBeau MM, et al. International scoring system for evaluating prognosis in myelodysplastic syndromes. Blood 1997;89:2079.

[b] *Data from* Malcovati L, Germing U, Kuendgen A, et al. Time-dependent prognostic scoring system for predicting survival and leukemic evolution in myelodysplastic syndromes. J Clin Oncol 2007;25:3503. (*From* Cazzola M, Malcovati L. Risk-adapted treatment of myelodysplastic syndromes. Hematology Education 2009;3:181.)

A NEW RISK MODEL IN MYELODYSPLASTIC SYNDROME THAT ACCOUNTS FOR EVENTS NOT CONSIDERED IN THE ORIGINAL INTERNATIONAL PROGNOSTIC SCORING SYSTEM

Kantarjian and coworkers[22] have recently proposed a new risk model for patients with MDS and chronic myelomonocytic leukemia (CMML) that refines the prognostic precision of the IPSS and is applicable to all such patients at any time during the course of the disease and irrespective of previous treatments. These authors included in the new model all the factors identified as significant by multivariate analysis in the study group (ie, performance status, age, platelet count, hemoglobin, bone marrow blasts, white blood cell count, and karyotype). The new MDS prognostic model divided patients into four prognostic groups with significantly different outcomes.

THE IMPACT OF COMORBIDITIES ON SURVIVAL OF PATIENTS WITH MYELODYSPLASTIC SYNDROMES AND THEIR ELIGIBILITY TO ALLOGENEIC STEM CELL TRANSPLANTATION

As underscored previously, myelodysplastic syndromes occur mainly in older persons and this will occur increasingly in the future. In fact, the proportion of people more than 65 years of age is expected to double in the next 40 years, and therefore the number of newly diagnosed MDS is likely to increase accordingly.[23] Aging is associated with an increased risk for developing comorbidity, and a high prevalence of comorbidity was recently reported in patients with MDS, suggesting that this is emerging as a relevant clinical problem in these patients.[24]

Sorror and colleagues[25] found that comorbidity predicts posttransplantation outcome, and developed a Hematopoietic Cell Transplantation Comorbidity Index (HCT-CI) as a tool that captures pretransplant comorbidities and can be used in predicting outcomes and stratifying patients. This tool was employed in subjects with MDS and AML to stratify and compare patients conditioned with nonmyeloablative or myeloablative regimens.[26] This study showed that patients with low comorbidity scores may be candidates for prospective randomized trials comparing these two conditioning regimens regardless of disease status.

However, the previously mentioned study was conducted on a highly selected subset of patients with MDS eligible for allogeneic transplantation, and it is unclear whether the HCT-CI can be employed in the whole MDS patient population to predict clinical outcome outside the setting of transplantation.[24] Therefore, one of our primary tasks in the next few years should be the development of an MDS-specific comorbidity index that can be applied in the whole MDS patient population.

MOLECULAR MARKERS OF PROGNOSTIC SIGNIFICANCE

Several somatic mutations have been described in patients with MDS in the last few years, but most of them have been considered as nonspecific so far.[2] However, there have been recent developments in this field.

Acquired somatic mutations, including deletions, insertions, nonsense, and missense mutations of *TET2*, a putative tumor suppressor gene located at 4q24, were first identified by Delhommeau and colleagues[27] and Langemeijer and colleagues[28] following the findings of small deletions and acquired uniparental disomy at 4q24. *TET2* mutations occur early during disease evolution and generally precede *JAK2* (V617F) in myeloid neoplasms that have mutations in both genes.

A preliminary report indicates that *TET2* mutations are a favorable prognostic factor in MDS.[29] In fact, multivariable analysis including age, IPSS, and transfusion requirement demonstrated that *TET2* mutation was an independent factor of favorable prognosis. The survival advantage resulted at least in part from a lower propensity to leukemic evolution in patients who are mutated. By contrast, in a cohort of subjects with CMML,[30] *TET2* mutations were associated with a trend to significantly lower survival, which reached significance in subjects with CMML1 according to the WHO classification.[31] The reasons for this discrepancy are unclear.

In a study on subjects who have refractory anemia with ringed sideroblasts associated with marked thrombocytosis, the authors found that *JAK2* and *MPL* mutations did not have any independent effect on survival.[32]

We are just starting to define the molecular basis of MDS, and in the next few years the molecular parameters might be incorporated in novel prognostic models.

WORLD HEALTH ORGANIZATION PROGNOSTIC SCORING SYSTEM-BASED RISK-ADAPTED TREATMENT STRATEGY

Several therapeutic tools have been proposed in the last decades for myelodysplastic syndromes, but only few survived the evidence-based criteria of efficacy.[1,33,34] They include supportive care, hematopoietic growth factors, lenalidomide, antithymocyte globulin (ATG), azacitidine, decitabine, and allogeneic stem cell transplantation.

The authors base risk-adapted strategy on the WPSS as summarized in **Table 4**. The inclusion of comorbidities in clinical decision making is likely to improve this strategy in the near future.

Table 4
WPSS-based risk-adapted treatment strategy for myelodysplastic syndromes

WPSS Risk-Group Defined as Indicated in Table 2	Therapeutic Options
Very low risk	Watchful-waiting strategy. These patients include those with refractory anemia, or refractory anemia with ringed sideroblasts, or myelodysplastic syndrome with isolated deletion (5q) and no transfusion requirement. Their median life expectancy is greater than 10 years (see **Table 2**), and as long as the disease remains stable these patients do not need any treatment and can be just followed regularly.
Low risk	Patients with multilineage dysplasia or intermediate risk cytogenetics without symptomatic cytopenia may be just followed without any specific treatment (watchful-waiting strategy). However, frequent controls (every 3 months) are needed in these patients as the 1-year risk of disease progression is 25% (see **Fig. 2**). Patients who are transfusion-dependent can be treated with recombinant human erythropoietin; responsive patients are those with inadequate endogenous erythropoietin productions (serum erythropoietin levels lower than 100 to 200 mU/mL) and low need for blood transfusion (< two units per month). Patients who fail to respond to recombinant human erythropoietin may be considered for more aggressive treatments. Those who are given regular blood transfusion should also receive iron chelation therapy. Patients who are transfusion-dependent with MDS associated with deletion (5q) may respond to lenalidomide treatment with abolishment of transfusion requirement. In 2005, the US Food and Drug Administration approved lenalidomide for the treatment of patients with transfusion-dependent anemia caused by low- or intermediate-1-risk MDS associated with a deletion 5q cytogenetic abnormality with or without additional cytogenetic abnormalities. In 2008, the European Medicines Agency Committee for Medicinal Products for Human Use adopted a negative opinion, recommending the refusal of marketing authorization for lenalidomide intended for treatment of patients who are transfusion-dependent with MDS associated with del(5q). Patients with hypoplastic MDS who are less than 60 years of age may be treated with antithymocyte globulin of horse origin (h-ATG) and cyclosporine A.
Intermediate, high, and very high risk	Fit patients aged up to 65 years with intermediate to very high WPSS risk are candidates for allogeneic stem cell transplantation. Patients who are not eligible for allogeneic stem cell transplantation may be treated with azacitidine (Europe and United States) or decitabine (United States). Patients who are not eligible for allogeneic stem cell transplantation or do not respond to azacitidine may be considered for experimental treatments (clinical trials). Patients who do not fit into previous groups are given supportive therapy (regular red cell transfusion).

(From Cazzola M, Malcovati L. Risk-adapted treatment of myelodysplastic syndromes. Hematology Education 2009;3:181.)

REFERENCES

1. Cazzola M, Malcovati L. Myelodysplastic syndromes–coping with ineffective hematopoiesis. N Engl J Med 2005;352:536.
2. Tefferi A, Vardiman JW. Myelodysplastic syndromes. N Engl J Med 1872;361: 2009.
3. Cazzola M, Malcovati L. Risk-adapted treatment of myelodysplastic syndromes. Hematology Education 2009;3:181.
4. Bennett JM, Catovsky D, Daniel MT, et al. Proposals for the classification of the myelodysplastic syndromes. Br J Haematol 1982;51:189.
5. Vardiman JW, Harris NL, Brunning RD. The World Health Organization (WHO) classification of the myeloid neoplasms. Blood 2002;100:2292.
6. Brunning RD, Orazi A, Germing U, et al. Myelodysplastic syndromes/ neoplasms, overview. In: Swerdlow SH, Campo E, Harris NL, editors. WHO classification of tumours of hamatopoietic and lymphoid tissues. Lyon (France): IARC; 2008. p. 88.
7. Bennett JM, Orazi A. Diagnostic criteria to distinguish hypocellular acute myeloid leukemia from hypocellular myelodysplastic syndromes and aplastic anemia: recommendations for a standardized approach. Haematologica 2009;94:264.
8. Della Porta MG, Malcovati L, Boveri E, et al. Clinical relevance of bone marrow fibrosis and CD34-positive cell clusters in primary myelodysplastic syndromes. J Clin Oncol 2009;27:754.
9. Greenberg P, Cox C, LeBeau MM, et al. International scoring system for evaluating prognosis in myelodysplastic syndromes. Blood 1997;89:2079.
10. Sanz GF, Sanz MA, Greenberg PL. Prognostic factors and scoring systems in myelodysplastic syndromes. Haematologica 1998;83:358.
11. Vardiman JW, Thiele J, Arber DA, et al. The 2008 revision of the World Health Organization (WHO) classification of myeloid neoplasms and acute leukemia: rationale and important changes. Blood 2009;114:937.
12. Malcovati L, Porta MG, Pascutto C, et al. Prognostic factors and life expectancy in myelodysplastic syndromes classified according to WHO criteria: a basis for clinical decision making. J Clin Oncol 2005;23:7594.
13. Malcovati L. Impact of transfusion dependency and secondary iron overload on the survival of patients with myelodysplastic syndromes. Leuk Res 2007;31(Suppl 3):S2.
14. Kao JM, McMillan A, Greenberg PL. International MDS risk analysis workshop (IMRAW)/IPSS reanalyzed: impact of cytopenias on clinical outcomes in myelodysplastic syndromes. Am J Hematol 2008;83:765.
15. Groenveld HF, Januzzi JL, Damman K, et al. Anemia and mortality in heart failure patients a systematic review and meta-analysis. J Am Coll Cardiol 2008;52:818.
16. Cazzola M, Barosi G, Gobbi PG, et al. Natural history of idiopathic refractory sideroblastic anemia. Blood 1988;71:305.
17. Malcovati L, Della Porta MG, Cazzola M. Predicting survival and leukemic evolution in patients with myelodysplastic syndrome. Haematologica 2006; 91:1588.
18. Schafer AI, Cheron RG, Dluhy R, et al. Clinical consequences of acquired transfusional iron overload in adults. N Engl J Med 1981;304:319.
19. Malcovati L, Germing U, Kuendgen A, et al. Time-dependent prognostic scoring system for predicting survival and leukemic evolution in myelodysplastic syndromes. J Clin Oncol 2007;25:3503.
20. Cutler CS, Lee SJ, Greenberg P, et al. A decision analysis of allogeneic bone marrow transplantation for the myelodysplastic syndromes: delayed

transplantation for low-risk myelodysplasia is associated with improved outcome. Blood 2004;104:579.

21. Alessandrino EP, Della Porta MG, Bacigalupo A, et al. WHO classification and WPSS predict posttransplantation outcome in patients with myelodysplastic syndrome: a study from the Gruppo Italiano Trapianto di Midollo Osseo (GITMO). Blood 2008;112:895.

22. Kantarjian H, O'Brien S, Ravandi F, et al. Proposal for a new risk model in myelodysplastic syndrome that accounts for events not considered in the original International Prognostic Scoring System. Cancer 2008;113:1351.

23. National Cancer Institute. Surveillance EaERSR-A-AIRB, Bethesda, Maryland, National Cancer Institute. Available at: http://www.seer.cancer.gov. Accessed October, 2009.

24. Zipperer E, Pelz D, Nachtkamp K, et al. The hematopoietic stem cell transplantation comorbidity index is of prognostic relevance for patients with myelodysplastic syndrome. Haematologica 2009;94:729.

25. Sorror ML, Maris MB, Storb R, et al. Hematopoietic cell transplantation (HCT)-specific comorbidity index: a new tool for risk assessment before allogeneic HCT. Blood 2005;106:2912.

26. Sorror ML, Sandmaier BM, Storer BE, et al. Comorbidity and disease status based risk stratification of outcomes among patients with acute myeloid leukemia or myelodysplasia receiving allogeneic hematopoietic cell transplantation. J Clin Oncol 2007;25:4246.

27. Delhommeau F, Dupont S, Della Valle V, et al. Mutation in TET2 in myeloid cancers. N Engl J Med 2009;360:2289.

28. Langemeijer SM, Kuiper RP, Berends M, et al. Acquired mutations in TET2 are common in myelodysplastic syndromes. Nat Genet 2009;41:838.

29. Kosmider O, Gelsi-Boyer V, Cheok M, et al. TET2 mutation is an independent favorable prognostic factor in myelodysplastic syndromes (MDSs). Blood 2009; 114:3285.

30. Kosmider O, Gelsi-Boyer V, Ciudad M, et al. TET2 gene mutation is a frequent and adverse event in chronic myelomonocytic leukemia. Haematologica 2009; 94:1676.

31. Orazi A, Bennet JM, Germing U, et al. Chronic myelomonocytic leukaemia. In: Swerdlow SH, Campo E, Harris NL, editors. WHO classification of tumours of haematopoietic and lymphoid tissues. Lyon (France): IARC; 2008. p. 76.

32. Malcovati L, Della Porta MG, Pietra D, et al. Molecular and clinical features of refractory anemia with ringed sideroblasts associated with marked thrombocytosis. Blood 2009;114:3538.

33. Alessandrino EP, Amadori S, Barosi G, et al. Evidence- and consensus-based practice guidelines for the therapy of primary myelodysplastic syndromes. A statement from the Italian Society of Hematology. Haematologica 2002;87:1286.

34. Bowen D, Culligan D, Jowitt S, et al. Guidelines for the diagnosis and therapy of adult myelodysplastic syndromes. Br J Haematol 2003;120:187.

Patient Selection for Transplantation in the Myelodysplastic Syndromes

Corey Cutler, MD, MPH, FRCP(C)

KEYWORDS

• Stem cell transplantation • Myelodysplastic syndromes
• Allogeneic

Allogeneic hematopoietic stem cell transplantation remains the only known curative procedure for the myelodysplastic syndromes (MDS). MDS is currently the third most common indication for allogeneic stem cell transplantation as reported to the Center for International Blood and Marrow Transplantation Research (CIBMTR).[1] Comparative registry analyses have documented the benefit of transplantation over conventional supportive and disease-modifying therapeutics[2]; however, this should not be interpreted as an indication for transplantation in all patients. Because the median age at diagnosis for MDS is in the late seventh decade of life, despite the curative potential, transplantation is not undertaken routinely, and careful consideration must be made regarding the appropriateness of the transplant recipient. This article focuses on appropriate patient selection for transplantation for MDS.

TIMING OF TRANSPLANTATION

The timing of transplantation has always been a topic of discussion for patients and clinicians alike. From both the patient's and physician's perspective, faced with the uncertainty of transplantation outcomes but the certainty of eventual MDS disease progression, decisions often are made based on patient preference. Supporting these decisions are several single or multi-institution experiences that demonstrated improved outcomes with earlier transplantation. The inherent bias in these types of analyses is that patients and physicians self-select for early transplantation. This bias, although recognized, often is overlooked, because patients who choose early transplantation identify with those included in the analysis to justify their decision.

Most analyses that have examined the timing of transplantation for MDS have involved patients who underwent myeloablative procedures. For instance, the Seattle

Harvard Medical School, Dana-Farber Cancer Institute, 44 Binney Street, D1B13, Boston, MA 02115, USA
E-mail address: corey_cutler@dfci.harvard.edu

Hematol Oncol Clin N Am 24 (2010) 469–476
doi:10.1016/j.hoc.2010.02.006   hemonc.theclinics.com
0889-8588/10/$ – see front matter © 2010 Elsevier Inc. All rights reserved.

group presented results of targeted busulfan therapy in patients undergoing related or unrelated donor transplantation and examined the results based on the international prognostic scoring system (IPSS).[3] Although patients were enrolled prospectively on a targeted busulfan treatment program, the decision to undergo transplant was based upon physician and patient preference. As predicted, results correlated with IPSS stage, and suggested that outcomes were improved with transplantation at an earlier stage of disease. There were no relapses among the patients in the lowest IPSS score group, whereas the relapse rate was 42% for patients in the highest IPSS category. As a consequence, survival was 80% in the lowest IPSS risk group, but under 30% for patients in the high IPSS category.

de Witte and colleagues[4] examined outcomes of transplantation for patients with refractory anemia or refractory anemia and ringed sideroblasts. This analysis studied transplant outcomes in 374 patients who underwent transplantation from either matched, sibling, or unrelated donors. Both standard myeloablative and reduced-intensity conditioning regimens were used as deemed appropriate by the treating physician in this retrospective review. Unfortunately, fewer than half of the patients had sufficient information available to calculate IPSS risk scores, and therefore outcomes stratified on this basis were not reliable. One other shortcoming of this analysis was that transplantation procedures spanned over a decade, and inherent differences in transplantation technology were evident with improving overall survival with more recent transplantation. Although factors such as conditioning intensity, stem cell source, and donor status did not affect outcome, the authors noted a significant association between year of transplantation, recipient age, and most relevant here, duration of identified myelodysplastic disease as being important predictors of overall survival. None of these factors were associated with relapse-free survival in multivariable analysis. The authors therefore suggested that earlier transplantation was associated with improved transplantation outcome. Again, this should not be interpreted as a recommendation for early transplantation in individuals with otherwise low risk MDS, because the authors did not compare outcomes for cohorts of patients who chose supportive care alone with those who chose transplantation.

To address the shortcomings of these and other biased retrospective analyses, the author and colleagues generated a Markov decision model to best understand how treatment decisions would affect overall outcome in large cohorts of patients with newly diagnosed MDS.[5] The decision model was developed to determine if transplantation at the time of initial diagnosis, transplantation delayed a fixed number of years, or transplantation at the time of leukemic transformation was the optimal usage strategy for transplantation. Using data from several large, nonoverlapping databases, the author and colleagues demonstrated that the optimal treatment strategy for patients with low- and intermediate-1 IPSS disease categories was to delay transplantation until the time of leukemic progression. Immediate transplantation was recommended for patients with intermediate-2 and high-risk IPSS scores. These recommendations were stable when adjustments for quality of life were incorporated also. One of the shortcomings of this analysis was the inability to provide treatment decision guidance at other clinically relevant time points for patients not undergoing immediate transplantation. Although not formally tested, other important clinical events, such as a new transfusion requirement, recurrent infections, or recurrent bleeding episodes, certainly could be considered triggers to move on to transplantation.

In addition to identifying clinically relevant events that might trigger transplantation, there may be certain subgroups of patients with low- or intermediate-1 risk myelodysplasia in whom early transplantation may offer a survival advantage. As such, other prognostic systems may be of some utility.

Investigators at the MD Anderson Cancer Center analyzed the outcomes of 865 patients with low- or intermediate-1 IPSS risk disease referred to their center between 1976 and 2005.[6] Using regression techniques, the authors were able to further subdivide patients based on the degree of thrombocytopenia, patient age, cytogenetics, age, and marrow blast count into three groups of patients with clinically different clinical outcomes. It is important to consider that the MD Anderson model used clinical data collected at the time of referral, whereas the IPSS model used data collected at the time of patient diagnosis for modeling.

To determine if the clinical factors identified in the MD Anderson model added additional information when applied to the IPSS cohort of patients, the author and colleagues applied this algorithm to patients in the original IPSS cohort. Using the MD Anderson scoring system, 136 low- and intermediate-1 risk patients aged 18 to 60 years could be subclassified further into prognostically relevant subgroups. Collapsing the MD Anderson scores (because of small patient numbers) allowed the identification of two distinct patient subgroups within the low- and intermediate-1 risk groups. These groups had median survivals of 141.2 months and 55.2 months ($P = .012$, **Fig. 1**). Importantly, these two subgroups were not simply representative of the original low- and intermediate-1 IPSS risk groups. In fact, one third of the intermediate-1 risk patients were grouped into the higher risk group with the MD Anderson score, whereas all of the low-risk patients by IPSS remained in the low-risk group with the MD Anderson system. Thus, it is possible that some patients with higher-risk intermediate-1 IPSS scores may benefit from earlier, more aggressive intervention, including transplantation, although this requires formal testing either in a mathematical model or in a prospective clinical trial.

The MD Anderson Scoring system includes two gradations of thrombocytopenia ($<50 \times 10^9$/L and 50–200×10^9/L) but only one classification for anemia (hemoglobin less than 10 g/dL), which does not reliably capture red cell transfusion requirement. Transfusion frequency, and its sequelae, particularly iron overload, have recently both been demonstrated to be important prognostic factors in MDS transplant outcomes. For example, Platzbecker and colleagues[7] compared the outcomes of patients who were and were not transfusion-dependent at the time of transplantation.

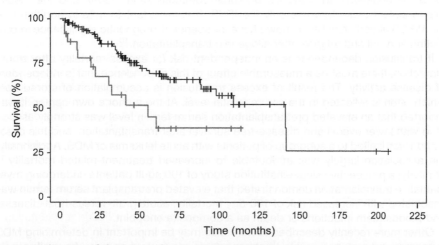

Fig. 1. Application of the MD Anderson Scoring System to IPSS low- and intermediate-1risk patients.

Even though patients in the transfusion-dependent group had more low-risk features compared with the transfusion-independent group, overall survival was inferior in this group, with a 3-year overall survival of 49% compared with 60% in the transfusion-independent group ($P = .1$).

Because transfusion dependency appears to have prognostic importance, it should be considered in choosing patients for transplantation. As a result of the evolving role that transfusion support plays in determining prognosis, the Pavia group examined a cohort of patients stratified by the IPSS classification system, to determine the relevance of the World Health Organization (WHO) classification among different IPSS groups. The new WHO classification system for myelodysplastic disorders clearly identifies patients into distinct prognostic categories.[8] For patients with low- and intermediate-1 risk IPSS scores, the WHO histologic classification scheme was able to significantly differentiate survival among the different histologic subtypes within each IPSS range.[8] Patients in higher IPSS categories did not have significantly different survival outcomes when some stratified by WHO histology. More importantly, in the same analysis, the authors were able to demonstrate a significant effect on survival based on the requirement for transfusion support. As would be expected, outcomes in patients with higher-grade myelodysplasia were affected less by transfusion requirement then were patients with less advanced WHO histologies. As a result of the demonstration of the impact of transfusion even among WHO stratified patients, the impact of transfusion requirement then was incorporated into the newer WHO Prognostic Scoring System (WPSS).[9] In this system, the impact of regular transfusion requirement (defined as requiring at least one transfusion every 8 weeks in a 4-month period) was given the same regression weight as progressing from favorable to intermediate cytogenetics, or from intermediate to unfavorable cytogenetics. In contrast to the initial IPSS publication, which carries prognostic information only at the time of initial MDS diagnosis, this model was time-dependent, such that patients could be re-evaluated continually with this scoring model, and updated prognostic information could be generated at any time point in the patient's treatment course. As such, the development of new cytogenetic changes, or the development of an ongoing transfusion need would add usable information that would help guide treatment decisions, including those that affect transplantation. A formal decision analysis using the WPSS is underway (M. Cazzola, personal communication, 2009), and the results may supplant those that use only the IPSS. It is important to note in addition that the WPSS already has been shown have independent prognostic significance in predicting survival and relapse after allogeneic transplantation.[10]

If transfusion dependence is an independent risk for excess mortality after transplantation, there must be a measurable effect of this dependence that is independent of disease activity. The result of excess transfusion is accumulation of stored iron, which often is reflected in the serum ferritin level. At the author's own center, it was reported that an elevated pretransplantation serum ferritin level was strongly associated with lower overall and disease-free survival after transplantation, and this association was limited to a subgroup of patients with acute leukemia or MDS. Additionally, the association largely was attributable to increased treatment-related mortality.[11] Similarly, a prospective single-institution study of 190 adult patients undergoing myeloablative transplantation demonstrated that elevated pretransplant serum ferritin was associated with increased risk of 100-day mortality, acute graft-versus-host-disease, and bloodstream infections or death as a composite endpoint.[12]

Other more recently described factors also may be important in determining MDS outcome, and may help guide treatment decisions toward or away from allogeneic stem cell transplantation. For example, Haase and colleagues[13] recently analyzed individual cytogenetic changes in over 2000 individuals with MDS. They identified several previously identified favorable cytogenetic changes that were associated with median survivals that ranged from 32 to 108 months, with some subgroups having survivals that were not reached. In addition, novel individual cytogenetic changes that were associated with an intermediate prognosis were identified that were not addressed in the IPSS analysis. At an even finer level, molecular prognostication may hold even more information than cytogenetics. Mills and colleagues[14] recently described a gene expression profile methodology to accurately predict the risk of transition from MDS to acute myeloid leukemia. This model was able to accurately differentiate groups of patients with a time to transformation greater than or less than 18 months, and this model was more powerful at predicting time to leukemic transformation and overall survival when compared with the IPSS scoring system. This gene expression profile needs to be tested in a prospective trial where it is used to help guide therapy to determine if it truly is effective.

COMORBIDITY AND CONDITIONING INTENSITY

It is known that comorbidity increases the likelihood of adverse outcomes in medicine and in hematologic malignancies, although the recognition that comorbidity scores may be useful in the latter scenario only recently has been noted.[15] Several comorbidity scores have been developed to help provide prognostic information in myeloid malignancies. In MDS, the Hematopoietic Cell Transplantation Comorbidity Index (HCT-CI), developed by Sorror and colleagues,[16] has been shown to carry prognostic value even in patients with MDS not undergoing transplantation.[17] Sorror and colleagues[18] demonstrated that the HCT-CI has specific prognostic utility in a group of patients undergoing transplantation for acute myeloid leukemia and MDS. In this analysis, the patients were divided into four separate groups, with each group being defined on the basis of comorbidity and malignant disease risk. Within each of the four risk groups, patients who underwent myeloablative and reduced intensity conditioning (RIC) transplantation were compared with each other. In each of the four groups, the RIC arm experienced a higher rate of relapse; however, the treatment-related mortality rates were all lower when compared with the myeloablative arm. As a result, disease-free survival and overall survival were similar between conditioning arms in all four groups.

The effects of elevated ferritin levels largely are limited to patients undergoing myeloablative transplantation; however, an elevated ferritin level should be considered a comorbid factor. As such, ferritin levels could influence the decision to pursue full-intensity or reduced-intensity transplantation. Optimally, if myeloablative transplantation is planned, proceeding to transplantation before the accumulation of a critical amount of iron should be pursued, or alternatively, chelation therapy before transplantation can be considered, although this latter approach has not yet been demonstrated to be effective in prospective clinical trials.

The consideration of comorbidity before transplantation is even more relevant now that RIC transplantation has been shown to be effective in the treatment of MDS.[19] There are several analyses that have compared RIC transplantation with conventional myeloablative transplantation, and most of them suggest similar outcomes. For example, at author's center, the outcomes of 136 patients with MDS or acute myelogenous leukemia were compared when stratified by conditioning regimen intensity.[20] Overall survival at 2 years was the same for individuals undergoing RIC transplantation as for those who received myeloablative conditioning. The causes of treatment failure, however, were significantly different, with more relapse in the RIC group, but higher treatment-related mortality in the myeloablative group, as anticipated. A larger analysis with similar results was presented by Martino and colleagues[21] on behalf of the European Group for Blood & Marrow Transplantation (EBMT). Finally, a retrospective CIBMTR review of the outcomes of 550 patients aged 50 years or older who underwent matched sibling donor transplantation demonstrated no difference in myeloablative and RIC outcomes.[1] None of these studies adjusted for comorbidity, and it is almost a certainty that if reanalyzed, the RIC cohorts would contain a higher proportion of patients with advanced comorbidities. Nonetheless, with similar outcomes, some patients now have opted for earlier RIC transplantation, even without comorbidity, because treatment-related morbidity and mortality after this procedure are lower than after traditional myeloablative transplantation.

The optimal timing of RIC transplantation therefore needs to be addressed in some form of prospective clinical trial, or in the absence of the feasibility of this approach, with mathematical Markov modeling. The issues surrounding the timing of RIC transplantation are more complex now that there are several US Food and Drug Administration-approved treatment options that can reduce transfusion dependence and even increase overall survival in transfusion-dependent patients.[22] A formal decision analysis examining the evolving role of transplantation in the context of the availability of DNA hypomethylating therapy therefore has been started through the CIBMTR (Study LK0802, J. Koreth and C. Cutler, PIs).

SUMMARY

Appropriate patient selection for transplantation is the first step in maximizing outcomes after transplantation for MDS. Because new therapeutics offer significant palliation and provide symptom control, the decision to pursue transplantation is not undertaken lightly. However, for younger patients, in whom an MDS-related death is very likely, early transplant generally is recommended. Several factors influence the decision to undergo transplantation, and many of these revolve around prognostic indicators that are evolving constantly. The goal of these systems is to identify patients in whom transplantation outcomes are likely to exceed nontransplant outcomes. This balance is most relevant in older patients in whom RIC transplantation is indicated, and where the optimal timing of transplantation has not yet been defined.

REFERENCES

1. Cibmtr. Report on state of the art in blood and marrow transplantation. Available at: http://www.cibmtr.org/SERVICES/Observational_Research/Summary_Slides/index.html. Accessed 2009.
2. Nachtkamp K, Kundgen A, Strupp C, et al. Impact on survival of different treatments for myelodysplastic syndromes (MDS). Leuk Res 2009;33:1024–8.
3. Deeg HJ, Storer B, Slattery JT, et al. Conditioning with targeted busulfan and cyclophosphamide for hemopoietic stem cell transplantation from related and unrelated donors in patients with myelodysplastic syndrome. Blood 2002;100:1201–7.
4. de Witte T, Brand R, Van Biezen A, et al. Allogeneic stem cell transplantation for patients with refractory anaemia with matched related and unrelated donors: delay of the transplant is associated with inferior survival. Br J Haematol 2009;146:627–36.
5. Cutler CS, Lee SJ, Greenberg P, et al. A decision analysis of allogeneic bone marrow transplantation for the myelodysplastic syndromes: delayed

transplantation for low-risk myelodysplasia is associated with improved outcome. Blood 2004;104:579–85.

6. Garcia-Manero G, Shan J, Faderl S, et al. A prognostic score for patients with lower risk myelodysplastic syndrome. Leukemia 2008;22:538–43.

7. Platzbecker U, Bornhauser M, Germing U, et al. Red blood cell transfusion dependence and outcome after allogeneic peripheral blood stem cell transplantation in patients with de novo myelodysplastic syndrome (MDS). Biol Blood Marrow Transplant 2008;14:1217–25.

8. Malcovati L, Porta MG, Pascutto C, et al. Prognostic factors and life expectancy in myelodysplastic syndromes classified according to WHO criteria: a basis for clinical decision making. J Clin Oncol 2005;23:7594–603.

9. Malcovati L, Germing U, Kuendgen A, et al. Time-dependent prognostic scoring system for predicting survival and leukemic evolution in myelodysplastic syndromes. J Clin Oncol 2007;25:3503–10.

10. Alessandrino EP, Della Porta MG, Bacigalupo A, et al. WHO classification and WPSS predict post-transplantation outcome in patients with myelodysplastic syndrome: a study from the Gruppo Italiano Trapianto di Midollo Osseo (GITMO). Blood 2008;112:895–902.

11. Armand P, Kim HT, Cutler CS, et al. Prognostic impact of elevated pretransplantation serum ferritin in patients undergoing myeloablative stem cell transplantation. Blood 2007;109:4586–8.

12. Pullarkat V, Blanchard S, Tegtmeier B, et al. Iron overload adversely affects outcome of allogeneic hematopoietic cell transplantation. Bone Marrow Transplant 2008;42:799–805.

13. Haase D, Germing U, Schanz J, et al. New insights into the prognostic impact of the karyotype in MDS and correlation with subtypes: evidence from a core dataset of 2124 patients. Blood 2007;110:4385–95.

14. Mills KI, Kohlmann A, Williams PM, et al. Microarray-based classifiers and prognosis models identify subgroups with distinct clinical outcomes and high risk of AML transformation of myelodysplastic syndrome. Blood 2009;114:1063–72.

15. Della Porta MG, Malcovati L. Clinical relevance of extrahematologic comorbidity in the management of patients with myelodysplastic syndrome. Haematologica 2009;94:602–6.

16. Sorror ML, Maris MB, Storb R, et al. Hematopoietic cell transplantation (HCT)-specific comorbidity index: a new tool for risk assessment before allogeneic HCT. Blood 2005;106:2912–9.

17. Zipperer E, Pelz D, Nachtkamp K, et al. The hematopoietic stem cell transplantation comorbidity index is of prognostic relevance for patients with myelodysplastic syndrome. Haematologica 2009;94:729–32.

18. Sorror ML, Sandmaier BM, Storer BE, et al. Comorbidity and disease status based risk stratification of outcomes among patients with acute myeloid leukemia or myelodysplasia receiving allogeneic hematopoietic cell transplantation. J Clin Oncol 2007;25:4246–54.

19. Oliansky DM, Antin JH, Bennett JM, et al. The role of cytotoxic therapy with hematopoietic stem cell transplantation in the therapy of myelodysplastic syndromes: an evidence-based review. Biol Blood Marrow Transplant 2009; 15:137–72.

20. Alyea EP, Kim HT, Ho V, et al. Impact of conditioning regimen intensity on outcome of allogeneic hematopoietic cell transplantation for advanced acute myelogenous leukemia and myelodysplastic syndrome. Biol Blood Marrow Transplant 2006;12:1047–55.

21. Martino R, Iacobelli S, Brand R, et al. Retrospective comparison of reduced-intensity conditioning and conventional high-dose conditioning for allogeneic hematopoietic stem cell transplantation using HLA-identical sibling donors in myelodysplastic syndromes. Blood 2006;108:836–46.

22. Fenaux P, Mufti GJ, Hellstrom-Lindberg E, et al. Efficacy of azacitidine compared with that of conventional care regimens in the treatment of higher-risk myelodysplastic syndromes: a randomised, open-label, phase III study. Lancet Oncol 2009;10:223–32.

Index

Note: Page numbers of article titles are in **boldface** type.

A

Acute myelogenous leukemia (AML), epigenetic changes in MDS leading to, **317–330**
    innate immune signaling in MDS, **343–359**
    prognostic classification and risk assessment in MDS, **459–468**
Age, in risk assessment for hematopoietic stem cell transplantation for MDS, 410
Anemia, prognostic classification and risk assessment in MDS, **459–468**
Animal models, mouse models of MDS, **361–375**
Antithymocyte globulin (ATG), treatment of MDS based on, 335–337
Arid4a deficiency, in mouse models of MDS, 367
ASXL1 gene mutations, in MDS, 302
Autologous hematopoietic stem cell transplantation, for MDS, 415
Azacitidine, hypomethylating therapy of MDS with, **389–406**

B

BCL-2, in mouse models of MDS, 366
Belinostat (PXD101), MDS therapy with, 429
Bone marrow destruction, model for immunologically mediated, in MDS, 332–334

C

Cancer, DNA methylation changes in, 319–320
    epigenetic therapy of, 323–324
CBL gene mutations, in MDS, 303
Characteristics, clinical, of MDS, 288–289
Chemotherapy, induction, prior to hematopoietic stem cell transplantation for MDS, 411–412
Chromosomal amplifications, in MDS, 297–298
Chromosomal deletions, in MDS, 297–298
Chronic myelomonocytic leukemia (CMML), risk stratification for, 452–454
Classification, of MDS, **443–457**
    diagnostic criteria, 444–445
    other MDS groups, 449–450
    pathologic classifications, 445–449
        FAB, 445–447
        WHO, 447–449
    prognostic, of MDS, **459–468**
        dynamic prognostic assessment, 462–464
        impact of comorbidities on survival, 464–465
        molecular markers of prognostic significance, 465
        new model for, 464
        treatment strategy based on WHO scoring system, 465–466
        WHO classification-based prognostic scoring system, 461–462

Hematol Oncol Clin N Am 24 (2010) 477–485
doi:10.1016/S0889-8588(10)00043-2
0889-8588/10/$ – see front matter © 2010 Elsevier Inc. All rights reserved.

hemonc.theclinics.com

Moving?

Make sure your subscription moves with you!

To notify us of your new address, find your **Clinics Account Number** (located on your mailing label above your name), and contact customer service at:

Email: journalscustomerservice-usa@elsevier.com

800-654-2452 (subscribers in the U.S. & Canada)
314-447-8871 (subscribers outside of the U.S. & Canada)

Fax number: 314-447-8029

**Elsevier Health Sciences Division
Subscription Customer Service
3251 Riverport Lane
Maryland Heights, MO 63043**

ELSEVIER

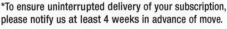

Printed and bound by CPI Group (UK) Ltd, Croydon, CR0 4YY

03/10/2024

01040459-0001